Donald E. Greydanus, Gabriel Kaplan, Dilip R. Patel, and Joav Merrick (eds.)
Substance Abuse in Adolescents and Young Adults

Health, Medicine and Human Development

Health is a key component of human development, growth, and quality of life. The Health, Medicine and Human Development book series aims to provide a public forum for book publications from a multidisciplinary group of researchers, practitioners, and clinicians for an international professional forum interested in the broad spectrum of health, medicine, and human development. We welcome research on a wide variety of substantive areas that will promote and impact healthy human development including prevention, intervention, and care also among people in vulnerable conditions.

Edited by
Joav Merrick

Bricker JT, Omar HA, Merrick J, eds.
Adults with Childhood Illnesses: Considerations for Practice.
Berlin: De Gruyter, 2011.
ISBN 978-3-11-025521-8
e-ISBN 978-3-11-025568-3

Derevensky JL, Shek D, Merrick J, eds.
Youth Gambling: The Hidden Addiction.
Berlin: De Gruyter, 2011.
ISBN 978-3-11-025520-1
e-ISBN 978-3-11-025569-0

Greydanus DE, Patel DR, Omar HA, Feucht C, Merrick J, eds.
Adolescent Medicine: Pharmacotherapeutics in General, Mental and Sexual Health.
Berlin: De Gruyter, 2012.
ISBN 978-3-11-025522-5
e-ISBN 978-3-11-025570

Greydanus DE, Patel DR, Omar HA, Feucht C, Merrick J, eds.
Adolescent Medicine: Pharmacotherapeutics in Medical Disorders.
Berlin: De Gruyter, 2012.
ISBN 978-3-11-027580-3
e-ISBN 978-3-11-027636-7

Tareen RS, Greydanus DE, Jafferany M, Patel DR, Merrick J, eds.
Pediatric Psychodermatology: A Clinical Manual of Child and Adolescent Psychocutaneous Disorders.
Berlin: De Gruyter, 2012.
ISBN 978-3-11-027387-8
e-ISBN 978-3-11-027393-9

Substance Abuse in Adolescents and Young Adults

A Manual for Pediatric and Primary Care Clinicans

Edited by
Donald E. Greydanus, Gabriel Kaplan, Dilip R. Patel,
and Joav Merrick

DE GRUYTER

Editors

Donald E. Greydanus, MD, Dr. HC (Athens),
Professor and Chair
Program Director
Department of Pediatric and Adolescent Medicine
Western Michigan University
School of Medicine
Kalamazoo, MI
United States of America
Donald.Greydanus@med.wmich.edu

Gabriel Kaplan, MD, DFAPA
Clinical Associate Professor of Psychiatry
Rutgers New Jersey Medical School
Newark, NJ
United States of America
drgkaplan@gmail.com

Dilip R. Patel, MD, FAAP, FSAM, FAACPDM, FACSM
Western Michigan University
School of Medicine
Kalamazoo, MI
United States of America
Dilip.Patel@med.wmich.edu

Joav Merrick, MD, MMedSc, DMSc
Ministry of Social Affairs and Social Services
National Institute of Child Health and Human Development
Jerusalem
Israel
jmerrick@zahav.net.il

ISBN 978-3-11-031301-7
e-ISBN 978-3-11-031138-9

Library of Congress Cataloging-in-Publication Data
A CIP Catalog record for this book has been applied for at the Library of Congress.

Bibliographic information published by the Deutsche Nationalbibliothek
The Deutsche Nationalbibliothek lists this publication in the Deutsche Nationalbibliografie; detailed bibliographic data are available in the Internet at http://dnb.dnb.de.

Typesetting: Apex CoVantage
Printing: Hubert & Co. GmbH & Co. KG, Göttingen
Cover image: iStockphoto/Thinkstock

∞ Printed on acid-free paper
Printed in Germany
www.degruyter.com

Dedication

Donald E. Greydanus. I dedicate this book to my parents – John S. and Margaret E. Greydanus, who sacrosanctly and sacerdotally taught me joie de vivre apart from caustic chemicals. From my loving parents, I learned nam et ipsa scientia potestas est. Requiescat in pace cum Deo.

Gabriel Kaplan. I dedicate this book to my parents Drs. Ana and Alberto Kaplan who have not stopped helping patients yet; and to my children Aaron, Yonatan, Ilan, and Arielle who will start helping patients soon.

Dilip R. Patel. I dedicate this book to my lovely wife, Ranjan, and wonderful son, Neil, for their years of love and support.

Joav Merrick. I dedicate this book to my wife and children for their support.

Contents

Author Index

Sarah Ann Anderson, PhD
Department of Pharmacology and Systems Biology
Mount Sinai School of Medicine, New York, NY
United States of America
Chapter 11

Jeffrey Berman, MD
Director, Evergreen Substance Abuse Services
Bergen Regional Medical Center
Paramus, NJ 07652
United States of America
jberman@bergenregional.com
Chapter 22

Oscar G. Bukstein, MD, MPH
Professor of Psychiatry, Chief
Division of Child and Adolescent Psychiatry
Department of Psychiatry and Behavioral Sciences
University of Texas at Houston
1941 East Road
Houston, TX 77054
United States of America
oscar.g.bukstein@uth.tmc.edu
Chapter 9

Joseph L. Calles, Jr., MD
Associate Professor of Psychiatry
Western Michigan University School of Medicine
Director, Child and Adolescent Psychiatry
Psychiatry Program, Western Michigan University School of Medicine
1722 Shaffer Rd., Suite 3
Kalamazoo, MI 49048
United States of America
joseph.calles@med.wmich.edu
Chapters 10 and 19

Jonathan P. Caulkins, PhD
Professor of Operations Research and Public Policy
Heinz College, Carnegie Mellon University
5000 Forbes Ave., Hamburg Hall
Pittsburgh, PA 15213–3890
United States of America
caulkins@andrew.cmu.edu
Chapters 20 and 21

Colleen Dodich, MD
Assistant Professor
Department of Pediatric and Adolescent Medicine
Western Michigan University School of Medicine
1000 Oakland Drive, D48G
Kalamazoo, MI 49008–1284
United States of America
colleen.dodich@med.wmich.edu
Chapters 12 and 18

Aaron Ellington, PhD
Division of Child & Adolescent Psychiatry
University Hospitals Case Medical Center
577 Vinita Avenue
Akron, OH 44320
Chapter 14

Robert L. Findling, MD, MBA
Director, Child & Adolescent Psychiatry
The Johns Hopkins Hospital
Bloomberg Children's Center

1800 Orleans Street
Suite 12344A
Baltimore, MD 21287
RFindli1@jhmi.edu
Chapter 14

Donald E. Greydanus, MD, Dr. HC (Athens)
Professor and Chair
Program Director
Department of Pediatric and Adolescent Medicine
Western Michigan University
School of Medicine
Kalamazoo, MI
United States of America
Donald.Greydanus@med.wmich.edu
Chapters 1 (Introduction), 8, and 17

Megan M. Greydanus, BFA
Graphic Designer
Hollywood, CA
United States of America
mgreydanus@gmail.com
Chapter 8

Elizabeth K. Hawver, LMSW, CAADC
Community Healing Center
Kalamazoo, MI 49008
United States of America
Chapter 8

John L. Hertzer, MD
Division of Child & Adolescent Psychiatry
University Hospitals Case Medical Center
W.O. Walker Building
10524 Euclid Avenue Suite 1155
Cleveland OH 44106
United States of America
Chapter 14

Danielle Hirsch, MD, MPH
Department of Pediatric and Adolescent Medicine
Western Michigan University School of Medicine
Kalamazoo, MI
United States of America
Chapter 7

Ray Chih-Jui Hsiao, MD
Co-Director, Adolescent Substance Abuse Program
Seattle Children's Hospital
4800 Sand Point Way NE, M/S W3636, P.O. Box 5371
Seattle, WA 98105
United States of America
rhsiao@uw.edu
Chapter 13

Iliyan Ivanov, MD
Assistant Professor, Psychiatry
Mount Sinai School of Medicine
New York
241 West 97th Street, 2N
New York, NY 10025
United States of America
iliyan.ivanov@mssm.edu
Chapter 11

Brandon Johnson, MD
Mount Sinai School of Medicine
New York, NY
United States of America
Chapter 16

Gabriel Kaplan, MD, DFAPA
Clinical Associate Professor of Psychiatry
Rutgers New Jersey Medical School
Newark, NJ
United States of America
drgkaplan@gmail.com
Chapters 1 (Introduction) and 6

Anna Kasunic, MS
Heinz College
Carnegie Mellon University
Pittsburgh, PA
United States of America
Chapters 20 and 21

Mark Kleiman, PhD
University of California Los Angeles
Los Angeles, California
United States of America
Chapter 21

Michael A. C. Lee, MS
Heinz College
Carnegie Mellon University
Pittsburgh, PA
United States of America
Chapters 20 and 21

Marc Lener, MD
Department of Psychiatry
Mount Sinai School of Medicine
New York, NY
United States of America
Chapter 11

Michael R. Liepman, MD
Department of Psychiatry
Western Michigan University School of Medicine
Kalamazoo, MI
United States of America
Chapters 2 and 5

Joav Merrick, MD, MMedSc, DMSc
Ministry of Social Affairs and Social Services
National Institute of Child Health and Human Development
Jerusalem
Israel
jmerrick@zahav.net.il
Chapter 1 (Introduction)

Kristin A. Miselis, MD
Department of Psychiatry and Behavioral Sciences
University of Washington School of Medicine
Seattle, WA
United States of America
Chapter 13

Angela Nash, MSN, APRN, CPNP-PC
The University of Texas
Health Science Center at Houston
School of Nursing
Houston, TX
United States of America
Chapter 9

Ahsan Nazeer, MD
Associate Professor
Department of Psychiatry
Western Michigan University School of Medicine
1717 Shaffer Street, Suite 010
Kalamazoo, MI 49048–1623
United States of America
ahsan.nazeer@med.wmich.edu
Chapters 2 and 5

Jeffrey Newcorn, MD
Associate Professor of Psychiatry
241 West 97th Street, 2N
Mount Sinai Medical School
New York, NY
United States of America
jeffrey.newcorn@mssm.edu
Chapter 16

Sherry Pancost, MA
Behavioral/Developmental Pediatrics, Department of Pediatric and Adolescent Medicine
Western Michigan University School of Medicine
Kalamazoo, MI
United States of America
Chapter 4

Michael Paolello
Bergen Regional Medical Center
Paramus, NJ
United States of America
Chapter 22

Dilip R. Patel, MD, FAAP, FSAM, FAACPDM, FACSM
Western Michigan University
School of Medicine
Kalamazoo, MI
United States of America
Dilip.Patel@med.wmich.edu
Chapters 1 (Introduction), 7, and 17

Shalin Patel, MD
Department of Pediatric and Adolescent Medicine
Western Michigan University School of Medicine
Kalamazoo, MI
United States of America
Chapter 18

Helen D. Pratt, PhD
Director
Behavioral/Developmental Pediatrics, Department of Pediatric and Adolescent Medicine
Western Michigan University School of Medicine
1000 Oakland Drive, D48G
Kalamazoo, MI 49008–1284
United States of America
helen.pratt@med.wmich.edu
Chapter 4

Brieana M. Rowles, MA
Regulatory Specialist, Clinical Research Services
UPMC CancerCenter
5150 Centre Avenue, Suite 301
Pittsburgh, PA 15232
United States of America
rowlesbm@upmc.edu
Chapter 14

Monika Siedlarz, MD
Department of Pediatric and Adolescent Medicine
Western Michigan University School of Medicine
Kalamazoo, MI
United States of America
Chapter 12

Ruqiya Shama Tareen, MD
Associate Professor of Psychiatry
Director of Women's Behavioral Health
Department of Psychiatry
Western Michigan University School of Medicine
1717 Shaffer Road
Kalamazoo, MI 49048
United States of America
shama.tareen@med.wmich.edu
Chapter 15

Andrew R. Tarr, BS
3450 North Lake Shore Drive
Apartment #1607
Chicago, IL 60657
United States of America
Chapter 14

Helga V. Toriello, PhD
Director
Clinical Genetics
Spectrum Health Hospitals
25 Michigan St., Suite 2000
Grand Rapids, MI 49503
United States of America
helga.toriello@spectrumhealth.org
Chapter 3

Christopher K. Varley, MD
Department of Psychiatry and
Behavioral Sciences
University of Washington School of
Medicine
Seattle, WA
United States of America
Chapter 13

Amanda Williams, MD
Department of Pediatric and Adolescent
Medicine
Western Michigan University School of
Medicine
Kalamazoo, MI
United States of America
Chapter 18

David Bennett

Foreword

Adolescence is the life stage in which experimentation with substance abuse – especially alcohol, cannabis, and nicotine – usually begins. For most young people, trying alcohol and other drugs (including prescribed medications) is unlikely to result in long-term harm, but immediate risk is ever present, even on a single occasion. Unfortunately, accidents and violence, mental impairment, legal issues, unwanted sexual activity, damaged reputation, missing study or work, or on rare occasions, even death can result.

Ongoing substance abuse is particularly concerning, with complications including mental health problems (in particular anxiety, depression, and sleep disorders), infections with blood-borne infections, damage to organs (i.e., liver, heart, and brain), and increased risk of cancers as well as other serious health conditions.

It is therefore timely to focus on what is currently happening in this often vexing and complex area of adolescent/young adult health care. Substance abuse does not occur in isolation – it is mediated by an amalgam of individual, interpersonal, and societal factors. Predictors for initiation of substance use in adolescence, for example, include intrauterine assaults and genetic predispositions, temperament and personality, familial substance abuse, family conflict, and poor parenting. Some populations of young people are particularly at risk.

Fortunately, much is also known about factors protecting against risk behaviors, such as a warm, nurturing parenting style with judicious monitoring of behavior and fair rule setting, especially in the vulnerable early teenage years. Adolescents yearn for social acceptance and a sense of belonging and are less likely to engage with drugs when they feel supported and cared about as well as being well connected to family, school, and (hopefully) non-drug-taking peers. Contemporary treatment approaches, whether psychopharmacological or psychotherapeutic, reflect these new understandings.

Clinicians dealing with young people not uncommonly feel poorly equipped to inquire about drug taking or to know how best to respond if such disclosures are forthcoming including where to turn for help. There is evidence in Australia, for example, that doctors are not taking up opportunities to target problematic alcohol and tobacco use, a situation that is likely to be true in other countries as well. This practical manual sets the scene by providing up-to-date, evidence-based information in support of optimal clinical practice. A wide variety of aspects of substance abuse are covered, and I congratulate the editors and authors for developing this treatise on such an important and timely topic.

Clinical Professor David Bennett, AO, FRACP, FSAHM
University of Sydney
Clinical Director (Medical) – Priority Populations
Sydney Children's Hospitals Network and Senior Clinical Advisor and Director, Youth Health and Wellbeing, NSW Kids and Families
Sydney, Australia
david.bennett@health.nsw.gov.au

Abbreviations

2-AG	2-arachidonoyl glycerol
5-Me-DIPT	5-methoxydimethyltryptamine
AAS	anabolic-androgenic steroids
ADHD	attention-deficit/hyperactivity disorder
AEA	arachidonoyl ethanolamide
AmED	alcohol mixed with an energy drink
AMT	alpha-methyltryptamine
ASSIST	Alcohol, Smoking and Substance Involvement Screening Test
ATP	adenosine triphosphate
AUD	alcohol use disorder
AUDIT	Alcohol Use Disorders Identification Test
BAC	blood alcohol concentration
BD	1,4-butanediol
BDNF	brain-derived neurotrophic factor
BI	brief intervention
BMI	brief motivational intervention
BPD	bipolar disorder
BTCP	1-bensothiophenyl cyclohexylpiperidine
BZP	benzodiazepine
BZP	benzylpiperazine
CAGE	cut down, annoyed, guilty, eye opener
CB	cannabinoid
CBC	complete blood count
CBD	cannabidiol
CBG	cannabigerol
CBT	cognitive behavioral therapy
CD	conduct disorder
CM	contingency management
CNR1	cannabis receptor-1 gene
CNS	central nervous system
CNV	copy number variations
COI	cost of illness
COPD	chronic obstructive lung disease
CRA	community reinforcement approach
CRH	cortisol-releasing hormone
CSF	cerebrospinal fluid
CT	computerized tomography
CUD	cannabis use disorder
DA	dopamine

DArgic	dopaminergic
DAST	Drug Abuse Screen Test
DAT	DA transporter
DHEA	dihydroepiandrostenedione
DMT	N, N-dimethyltryptamine
DPH	diphenhydramine
DXM	dextromethorphan
ECG	electrocardiogram
EPO	erythropoietin
FAS	fetal alcohol syndrome
FHS	follicle stimulating hormone
GABA	γ-aminobutyric acid
GAD	generalized anxiety disorder
GBL	gamma butyrolactone
GHB	γ-hydroxybutyric acid or gamma hydroxybutyrate
GI	gastrointestinal
GWAS	genome-wide association studies
HCG	human chorionic gonadotropin
HDAC	histone deacetylase
hGH	human growth hormone
HPA	hypothalamic-pituitary axis
HTG	hypertriglyceridemia
IM	intramuscularly
IUGR	intrauterine growth restriction
IV	intravenous, intravenously
LH	luteinizing hormone
LSD	lysergic acid diethylamide
LTD	long-term depression
LTP	long-term potentiation
MAO	monoamine oxidase
MAS	mixed amphetamine salts
MBDB	N-methyl-1,3-benzodioxolylbutanamine
MCD	meso-corticolimbic dopamine
mCPP	meta-chlorophenylpiperazine
MDA	methylenedioxyamphetamine or 3,4-methylenedioxyamphetamine
MDD	major depressive disorder
MDEA	methylenedioxyethylamphetamine or 3,4-methylenedioxy-N-ethylamphetamine
MDFT	multidimensional family therapy
MDMA	3,4-methylenedioxy-N-methylamphetamine or 3,4-methylenedioxymethamphetamine
MDPV	3,4-methylenedioxypyrovalerone

MeOPP	1-(4-methoxyphenyl)piperazine
MET	motivation enhancement therapy
MI	motivational interviewing
MMT	methadone maintenance treatment
MRI	magnetic resonance imaging
MXE	methoxetamine
NAC	N-acetylcysteine
NAc	nucleus accumbens
nAChR	nicotinic-subtype acetylcholine receptors or nictotinic cholinergic receptors
NAS	neonatal abstinence syndrome
NMDA	N-methyl-D-aspartate
NMUPD	nonmedical use of prescription drugs
NRT	nicotine replacement therapy
OCD	obsessive compulsive disorder
OROS-MPH	osmotic-release methylphenidate
OTC	over-the-counter
P2P	phenyl-2-propanone
PCP	phencyclidine
PDV	physical dating violence
PET	positron emission tomography
PFC	prefrontal cortex
PGB	pregabalin
PMA	paramethoxyamphetamine
PMK	3,4-methylenedioxyphenylpropan-2-one
PPD	postpartum depression
PTSD	posttraumatic stress disorder
QALY	quality-adjusted life year
RP	relapse prevention
SARMs	selective androgen receptor moderators
SBIRT	screening, brief intervention, and referral to treatment
SID	substance-induced disorder
SIDS	sudden infant death syndrome
SNP	single nucleotide polymorphism
SNRI	serotonin-norepinephrine reuptake inhibitor
SPECT	single-photon emission computed tomography
SR	sustained release
SSRI	selective serotonin reuptake inhibitor
STI	sexually transmitted infection
SUD	substance use disorder
TB	tuberculosis
TFMPP	trifluoromethylphenylpiperazine

THC	tetrahydrocannabinol
TPP	tegmental pedunculo-pontine
UDS	urine drug screen
VMAT	vesicular monoamine transporter
VPA	valproic acid
VTA	ventral tegmental area
WTP	willingness to pay

1 Introduction: Substance abuse in adolescents and young adults

Donald E. Greydanus, Gabriel Kaplan,
Dilip R. Patel, and Joav Merrick

Cannabis sativa and Papaver somniferum: Plants of Paradise that produce a vicious viniculum between ancient and modern homo sapiens:

> "On a bright morning they have fixed,
> To seek the plain that southward lies,
> Then from her task of twisting hemp,
> See dancing through the mart she hies"

– She King, *Book of Ancient Poetry*, China, 2350 BCE

Homo sapiens sapiens emerged over 200,000 years ago and the flexuous, precarious journey of this species is nebulous, since writing only developed in southern Mesopotamia in the 4th millennium BCE (1,2). One aspect about these early humans that seems clear is they possessed a predatory, puerile central nervous system wired for seeking pleasure and foudroyant experiences. Perhaps the first recorded incident of humans seeking ultimate joy was the willingness to receive knowledge that would lead to happiness, as found in the Genesis 3:6 account of Eve and then Adam (in Hebrew *ha-adam*, or "mankind") consuming the forbidden fruit (in Hebrew *p'ri*) from the tree (in Hebrew *etz* or *Ha-etz*) of the knowledge of good and evil. They failed to first partake of the fruit (in Hebrew *ruach*, or spirit that provides eternal life) from the tree of life, and the consequences were disastrous for them, and for others, in this recording of the Fall of Man because a Cadmean curse resulted. They, of course, did not appreciate the tenacious puissance of consuming the wrong product; indeed, seeking and partaking of "fruits" or various epinosic and edacious chemicals, including those from natural plants, for various levels of joy and avoiding healthy plants has proved to be cimmerianly cataclysmic for human beings ever since.

There are many hallucinogenic and euphoria-inducing plants that have been available to humans for thousands of years. Some of them include *Datura stramonium, Datura candida, Amanita muscaria, Atropa belladonna, Rivea corymbosa, Pancreatium trianthum, Hyoscyamus niger, Erythroxylon coca, Papaver somniferum*, and many others. Each has induced its own unique jeremiad with promises of joy that end as an oubliette with a trap door of addiction and potential death. However, one could speculate that one of the most classic apolaustic drugs was the marijuana plant, which has been smoked for unknown millennia. The first worn fabric may have been woven from the hemp plant and dates back to 7,000–8,000 BCE, while use of hemp seeds as food has been noted in China by 6,000 BCE (3,4).

The first classifier of medicinal herbs was the Chinese emperor Shen-Nung (2737 BCE), and there is a classic painting of this emperor holding leaves of Ephedra (*ma-chuang*) (5). Humans turned to what was around them and found plants that proved useful for improving health as well as inducing euphoria. Shen-Nung, the red emperor who is the father of Chinese medicine, taught his Chinese subjects to grow *ma* (hemp) to make hempen cloth and, as noted, it was later used as a food product (6). His classic work, *Pen Ts'ao*, became a *Materia Medica* on various products, including the *dioecious cannabis* (4). Even today cannabis can be part of food products for humans and animals (7).

The hemp plant probably came from the Himalayas to ancient China and later to the entire world. The Hindu sacred text *Arthava-Veda* refers to cannabis as "Sacred Grass" and lists it as one of its five sacred plants; cannabis was used as offerings to the Hindu god Shiva, and was used as medication in India as early as 1200 BCE (3). Herodotus writes of the use of cannabis by the Scythians in 430 BCE (8). A tomb was found in China that contains marijuana and dates back to 700 BCE (9). The consummate Chinese cognoscenti, Confucius (551–479 BCE), compiled Chinese classics that included citations about cultivating and consuming cannabis crops.

Hallucinogenic-huffing bowls have been found in various parts of the world that are over 2,500 years old. Historians tell us of the Ebers Paprus (1550 BCE) from ancient Egypt, which was a 110-page scroll recording of over 700 formulas and remedies of mineral, vegetable, and animal origins (10,11). The history of opium poppy seed consumption dates back at least to ancient Egypt; the opium poppy seed was used as a food product long before its narcotic and soporific effects were fully appreciated (12). Athletes of the ancient Olympics (776 BC–393 AD) were known to consume various chemicals to aid in victory, and these chemicals included mushrooms, figs, and opioids that contained stimulants such as strychnine (13).

Ale is one of oldest liquids produced by humans, dating back to the 5th millennium BCE; beer dates back to at least 3000 BCE (14). The Old Testament notes that wine "gladdens" the heart (Psalm 104:15) but also warns of the dangers of overuse of alcohol (Proverbs 20:1, 10th century BCE), including poverty, strife, and injustice (Proverbs 23:20–21; 23:29–30; 31:4–5). Wine was prominently mentioned in the New Testament in the first century AD, such as its use at weddings (John 2:3) or association with drunkenness and debauchery (Ephesians 5:18). Moderation in wine drinking was also linked to improved health (1 Timothy 5:23).

The pioneer of surgical anesthesia was Hua Tue (190 AD), who used a formula called *ma-fei-san* (bubbling wine) that most likely contained medical cannabis (9). In the Roman civilization, the Greek physician to the Romans, Dioscorides, in 70 AD, wrote *Materia Medica*, which discussed cannabis as a material to make strong rope and as treatment of ear aches as well as decreased libido (4). This publication was an influential medical treatise for the next 1500 years. Galen (129–200 AD), another Greek who was a physician to the Romans, commented on a pot-seed dessert consumed by Romans and noted that an overdose of this substance could “affect the head by sending to it a warm and toxic vapor” (4).

Cannabis became a popular product in the Middle East in the 12th century and thereafter spread to other parts of the world (15). Li Shi Chen (1517–1593) became a medical textbook writer in China and rewrote as well as updated classic Chinese medical texts; in his “The Great Herbal of Medicine” he includes use of medical cannabis (9). Indeed, the use of medicinal cannabis may date back to ancient China, as far back as 4,000 BCE (9). The French and British cultivated cannabis in early America in Virginia and Plymouth in 1632 (16).

Of course, other drugs have emerged in the modern world with roots to the ancient. For example, ancient and native South American Indians were pleasured by the mild stimulant effects of chewing coca leaves from the plant *Erythroxylon coca*. This stimulant pleasure is similar to that of caffeine, which is utilized by billions of people in the 21st century. Life would have been safer if humans remained at an abecedarian knowledge of coca and simply chewed it. However, science complicated this issue. Albert Niemann (1834–1861), a PhD student, was given imported coca leaves by his supervisor (Dr. Friedrich Wöhler, 1800–1882) at the University of Göttingen in Germany with a request to study it. The obedient Niemann, in 1859, then was able to isolate an alkaloid he called *cocaine* and dutifully published his results in 1860 (17). His work of noesis earned him his doctoral degree, but his premature death in 1861 at age 27 prevented Dr. Niemann from seeing the death and carnage this extreme drug of euphoria would cause for countless millions of humans in the world of the 19th, 20th, and now 21st century (18).

Another deadly plant, tobacco, was first consumed by pre-Columbian American natives. These American Indians grew tobacco and developed ceremonial as well as medical uses for smoking this Trojan-horse product. It was introduced to Europe in the 16th century and was popularized by such figures as the French diplomat Jean Nicot, for whom nicotine was named. Use of tobacco was increased after the U.S. Civil War (1861–1865) by the overwhelming amount of tobacco grown in North Carolina and Virginia. Cyclopean and predatory promotion by the tobacco corporations and the movie industry increased the use of tobacco in the 20th century until the historic release of the first report of the Surgeon General’s Advisory Committee on Smoking and Health on January 11, 1964. This report by Luther L Terry, MD, identified the severe adverse effects of tobacco as a tenebrous product that first addicts the victim and later kills him or her with cancer or heart disease (19). The U.S. government has launched a major, ongoing campaign since then to educate the unwary public to the major dangers of tobacco, resulting in far fewer Americans addicted to tobacco in the 21st century in contrast to the previous century (20).

Despite current knowledge of the minacious nature of tobacco, the premature deaths of over 400,000 Americans each year from tobacco (5 million worldwide), the publicized prestidigitation of tobacco apologists, and the widespread global medical philippics on *Nicotiana tabacum*, this Plutonian product continues to be grown and promoted with the aid of governments, societies, and the truculent tobacco enterprise. In its 31st publication on tobacco by the U.S. Surgeon General's office, the government concludes that the threat on the health of youth and young adults remains real and unremitting (20). Indeed this plant turns our youth and young adults into helpless myrmidons who blindly smoke this chemical until they prematurely die years later from its relentless and well-known complications. In order to replace these large numbers of tabescent and dead people, younger humans are tragically and lubriciously targeted for tobacco addiction by a powerful, brummagem industry.

Thousands of years of searching for the perfect chemical to produce joie de vivre has resulted in many drugs of addiction that are available to humans. Just as cannabis is currently idolized by media stars and others as a condign chemical to enhance life, cocaine was at first praised as an ideal chemical to assist in amelioration of life's woes. For example, the well-known 19th-century English detective Sherlock Holmes was a classic cocaine addict, as fictionalized by the famous Scottish author and physician Sir Arthur Conan Doyle (1859–1930).

One could speculate that cocaine lead to sweeping changes in mental health management. An Austrian neurologist, Sigmund Freud (1859–1930), was an advocate of cocaine utilization to promote happiness, sexual pleasure, and health; indeed, he wrote a landmark, thrasonical paper of praise for cocaine in 1884 (21). However, sensible science began to arise with a published critique of Freud's praise of cocaine by Albert Erlenmeyer who criticized Freud's use of cocaine to treat morphine addiction and initiated the understanding of cocaine's adverse effects (22). Freud left his hometown of Vienna to escape this barrage of embarrassing criticism and reinvented his career in Paris as the father of psychoanalysis. Freud no longer advocated for the "wonders" of cocaine.

Another "wonder" drug, heroin, has also played a major yet treacherous role in the history of the world (18,23). Analgesic effects from chewing or swallowing Opium poppy seeds (*Papaver somniferum*) was written about in both Egyptian and Roman texts of the past centuries. However, it was not until 1806 that a German pharmacist's assistant, Friedrich Wilhelm Adam Sertürner (1783–1841), identified morphine in attempts to chemically find the part of opium that induced sopor. It was called *morphine* after Morpheus, the Greek god of dreams, and Sertürner spent many years studying the effects of this sleep-inducing agent on himself and others. Reliable syringes were developed in Edinburgh in 1853 and the intravenous delivery of these drugs has exploded ever since. Control of opium became part of the 19th-century Opium Wars between the Qing Dynasty in China and the British as well as the French empires from 1839 to 1842, and then the United States from 1856 to 1859 (24).

Much like cocaine, the use of morphine was touted as a cure for various conditions until the true minacious effects of addiction were realized. Morphine was liberally used for injured soldiers in the U.S. Civil War and wounded veterans were sent home with morphine and hypodermic needles. A London chemist, C.R. Alder Wright, identified diacetyl-morphine in 1874 as he sought a nonaddictive derivation of morphine. A chemist at the Bayer laboratories, Heinrich Dreser, found that Wright's discovery had remarkable analgesic properties and also appeared to improve pulmonary problems. Bayer then marketed it in 1898 as a sedative, anti-tussive medication and named diacetyl-morphine with the term *heroin* for its "heroic" property of analgesia. Bayer stopped heroin production in 1913 due to its addictive, precarious potential and focused on his other product – aspirin.

There were an estimated one-quarter of a million morphine/heroin addicts in the United States in the early 1900s. Addictive chemicals such as morphine and cocaine were unregulated and available without prescription from physicians as well as from drugstores, traveling salesmen, and even via the mail. Dr. William Halsted (1850–1922), notable John Hopkins surgeon and contemporary of Freud, started his cocaine addiction as he introduced regional anesthesia with this compound. Years later, he was to exchange the use of cocaine for morphine (25).

As the major problem of drug addiction was slowly realized, legal measures against drugs were gradually developed in the United States. Opium establishments (so-called dens) were outlawed in San Francisco in 1875, but the first national drug law was not established until 1906 with the Pure Food and Drug Act, which ordered accurate labeling of patent chemicals that contained various drugs and started regulation for such drugs as alcohol, opiates, cocaine, and cannabis.

Finally, in 1914, critical doses of opiates and cocaine were restricted to licensed physicians and pharmacies; this law was called the Harrison Narcotic Act. At this time heroin was fully banned and physicians were not allowed to legally prescribe narcotics even as part of a maintenance program for addicts. Alcohol came under regulation as well, even though this chemical had been well-known for thousands of years and mentioned in various biblical texts. The United States officially prohibited alcohol in 1919 (through the Eighteenth Amendment to the U.S. Constitution), but prohibition of alcohol was eventually repealed in 1933. Cannabis was well accepted in the United States for a time and was even grown by the leading forefathers of the country. However, the battle against cannabis intensified with the 1937 Marijuana Tax Act, which made it illegal to buy, sell, barter, or give away cannabis in the United States.

The 20th century also saw the rise of methamphetamine, a drug first synthesized as amphetamine in 1887 in Berlin, Germany, by Romanian chemist Lazar Edeleanu. Methamphetamine was developed from ephedrine by a Japanese chemist, Nagai Nagayoshi, in 1893; crystallized methamphetamine was synthesized by pharmacologist Akira Ogata in Japan in 1919 (26). Ephedrine had been isolated from the plant Ma-Huang (Ephedra) in 1887 by Nagayoshi Nagai. As with other now illicit drugs, methamphetamine was first hailed as a wonder drug and was used to treat narcolepsy, keep World War II fighter pilots awake, manage obesity as well as attention-deficit hyperactivity disorder, and even help assuage heroin addiction in the 20th century

(27). However, as with other devious and duplicitous drugs of addiction, its adverse effects were gradually recognized and it was identified as a controlled drug in the United States in the 1970s. Its fame has spread among the world of addiction and rural labs making this chemical (from ephedrine, pseudoephedrine, and anhydrous ammonia) have sprung up all over the United States since the 1990s.

The 20th century was characterized by each subsequent decade having an ebb and flow in drug addiction as well as marked by a fear that comprehensive drug education in children and youth would augment drug addiction. There was a dithyrambic explosion of drug use in the 1960s based on the so-called hippy and free-love generation. Cannabis remained a popular drug and the battle to make cannabis legal has been waged ever since with the a fortiori, accipitrine argument that marajuana is safe and good for the public to use. This vade mecum considers this eristic argument and other issues in the vast and complex phenomenon of substance abuse in adolescents and young adults.

Wars for control of drugs of addiction continue in the 21st century as war lords ruthlessly fight to gain the rewards of fortune in the multibillion-dollar drug trade. We have learned that drug addicts have a saturnine brain disorder that makes them seek their drugs of choice at any price even if this price leads to lifelong addiction, imprisonment, hospitalizations, poverty, high morbidity, and premature death (28–32). We have also learned that drugs of addiction and euphoria are numerous and even include medications that are prescribed by clinicians (33). We know about the link of substance experimentation and abuse with overall high-risk behavior in adolescents and young adults (34). We have learned that simply relying on abstinence-only education ("Just Say No!") and punishment with incarceration for drug use does not reduce or ameliorate the drug use and abuse epidemic in the world (35). Links between substance-use prevention and its impact on mental health treatment remain to be elucidated (36).

Drug addicts have rapacious needs that are often never satisfied. Youth must learn that drug dealers do not conduct an ecumenical, eidolonic, eleemosynary business but are esurient epigones and panjandrumic, Pecksniffian, peculating pied pipers often falsely and tragically idolized by the eristic media.

Thus, we desperately need guidance in learning how to prevent drug addiction in our youth and establish prevention programs to decrease the devastating toll it has and will take on billions of human beings in this century and beyond (37–39). We must be concerned about drug addiction and its tenebrous effect on our youth, including their alarming use of nonmedical analgesics (40). It is important to study youth in their communities and thus support more community-based research protocols (41). It is useful to know what is salubrious in substance abuse management as well as what is not salutary (42,43). We must not remain desipiently pococurante with respect to the Faustian dangers of drug addiction for our youth.

This effusive enchiridion on substance abuse in adolescents and young adults provides au courant information on this global, brobdingnagian, bunyanesque topic. We cover a wide variety of subjects within the paradigm of drug abuse and agree with the 21st-century message of integrating substance abuse management with primary care services (44). The editors thank the many experts who so graciously and lambently provided their time and knowledge in these areas. The editors hope that the readers of this treatise find useful and beneficial information that will help them in their work seeking to understand and ameliorate the negative effects of these plants of paradise and of other chemicals that are part of the drug addiction pharmacopoeia of the 21st century (45). We must not be seen as being fainéant with regard to helping our apolaustic youth in their agons with addictive chemicals. We must rescue our adolescents and young adults from their stygian journey of drug addiction and return them to a prelapsarian, supernal existence devoid of these caustic chemicals. There is simply nothing more important that adults of this world should do for their children. The Zeitgeist of the 21st century should be a spirit of true love for our youth marked by a renewed willingness to help our adolescents and young adults avoid a lifetime of maundering addiction.

I would rather have a life span of ten years with coca than one of ten million centuries without it.

– Paolo Mantegazza (1831–1910), Italian physiologist and neurologist (16)

References

1. McHenry HM. Human evolution. In: Ruse M, Travis J, eds. Evolution: The first four billion years. Cambridge, MA: Belknap Press, Harvard University Press, 2009:265.
2. Houston SD. The first writing: Script invention as history and process. Cambridge, MA: Cambridge University Press, 2004.
3. Milestones in the history of marijuana. Accessed 2012 Dec 01. URL: http://brainz.org/420-milestones-history-marijuana/
4. Abel EL. Marijuana. The first twelve thousand years. Accessed 2012 Dec 01. URL: http://druglibrary.org/schaffer/hemp/history/first12000/abel.thm
5. Grollman AP. Alternative medicine: the importance of evidence in medicine and medical evidence. Is there wheat among the chaff? Acad Med 2001;76(3):221–3.
6. Yearbook of the United States Department of Agriculture 1913;288.
7. Belda A, Peiró V, Seva E. The relationship between plants used to sustain finches (Fringillidae) and uses for human medicine in southeast Spain. Evid Based Complement Altern Med 2012; 2012:360913.
8. Rawlinson G. The Histories. Herodotus of Halicarnassus. 430 BC. Translated in 1858. Accessed 2012 Dec 01. URL: http://classics.mit.edu/Herodotus/history.html
9. Medical cannabis. A short graphical history of China. Accessed 2012 Dec 01. URL: http://antiquecannabisbook.com/chap2B/China/China.htm
10. Scholl R. Der Papyrus Ebers. Die grösste Buchrolle zur Heilkunde Altägyptens (Schriften aus der Universitätsbibliothek 7). Leipzig, Germany: Universitat von Leipzig, 2002. [German]

11. Greydanus DE, Patel DR, Feucht C, eds. Preface: Pediatric and adolescent psychopharmacology. Pediatric Clin North Am 2011;58(1):iii–iv.
12. Eddy NB. The history of development of narcotics. Law Contemp Prob 1957;22(1):22–5.
13. Greydanus DE, Feucht C. Performance-enhancing drugs and supplements. In: Patel DR, Greydanus DE, Baker RJ, eds. Pediatric practice: Sports medicine. New York, NY: McGraw Hill Medical. 2009:63–77.
14. History of beer. Accessed 2012 Dec 01. URL: http://en.wikipedia.org/wiki/history_of_beer
15. Escohotada A. A brief history of drugs. London: Park Street Press. 1999.
16. Courtwright DT. Forces of habit. Cambridge, MA: Harvard University Press. 2001.
17. Niemann A. Ueber eine neue organische Base in den Cocablättern. Archiv der Pharmazie 1860;153(2):129–256. [German]
18. Greydanus DE, Patel DR. The adolescent and substance abuse: Current concepts. Disease-a-Month 2005;51(7):387–432.
19. United States. Surgeon General's Advisory Committee on Smoking and Health United States. Rockville, MD: Public Health Service, Office Surgeon General Luther Terry Surgeon General Report, 1964.
20. Preventing tobacco use among youth and youth adults. A report of the Surgeon General. Rockville, MD: US Department Health Human Services, Public Health Office, Office of the Surgeon General, 2012.
21. Freud S. Über Coca. Centralblatt für die ges Therapie 1884;2:289–314. [German]
22. Koelbing HM. Cocaine addiction 100 years ago. A. Erlenmeyer: Uber cocainsucht. [Deutsch] Medizinal Zeitung 31 Mai 1886. Schweiz Rundsch Med Prax 1986;75:1565–8.
23. Accessed 2012 Dec 01. URL: www.narconon.org/drug-information/heroin-history.html
24. Waley A. The opium war through Chinese eyes. London: Allen Unwin, 1958; Reprinted Stanford, CA: Stanford University Press, 1968.
25. Toledo-Pereyra LH: Vignettes on surgery, history and the humanities. Austin, Texas: Landes Bioscience, 2005.
26. Accessed 2012 Dec 01. URL: http://en.wikipedia.org/wiki/Methamphetamine
27. Greydanus DE, Pratt HD. Attention-deficit/hyperactivity disorder in children and adolescents: interventions for a complex costly clinical conundrum. Pediatr Clin North Am 2003;50:1049–92.
28. Hanion CA, Canterberry M. The use of brain imaging to elucidate neural circuit changes in cocaine addiction. Subst Abuse Rehabil 2012;3(1):115–28.
29. de Los Rios F, Kleindorfer DO, Khoury J, Broderick JP, Moomaw CJ, Adeove O, et al. Trends in substance abuse preceding stroke among young adults: a population-based study. Stroke 2012; 43(12):3179–83.
30. Jouanjus E, Pourcel J, Saivin S, Molinier L, Lapeyre-Mestre M. Use of multiple sources and capture-recapture method to estimate the frequency of hospitalizations related to drug abuse. Pharmacoepidemiol Drug Saf 2012 May 02. doi: 10.1002/pds.3280.
31. Beletsky L, Rich JD, Walley AY. Prevention of fatal opioid overdose. JAMA 2012;308(18):1863–4.
32. Alexander GC, Kruszewski SP, Webster DW. Rethinking opioid prescribing to protect patient safety and public health. JAMA 2012;308(18):1865–6.
33. Currie CL, Wild TC. Adolescent use of prescription drugs to get high in Canada. Can J Psychiatry 2012;57(12):745–51.
34. McGuire J, Want B, Zhang L. Substance use and sexual risk behaviors among Mississippi public high school students. J Miss State Med Assoc 2012;53(10):323–8.
35. Brown JH, Clarey AM. The social psychology of disintegrative shaming in education. J Drug Educ 2012;42(2):229–53.
36. Salvo N, Bennett K, Cheung A, Chen Y, Rice M, Rush B, et al. Prevention of substance use in children/adolescents with mental disorders: a systematic review. J Can Acad Child Adolesc Psychiatry 2012; 21(4):245–252.

37. Kuehn BM. WHO documents worldwide need for better drug abuse treatment – and access to it. JAMA 2012;308(5):442–3.
38. Greydanus DE, Feucht C, Patel DR. Pharmacologic management of substance abuse disorders in adolescents: current concepts. In: Merrick J, ed. Child and adolescent health yearbook. New York: Nova Science, 2010:297–309.
39. Greydanus DE. Drug addiction and our youth. Int J Child Adolesc Health 2011;4(3):211–2.
40. Miech R, Bohnert A, Heard K, Boardman J. Increasing use of nonmedical analgesics among younger cohorts in the United States: a birth cohort effect. J Adolesc Health 2013;52(1):25–41.
41. Vaughn LM, Wagner E, Jacquez F. A review of community-based participatory research in child health. MCN Am J Matern Child Nurs 2013;38(1): 48–53.
42. Peloquin SM, Ciro CA. Self-development groups among women in recovery: client perceptions of satisfaction and engagement. Am J Occup Ther 2013; 67(1): 82–90.
43. Rucklidge JJ, Kaplan BJ. Broad-spectrum micronutrient formulas for the treatment of psychiatric symptoms: a systematic review. Expert Rev Neurother 2013;13(1):49–73.
44. Padwa H, Urada D, Antonini VP, Ober A, Crèvecoeur-MacPhail DA, Rawson RA. Integrating substance use disorder services with primary care: the experience in California. J Psychoactive Drugs 2012; 44(4):299–306.
45. Greydanus DE, Feucht C, Hawver EK. Substance abuse disorders. In: Greydanus DE, Patel DR, Omar HA, Feucht C, Merrick J, eds. Adolescent medicine: Pharmacotherapeutics in general, mental, and sexual health. Berlin: De Gruyter, 2012:157–99.

Section I: **Etiology and diagnosis**

2 Neurobiology of substance use disorders

Ahsan Nazeer and Michael R. Liepman

Substance use disorders pose a significant burden to communities and societies across the world. Primarily disorders with onset in childhood or adolescence, untreated substance use disorders typically progress into adulthood, growing in severity and becoming chronic, relapsing, and potentially fatal disorders. Resulting morbidities and sometimes mortality cause a staggering amount of medical and societal costs. Understanding the causes of addiction and underlying neurobiological processes is an active area of research. Most of the current knowledge is derived from preclinical studies and animal models of addiction. The following is a brief review of the mechanisms underlying the addiction process.

2.1 Introduction

Substance use disorders are characterized by a chronic remitting and relapsing course. Symptoms of tolerance and withdrawal are characteristics of physical dependence, but maladaptive patterns of behavior are key to the diagnosis of substance use disorders. In this chapter we briefly review the neurobiology of addictive disorders and for the sake of simplicity, the previously mentioned terms will be used interchangeably. Psychoactive substances act on the neuronal structures and processes that are important for the regulation of healthy mood, behavior, and motivation. Most of the current understanding of this cause and effect is derived from animal models of addiction. These models have been particularly helpful to demystify mechanisms at the neuronal and synaptic level during the acute phase of drug intake. With advancement in research techniques, animal models of chronic drug preference, self-administration, reward, cravings, tolerance development, and withdrawal are being developed in order to better understand the neuroadaptive mechanisms underlying long-term use. Use of genetic variants and characterization of receptor subtypes and interacting neuronal circuits have advanced our understanding of how addictive drugs work in the brain. More recently, the use of positron emission tomography (PET) and functional magnetic resonance imaging (fMRI) have provided critical insights into this highly complex neurocognitive loop. Progress in neurobiology is so rapid that we can only hope to capture a snapshot of today's view because what we know keeps changing.

2.2 General concepts

In the majority of cases, substance use starts either as a recreational activity or as a means to gain some perceived benefits from a particular drug (e.g., pain relief from prescription opioids, control of anxiety, anger, depression, or increasing energy or attention). With repeated intake, a maladaptive pattern of use and loss of control of consumption accompanies the transition to drug dependence. Seeking faster routes of administration, escalating doses, evolution of purpose for taking the drug, repetitive patterns of use, shifting social support networks to incorporate mostly other users, ease of access to drugs, abandoning healthy supports and activities, emotional stress, disregard of danger warnings, and lack of enforcement of safety procedures all play roles in facilitating the progression to harmful addictive use. At this stage, the individual's use becomes more habitual and continues despite ongoing adverse effects and deterioration in psychosocial functioning. From a clinical point of view, this use results in the emergence of complex behavioral problems that probably are a result of substance-induced neurochemical changes in the nervous system.

During the early days of addiction research, the brain reward system was considered the final common pathway in the addiction process. Recent research, however, has shown that the addiction models are more complex than can be explained by the reward model alone. In addition, it is important to understand that the effects of drugs on the reward system continue to play an important role in the overall understanding of the neurobiology of addiction (1). Numerous brain structures are involved in the circuitry of learning, motivation, reward, and pleasure. The caudate, putamen, globus pallidus, and amygdala constitute the basal ganglia. The caudate and putamen together are called the striatum. The nucleus accumbens (NAc) is associated with reward, motivation, and learning. The hippocampus in the limbic system has widely dispersed neuronal connections and plays a role in the development of dependence. Other areas of interest include: orbitofrontal cortex (inhibitory control), prefrontal cortex (executive control), and hypothalamic-pituitary-adrenal axis (associated with stress).

Given the importance of these areas in the regulation of behavior and emotion, it is no surprise that these structures have been the focus of intense scrutiny in substance abuse research. Particularly, dense connections between these areas and the forebrain, including mesolimbic and mesocortical DArgic pathways, have been considered central to the positive reinforcing effects of drugs. Although many consider that understanding how these areas interact with each other and the neurotransmitters involved are key to understanding the addiction model, the realities are quite complex. With ongoing research, the role of non-DArgic systems and deficits in the frontal cortex also are coming to the forefront.

Our understanding of personal genetics has revealed numerous mutations in genes for various structures in the brain, including receptors, transporters, and enzymes. Epigenetic processes also become involved with chronic exposure to high doses of drugs. Complex interactions between neurons modulate presynaptic and postsynaptic activities. Heavy repetitive exposures to certain drugs may generate signals to cell bodies to increase populations of receptors affecting levels of tolerance.

2.2.1 Dopamine

Dopamine (DA) was discovered by Nobel laureate Arvid Carlsson. DA, along with serotonin and epinephrine, is one of the most widely studied and researched neurotransmitters in the nervous system. It is involved in numerous key functions, including the regulation of fine motor movements, learning, motivation, and cognitive functioning. Numerous stimuli including food, sex, and addictive drugs increase intrasynaptic DA levels in the nucleus accumbens (NAc) via their effects on the ventral tegmental area (VTA) (2). It is now known that the NAc responds to the motivational aspect of the stimuli while the striatum is associated with behavioral execution. DA plays a vital role in this mechanism and the DA reward pathway has been the center of addiction research for several decades (3). However, it is worth noting that the underlying neurobiological mechanisms of reward and pleasure are especially complex, and DA does not appear to be the sole culprit in this pathway. It is noted from the fact that numerous noxious and novel stimuli can increase DA within the NAc without causing a reward or an addiction potential.

Acute DA release in the NAc also does not fully explain the desire and compulsions that arise when individuals are exposed to places, persons, and paraphernalia of drug use (triggers, cues). Other evidence comes from animal models with a hypo-DArgic genetic trait who, despite the DA signal blockage, continue to show pleasurable responses to sweet fluids (4). Another observation against DA being the sole neurotransmitter in addiction came from the observation that opiates, ethanol, nicotine, and cannabis appear to bypass the DArgic system while still maintaining part of their addiction potential.

It is worth noting that animal models of addiction have shown a variable pattern of DA neuronal firing that is as much dependent on cues to reward as to the reward itself. In these models, a reward causes firing in DA neurons, but as the animals learn the signals, response to reward habituates and firing occurs in response to the cues themselves (5–6). This pattern suggests extensive input from the cerebral cortex and interactions between the hippocampus, amygdale, and striatum, implicating complex pathways in this neurocircuitry of reward, craving, and habituation. With repeated stimuli, a homeostatic state is reached that is indicated by decreased DA response to such stimuli, a condition synonymous with tolerance in humans.

Numerous studies also have converged on the hypothesis that the previously mentioned cue-based neuronal firing is the cause of persistent drug use. This hypothesis is supported by the fact that most drug use and relapses follow exposure to environmental cues, including places of drug use, drug-using peers, and drug-related paraphernalia. These processes gradually lead to long-term changes and reorganization of neuronal circuitry. The candidate mechanisms underlying this neuronal reorganization are long-term potentiation (LTP) and long-term depression (LTD), the same processes that are also involved in long-term memory and learning.

So far, five DA receptors have been identified and are categorized into two different families.

2.2.1.1 D1, D5 receptors

These receptors are G-protein linked and stimulate cyclic AMP (adenosine monophosphate). They are located postsynaptically and are associated with reward and behavioral inhibition (7). Stimulants, cocaine, ethanol, and food stimulate D1 receptors. This activation causes numerous extra- and intracellular changes including induction of Fos in the NAc and caudate-putamen regions. Research is ongoing to identify the exact role of D1 receptors in the addiction process. In preclinical studies, an increased pattern of cocaine self-administration is found among animals that were exposed to a DA antagonist (8). This behavioral change can be explained by super-sensitivity of DA receptors in the NAc, an observation that suggests a role of D1 receptors in the addiction process.

2.2.1.2 D2, D3 receptors

These receptors also play a major role in the signaling of DA neurons. Studies using animal models have yielded complex results. Pharmacological blockade of D2 receptors leads to decreased response to morphine and ethanol (9). D2 receptors have two isoforms: D2L, which has postsynaptic effects, and D2S, which acts as presynaptic autoreceptor. Because of its inhibitory function as presynaptic autoreceptor, in genetically modified D2-negative mice administration of cocaine causes significant elevations in the striatum (10). positron emission tomography (PET) and single-photon emission computed tomography (SPECT) studies have shown decreased D2 density in frequent users of cocaine, heroin, and methamphetamine (11). Other studies have found an inverse correlation between the D2 receptor density and self-administration of cocaine (12). In human studies of ethanol and methylphenidate, individuals with fewer D2 receptors were found to require higher doses of these drugs in order to get the same response in comparison to individuals with higher D2 density in the NAc (13). Whether the decrease in D2 receptors is a predisposing event that causes drug addiction, is an area of ongoing research (14).

D3 receptors are mainly localized in the limbic region and are structurally similar to D2 receptors. In animal studies, pharmacological blockage of these receptors was found to reduce ethanol-seeking behavior, self-administration of ethanol, and reinstatement of cocaine- as well as nicotine-seeking behaviors (15–17).

2.2.2 Serotonin and norepinephrine

Serotonin (5-HT) is a neurotransmitter that is involved in numerous bodily functions including impulse control, sleep, appetite, sexual behaviors, and pain modulation. There are several varieties of serotonin receptors with some being excitatory and some inhibitory in their function. Most important among these in addiction research is 5-HT1B, which is widely distributed across the central nervous system (CNS) and is present on the terminal regions of DA and γ-aminobutyric acid (GABA) neurons. Stimulation of this receptor inhibits GABA release that in turn removes the inhibitory influence of GABAergic effects on the DA system. In genetically modified 5-HT1B-negative mice, reinforcing effects of cocaine were markedly reduced.

Norepinephrine (NE) is another neurotransmitter that is present in abundance in the CNS. It has widespread projections from the locus coeruleus, pons, and medulla to the hippocampus, hypothalamus, and amygdala. It plays a role in stress and arousal responses by its actions on α- and β-adrenergic receptors. During the early 1980s, animal models of self-administration (reward) have failed to show a role for NE in addiction research. However, in the 1990s, numerous other animal models emerged. Among them, the model of drug-induced locomotion proved critical to our understanding of neurobiology of drug addiction. Most drugs of abuse induce locomotor activity, which suggests sensitization that in turn is a sign of craving (18). By using different models of NE antagonism (prazosin, lesions of locus ceruleus), studies have shown NE to play an important role in psychostimulant-induced locomotion (19). On the other hand, increasing extracellular NE also increases the locomotor response to psychostimulants (20).

2.2.3 GABA

GABA is the main inhibitory neurotransmitter in the nervous system. It exerts its inhibitory effects by hyperpolarizing neurons. Three types of GABA receptors have been identified: A, B, and C. GABAA receptors also bind benzodiazepines and barbiturates. These are transmembrane ligand-gated ion channels that are mostly present in the postsynaptic membranes. Type A receptors play a vital role in the immediate and long-term effects of ethanol. Ethanol increases the ion influx by increasing the amount of time ion channels are in the open state and by decreasing their time in the closed state. GABAA receptor antagonists reduce self-administration of ethanol and cocaine (21). On the other hand, agents that potentiate the effects of GABAA receptors increase the self-administration of ethanol (22).

2.3 Neuropharmacology of specific drugs

In the following sections we review the mechanism of action of various common drugs of abuse.

2.3.1 Stimulants

Stimulants, including cocaine, amphetamines, and methylphenidate, exert their effects by increasing DA and NE levels in the respective synapses (see chapters 10, 11, and 16). Cocaine and methylphenidate block the presynaptic DA transporter (DAT), preventing DA reuptake from the synapses. This prolongs the availability of DA to postsynaptic DA receptors, enhancing postsynaptic neuron activity. Amphetamines, on the other hand, act as false substrates for DAT and are taken into the neuron instead of DA. Once inside the neuron, amphetamines again act as false substrates for vesicular monoamine transporter (VMAT) on the vesicles. These vesicles then release DA from vesicle to cytosol into the intrasynaptic cleft. Cocaine administration increases DA concentration and D1 receptor density in the striatum. This increased concentration in mesolimbic and mesocortical pathways is postulated to be responsible for the behavioral actions after cocaine administration. In animal studies, D1 receptor blockade in the NAc and the VTA reduce cocaine self-administration.

In human studies, the acute "high" response to cocaine is correlated with DAT occupancy and DA release in the NAc (23,24). On the other hand, clinical experience is not supportive of the previously mentioned DA hypothesis. This is mostly noted from the fact that the antipsychotic medications do not block the rewarding effects of DA or other stimulants. One possible explanation of this lack of effect is that stimulants, including cocaine, also exert their effects by acting on the NE neurons. This point is validated from animal studies in which DAT-deficient strains of mice appear to experience the rewarding effects of cocaine, suggesting an important role of other neurotransmitters in the neurobiology of reward and addiction (25).

NE, serotonin, and glutamate are other major neurotransmitter systems that are involved in the neurobiology of stimulant addiction. Cocaine administration increases NE activity by its action on the NE transporter. This increased plasma concentration of NE is correlated with the psychological effects of cocaine. Cocaine administration also increases extracellular serotonin concentration in the striatum and VTA by its effects on the serotonin transporter.

The exact role of serotonin in the reward pathway is unclear. Cocaine exerts its rewarding effects in serotonin transporter–deficient strains of mice whereas mice missing both DAT and serotonin transporters do not find cocaine rewarding (25). Human studies have failed to conceptualize a persistent role of serotonin in this pathway. Serotonin agonists (SSRIs), antagonists, or partial agonists all have reported to reduce the "high" and cravings of cocaine (26). Glutamate appears to play a role in relapse to cocaine (27). Acutely administered low-dose cocaine increases glutaminergic neuronal firing in the cortex and NAc, whereas higher doses inhibit this phenomenon. Cocaine also upregulates N-Methyl-D-aspartate (NMDA) receptors binding in the striatum and amygdala.

2.3.2 Alcohol

All drugs of abuse, including alcohol, enhance the release of DA within the mesolimbic and mesocortical pathways of the brain. Alcohol intake causes release of β-endorphins from the arcuate nucleus, which along with its effects on GABA and DA is thought to cause pleasurable effects after alcohol intake (see chapter 9). Acute intake of alcohol appears to increase the firing rate of midbrain DA neurons while chronic exposure leads to decreased excitability of these neurons. Other than DA, it is widely accepted that alcohol also acts by increasing inhibitory neurotransmission at GABA receptors and reducing excitatory transmission at glutamate neurons. Alcohol acts on presynaptic glutamate receptors and calcium channels to inhibit glutamate release. These initial effects on neurotransmitters and ion channels lead to a cascade of events that involve glycine, serotonin, and opioid systems.

Glutamate is a major excitatory neurotransmitter in the nervous system. AMPA (alpha-amino-3-hydroxy-5-methyl-4-isoxazolepropionic acid) and NMDA receptors are two ion channels that are associated with the glutamate system and are responsible for excitatory neurotransmission in the mechanisms of learning and memory. NMDA receptors are sensitive to alcohol while AMPA receptors show insensitivity. Inhibition of NMDA receptors in the prefrontal cortex may explain some of the sedative effects and cognitive deficits seen after alcohol use. These receptors also play a critical role in the regulation of DA in the nucleus accumbens. NMDA receptor antagonists increase the DA level in the NAc and this antagonism by alcohol can be one reason for its rewarding properties. These receptors also show increase in density in glutamatergic synapses after chronic alcohol consumption.

As noted previously, alcohol increases the blood level of certain opioids including β-endorphins. There is evidence that acetaldehyde, the first oxidative metabolite of ethanol, by competitive inhibition can interfere with removal of monoamine neurotransmitter aldehydes in the brain, leading to persistence of monoamine neurotransmitter aldehydes from cerebrospinal fluid (CSF). It has been demonstrated that mixing these monoamine aldehydes with monoamines facilitates chemical combinations known as tetrhydroisoquinolines, which are opioid agonists that can be blocked by opioid receptor antagonists (28–30). Naltrexone also blocks the rewarding effects of ethanol while increasing it sedative effects but not its neurological effects (31). These findings explain why the opioid antagonist naltrexone has been shown to be effective for the treatment of alcoholism.

2.3.3 Opioids

Opioids are natural and synthetic compounds that are related to natural opium and include heroin, morphine, codeine, methadone, hydrocodone, oxycodone fentanyl, tramadol, and pentazocine, among others (see chapters 10 and 16). So far, three different types of opioid receptors have been identified – mu, kappa, and delta – with several subtypes of the mu and kappa receptors identified. These receptors are abundant in the CNS, and are found in the amygdala, caudate, cortex, putamen, and thalamus. These are Gi-coupled transmembrane receptors and have a different affinity for endogenous peptides. β-endorphins are more selective for mu receptors, while dynorphins have more selectivity for kappa receptors. In opioid addiction, mu receptors are at the forefront of the research.

Numerous drugs, including heroin, morphine, and other opioid analgesics, are agonists of these receptors. Mu receptor agonists cause euphoria, analgesia, sedation, constipation, hypotension, respiratory depression, itching, nausea, and meiosis. Kappa receptor agonists may reverse the mu receptor actions, and cause dysphoria, delirium, dissociation, hallucinations, and possibly seizures. These receptors are quite sensitive to stress. Delta opioid receptors may produce mild analgesia, respiratory depression, and seizures in high doses.

Most of what we know about the neurobiology of opioid addiction has been derived from animal models. Different approaches have been used in these models, including self-administration of opioids, use of opioid antagonists to disrupt the reward pathway, and lesions in the critical areas that are thought to be involved in the addiction pathway. In mice models of opioid self-administration, numerous areas of interest have been identified, including ventral striatum (32), lateral septum (33), VTA, hippocampus, and periaqueductal gray. Increase in self-administration has been noticed after the injection of an opioid antagonist into the NAc and lateral hypothalamus. It is worth noting, however, that administration of an opioid antagonist into the VTA, a site that is considered one of the central areas in the reward pathway, failed to disrupt self-administration (34). The role of the mesolimbic DArgic system is also suggested, but more research is needed in this area. DA antagonists have no influence on the self-administration of opioids. However, opioids exert their reinforcing effects by increasing DA in the NAc, an effect that is thought to be the result of opioid-induced GABA inhibition (35).

2.3.4 Nicotine/tobacco

Tobacco continues to be the single largest cause of preventable morbidity and mortality in the Western world (36). In the United States, tobacco-related health problems cost about $75 billion per year in treatment expenditures (see chapter 7). Despite this awareness, tobacco use continues to increase all over the world.

Nicotine is a psychoactive substance that affects numerous neuronal pathways and neurotransmitter systems. Nicotine acts on neuronal nicotinic-subtype acetylcholine receptors (nAChR), which are widely distributed in the nervous system. These are ligand-gated ion channels that in the open stage permit cations to pass through the channel pores. Evidence suggests a role of the VTA and DA pathways in nicotine addiction. VTA contains numerous nAChR receptors and nicotine administration has been shown to activate DA signaling in the mesolimbic, mesocortical pathways, and increased DA release in nucleus accumbens. Continued activation of nAChR receptors leads to desensitization that partially explains the decreased rewarding effects of nicotine that a smoker experiences later in the day.

Other than acting on the DA system in the VTA, nicotine also effects the GABA system in a variety of ways. During the early phases of nicotine administration, it activates GABA neurons that in turn are inhibitory on the DA system. However, nAChRs of the GABA system desensitize rather quickly, leading to the removal of this inhibitory influence on the DA system. GABA agonists have been shown to decrease the self-administration of nicotine. This also corresponds to the activation of nAChRs on presynaptic glutamatergic neurons, leading to increased excitatory glutamatergic transmission to DArgic system. The VTA receives excitatory glutamatergic projections from the prefrontal cortex that modulate the activity of DA and GABA. The tegmental pedunculo-pontine (TPP) nucleus is a brain region that receives descending GABA projections from the VTA and sends ascending glutamatergic and cholinergic projections to the VTA. This area is associated with a non-DA-related reward system that seems to play an important role in the acute rewarding effects of opioids and nicotine.

It is important to recognize that the reward characteristics of tobacco products as nicotine delivery systems vary depending on the mode of entry into the body and whether acetaldehyde is combined with the nicotine. Smoking delivers both acetaldehyde and nicotine to the brain within seconds of inhalation. Acetaldehyde is also involved in the alcohol reward process (see earlier) and has been shown to enhance the addictive properties of smoking. Most heavy smokers (defined as 1–2 packs a day) consume from 200 to 400 rewarding puffs per day, the largest number of rewards of any known drug of abuse, accounting for the difficulty most smokers have in quitting. It should also be mentioned that most lifelong smokers begin smoking as adolescents, and 75% of those who smoke three cigarettes (30 puffs) will become committed lifelong smokers. Other forms of tobacco products, such as snuff and chewing tobacco, do not deliver acetaldehyde, yet many of the harmful constituents of tobacco are still present. Clearly smoking provides the most dangerous set of toxins, many resulting from combustion, including carbon monoxide, cyanide, formaldehyde, hydrogen sulfide, carcinogenic long-chain hydrocarbons (tar), and ashes. It is the reward pathways that reinforce the persistent ingestions despite noxious signals from the body to the contrary. Blockade of the alpha-4-beta-2 nicotinic cholinergic receptors by the partial agonist/antagonist varenicline removes the reward and lets the dysphoric effects of smoking speak for themselves (see chapter 7).

Nicotine delivery systems such as the gum, patch, and lozenge provide a slow nicotine delivery system devoid of acetaldehyde and the other 35,000 dangerous chemicals in tobacco smoke. The reduction in the reward both by eliminating the acetaldehyde and by spreading out and delaying the reward, reduces its ability to reinforce self-administration behavior and permits extinction. By diminishing the extent of the withdrawal syndrome, people trying to quit smoking find greater self-efficacy. If a smoking slip occurs, the occupancy of the nicotinic cholinergic receptors reduces the potency of the reward. Inhaled forms of nicotine delivery such as e-cigarettes and nicotine spray inhalers do provide harm avoidance, but do not delay the nicotine reward, hence keeping the enslavement of the smoker active.

Bupropion helps reduce the craving and response to smoking by its tendency to inhibit reuptake of DA and NE from synapses, causing enhanced and prolonged DArgic and noradrenergic activity, reducing the reward strength of nicotine and acetaldehyde-mediated opioids. Smokers may worry about weight gain, depression, and decreased concentration, symptoms commonly seen in withdrawal. Bupropion may be helpful in reducing these symptoms, especially if started several weeks before the quit date (37).

Many smokers evoke the stress-reducing anxiolytic properties of smoking as a reason why they cannot quit smoking right now. However, studies of stress in smokers revealed that the only stress that smoking relieves is the stress of nicotine withdrawal that is additive with any other stress they might be experiencing (38,39). Smokers smoke to maintain a steady nicotine level in the blood and CSF. Stress can increase adrenergic tone, thereby increasing heart rate, renal glomerular filtration, and excretion of nicotine. Every time the nicotine concentration drops below a certain level, craving surfaces, causing an urge to smoke; this increases during stress, causing increased consumption of cigarettes. By continuing to smoke, smokers increase their overall stress by adding recurrent nicotine withdrawal to their underlying anxiety.

2.3.5 Cannabinoids

Alcohol, nicotine, and marijuana are the most commonly used illicit drugs all over the world. Marijuana has a rich history and has for centuries been used as a legitimate medicine in some civilizations (see the introduction, chapter 1). In Western medicine, its role in appetite stimulation, pain management, and for the management of chemotherapy-induced nausea has been appreciated for some time. As noted previously, this is also a drug that has a significant abuse potential for the euphoric effects that it produces within minutes of its use.

So far, two cannabinoid receptors, CB1 and CB2, have been identified. Both are G protein coupled receptors. CB1 is predominantly found in the central and peripheral nervous system including the VTA, NAc, hippocampus, and amygdala, while CB2 is predominantly found in immune cells. It is interesting to note that other than modulating the abuse potential of marijuana, cannabinoid receptors also are involved in the rewarding potential of other drugs including alcohol, cocaine, and nicotine (40,41). CB1 receptors play a major role in the addiction of marijuana. CB1 antagonists reduce drug-seeking behavior in animal models (42).

Administration of tetrahydrocannabinol (THC) increases DA in the reward center, including NAc, striatum, and prefrontal cortex (43). This effect is considered a result of indirect action on glutamatergic and GABAergic neurons that modulate the DA system. Another interesting finding in this sequence has been the role of opioid receptors. It is shown that DA release after THC administration is not solely the result of CB1 receptor stimulation but that the opioid receptors also are involved in this cascade of events. Administration of the opioid antagonist naloxone blocks this effect (44), a finding that leads to the complex interaction of numerous neurotransmitters in the final pathway of cannabinoids effect.

2.4 Summary

Current research has advanced our knowledge from the basic concept of the DA reward system to a more complex understanding of intracellular signal transduction and the harmonious interactions of different areas of the nervous system. Much remains unknown, with more questions arising with every discovery. With passing years, models of addiction will be further refined that in turn will help to find successful treatment modalities for this population in need.

References

1. Koob GF, Le Moal M. Drug abuse: hedonic homeostatic dysregulation. Science 1997;278:52–8.
2. Yoshimoto K, McBride WJ, Lumeng L, Li T-K. Alcohol stimulates the release of dopamine and serotonin in the nucleus accumbens. Alcohol 1991;9:17–22.
3. Pettit HO, Justice Jr JB. Effect of dose on cocaine self administration behavior and dopamine levels in the nucleus accumbens. Brain Res 1991;539:94–102.
4. Robinson S, Sandstrom SM, Denenberg VH, Palmiter RD. Distinguishing whether dopamine regulates liking, wanting, and/or learning about rewards. Behav Neurosci 2005;199:336–41.

5. Hyman SE. Addiction: a disease of learning and memory. Am J Psychiatry 2005;162(8): 1414–22.
6. Hyman SE, Malenka RC. Addiction and the brain: the neurobiology of compulsion and its persistence. Nat Rev Neurosci 2001;2:695–703.
7. Goodman A. Neurobiology of addiction. An integrative review. Biochem Pharmacol 2008;75: 266–322.
8. Barone P, Tucci I, Parashos SA, Chase TN. Supersensitivity to a D-1 dopamine receptor agonist and subsensitivity to a D-2 receptor agonist following chronic D-1 receptor blockade. Eur J Pharmacol 1988;149:225–32.
9. Risinger FO, Freeman PA, Rubinstein M, Low MJ, Grandy DK. Psychopharmacology (Berlin) 2000; 152:343–50.
10. Welter M, Vallone D, Samad TA, Meziane H, Usiello A, Borrelli E. Absence of dopamine D2 receptors unmasks an inhibitory control over the brain circuitries activated by cocaine. *Proc Natl Acad Sci USA.* 2007;104:6840–5.
11. Volkow ND, Chang L, Wang GJ, Fowler JS, Ding Y-S, Sedler M, et al. Low level of brain dopamine D2 receptors in methamphetamine abusers: association with metabolism in the orbitofrontal cortex. Am J Psychiatry 2001;158:2015–21.
12. Nader MA, Morgan D, Gage HD, Nader SH, Calhoun TL, Buchheimer N, et al. PET imaging of dopamine D2 receptors during chronic cocaine self-administration in monkeys. Nat Neurosci 2006;9(8):1050–6.
13. Yoder KK, Kareken DA, Seyoum RA, O'Connor SJ, Wang C, Zheng Q-H, et al. Dopamine D2 receptor availability is associated with subjective responses to alcohol. Alcohol Clin Exp Res 2005; 29(6):965–70.
14. Volkow ND, Wang GJ, Fowler JS, Logan J, Gatley SJ, Wong C, et al. Reinforcing effects of psychostimulants in humans are associated with increases in brain dopamine and occupancy of D(2) receptors. J Pharmacol Exp Ther 1999;291:409–15.
15. Heidbreder CA, Andreoli M, Marcon C, Hutcheson DM, Gardner EL, Ashby CR. Evidence for the role of dopamine D3 receptors in oral operant alcohol self-administration and reinstatement of alcohol-seeking behavior in mice. Addict Biol 2007;12(1):35–50.
16. Cervo L, Cocco A, Petrella C, Heidbreder CA. Selective antagonism at dopamine D3 receptors attenuates cocaine-seeking behavior in the rat. Int J Neuropsychopharmacol 2007;10(2): 167–81.
17. Ross JT, Corrigall WA, Heidbreder CA, LeSage MG. Effects of the selective dopamine D3 receptor antagonist SB- 277011A on the reinforcing effects of nicotine as measured by a progressive-ratio schedule in rats. Eur J Pharmacol 2007;559(2/3):173–9.
18. Weinshenker D, Schroeder JP. There and back again: a tale of norepinephrine and drug addiction. Neuropsychopharmacology 2007;32:1433–51.
19. Salomon L, Lanteri C, Glowinski J, Tassin JP. Behavioral sensitization to amphetamine results from an uncoupling between noradrenergic and serotonergic neurons. Proc Natl Acad Sci USA 2006;103:7476–81.
20. Villégier AS, Drouin C, Bizot JC, Marien M, Glowinski J, Colpaert F, et al. Stimulation of postsynaptic alpha1b- and alpha2- adrenergic receptors amplifies dopamine-mediated locomotor activity in both rats and mice. Synapse 2003;50:277–84.
21. Nowak KL, McBride WJ, Lumeng L, Li T-K, Murphy JM. Blocking GABAA receptors in the anterior ventral tegmental area attenuates ethanol intake of the alcohol preferring P rat. Psychopharmacology 1998;139:108–16.
22. Boyle AE, Segal R, Smith BR, Amit Z. Bidirectional effects of GABAergic agonists and antagonists on maintenance of voluntary ethanol intake in rats. Pharmacol Biochem Behav 1993;46(1): 179–82.

23. Kimmel HL, O'Connor JA, Carroll FI, Howell LL. Faster onset and dopamine transporter selectivity predict stimulant and reinforcing effects of cocaine analogs in squirrel monkeys. Pharmacol Biochem Behav 2007;86:45–54.
24. Volkow ND, Fowler JS, Wang GJ, Baler R, Telang F. Imaging dopamine's role in drug abuse and addiction. Neuropharmacology 2009;56(Suppl 1):3–8.
25. Filip M, Frankowska M, Zaniewska M, Golda A, Przegalinski E. The serotonergic system and its role in cocaine addiction. Pharmacol Rep 2005;57:685–700.
26. Buydens-Branchey L, Branchey M, Fergeson P, Hudson J, McKerin C. Craving for cocaine in addicted users. Role of serotonergic mechanisms. Am J Addict 1997;6:65–73.
27. Gass JT, Olive MF. Glutamatergic substrates of drug addiction and alcoholism. Biochem Pharmacol 2008;75:218–65.
28. Deitrich RA. Tissue and subcellular distribution of mammalian aldehyde-oxidizing capacity. Biochem Pharmacol 1966;15:1911.
29. Collins MA, Bigdeli MG. Tetrahydroisoquinolines in vivo. I. Rat brain formation of salsolinol, a condensation product of dopamine and acetaldehyde, under certain conditions during ethanol intoxication. Life Sci 1975;16:585–601.
30. Yamanaka Y, Walsh MJ, Davis VE. Salsolinol, an alkaloid derivative of dopamine formed in vitro during alcohol metabolism. Nature 1970;227:1143–4.
31. Swift RM, Whelilhan W, Kuznetsov O, Buongiorno G, Hsuing H. Naltrexone-induced alterations in human ethanol intoxication. Am J Psychiatry 1994;151:1463–7.
32. David, V, Cazala, P. Anatomical and pharmacological specificity of the rewarding effect elicited by microinjections of morphine into the nucleus accumbens of mice. Psychopharmacology 2000;150:24–34.
33. Le Merrer J, Gavello-Baudy S, Galey D, Cazala P: Morphins self-administration into the lateral septum depends on dopaminergic mechanisms: Evidence from pharmacology and Fos neuroimaging. Behav Brain Res 2007;180(2):203–17.
34. Vaccarino FJ, Pettit HO, Bloom FE, Koob GF. Effects of intracerebroventricular administration of methyl naloxonium chloride on heroin self-administration in the rat. Pharmacol Biochem Behav 1985;23:495–8.
35. Johnson SW, North RA. Opioids excite dopamine neurons by hyperpolarization of local interneurons. J Neurosci 1992;12:483–8.
36. Annual smoking-attributable mortality, years of potential life lost, and economic costs-United States, 1995–1999. MMWR 2002;51:300–3.
37. Hurt RD, Sachs DPL, Glover ED, Offord KP, Johnston JA, Dale LC, et al. A comparison of sustained-release bupropion and placebo for smoking cessation. N Engl J Med 1997;337:1195–1202.
38. Schachter S, Silverstein B, Kozlowski LT, Herman CP, Liebling B. Studies of the interaction of psychological and pharmacological determinants of smoking IV. Effects of stress on cigarette smoking and urinary pH. J Experimental Psychol Gen 1977;106:24–30.
39. Schachter S, Silverstein B, Perlick D. Studies of the interaction of psychological and pharmacological determinants of smoking V. Psychological and pharmacological explanations of smoking under stress. J Experimental Psychol Gen 1977;106:31–40.
40. Mechoulam R, Parker L. Cannabis and alcohol–a close friendship. Trends Pharmacol Sci 2003; 24:266–8.
41. Forget B, Barthélémy S, Saurini F, Hamon M, Thiébot, MH. Differential involvement of the endocannabinoid system in short- and long-term expression of incentive learning supported by nicotine in rats. Psychopharmacology 2006;189:59–69.
42. Economidou D, Mattioli L, Cifani C, Perfumi M, Massi M, et al. Effect of the cannabinoid CB1 receptor antagonist SR-141716A on ethanol self-administration and ethanol-seeking behavior in rats. Psychopharmacology 2006;183:394–403.

43. Ng Cheong Ton JM, Gerhardt GA, Friedemann M, Etgen AM, Rose GM, Sharpless NS, et al. The effects of delta9- tetrahydrocannabinol on potassium-evoked release of dopamine in the rat caudate nucleus: an in vivo electrochemical and in vivo microdialysis study. Brain Res 1988;451: 59–68.
44. Tanda G, Pontieri FE, Di Chiara G. Cannabinoid and heroin activation of mesolimbic dopamine transmission by a common mu1 opioid receptor mechanism. Science 1997;276:2048–50.

3 Genetic influences on substance abuse disorders

Helga V. Toriello

This chapter is a review of some genetic influences on the development of substance use disorders in adolescents and young adults. Although there are many complex facets to substance abuse development, genetic factors appear to play an important role. Issues covered include shared environment and nonshared environment, comorbid psychiatric disorders, gene classes (i.e., dopamine, opioid, and serotonin), and genetic factors in specific addictions (i.e., alcohol, cannabis, tobacco, and cocaine). The influences of genetic factors will continue to be unraveled as the 21st century continues.

3.1 Introduction

Substance use disorders (SUD) are a significant public health problem in that the lifetime prevalence of alcohol dependence or abuse is 8%, the lifetime prevalence of illicit drug use is 2%–3% (1,2), and the lifetime prevalence of nicotine dependence is approximately 25% (3). The cause of these disorders is complex, but it is clear that SUD appear to "run in families," based on the observation that there is a higher frequency of SUD in family members compared to that in controls, and there is a higher frequency of SUD in close relatives compared to more distant relatives (4). Indeed, one family study found that the frequency of SUD in relatives was approximately eight times greater than the frequency in relatives of controls or psychiatric patients (5). But how much is attributable to environmental influences versus genetics? For many years, a number of approaches have been used to separate genetic from environmental effects.

Besides family studies, twin and adoption studies have been useful for demonstrating genetic influences on a particular trait. In twin studies, the concordance between monozygous twins is compared to the concordance between dizygous twins; if the monozygous twins are more alike (i.e., more often concordant) than are the dizygous twins, then that would indicate a genetic contribution to the phenotype. For example, for SUD in general, the concordance between monozygous twins has been found to be .63–.77, whereas for dizygous twins it was .44–.55 (6,7). In adoption studies, if there is a greater similarity between adoptees and their biologic parents than between adoptees and their adoptive parents, that would indicate that there is a genetic component to the phenotype as well (4). Further evidence for a biologic cause for a particular trait or behavior comes from animal studies. In the case of SUD, if laboratory animals voluntarily self-administer some drugs, then that observation provides evidence for a biologic basis for addiction (8).

Given these studies, the overwhelming evidence indicates that SUD are complex (multifactorial) traits as opposed to monogenic conditions (which are caused by pathogenic mutations with large effect and inheritance patterns that follow autosomal or X-linked, dominant or recessive modes). Complex traits are those presumed to occur because of gene-environment interaction. The genetic component is often referred to as the "heritability" of a trait, so that if a trait is said to have a heritability of .5, or 50%, it would indicate that 50% of the variance is attributable to genetic factors. Those genetic factors in turn are generally assumed to originate in multiple genes, each with a small effect, although this may not be universally true.

The environmental component can be further divided into shared environment and nonshared environment. For example, siblings raised in the same household have a shared environment. If one of those children, however, was injured in a motor vehicle accident, this would constitute a nonshared environmental effect. In addition, the steps in the progression from nonuse to drug dependence are likely under the influence of different degrees of genetic and environmental control. Evidence suggests that environmental factors have a greater influence on the initiation of drug use, whereas genetic factors become more important in the transition to the development of addiction (9,10).

So how are genetic studies done? In the past, linkage and association studies identified candidate genes that were likely to be related to a particular phenotype; research would follow looking for a higher frequency of variations in the genes of study subjects versus controls. The use of linkage and association studies, however, depended on an understanding of biologic mechanisms and precise definition of phenotypes. More recently, genome-wide association studies (GWAS) were developed to assay several hundred thousand to a million single nucleotide polymorphisms (SNPs) in populations as large as several thousand individuals. Studies further analyzed SNPs (which are variants usually caused by a single base pair change) and investigated differences between subjects and controls more thoroughly for relevance using various techniques. The basic assumption underlying the use of GWAS is that common diseases are caused by variants that are present in 1%–5% of the population (11).

3.2 Limitations

There are several limitations inherent to dissecting the genetic component of complex traits, particularly in terms of defining the phenotype (yes versus no, age of onset, severity, and so on). Put simply, "people become addicted or remain addicted (to alcohol) for different reasons" (12). Although the quote refers to alcohol dependence or abuse, the same holds true for other addictions. The presence of comorbidities can also make this endeavor difficult. It is known that individuals who abuse one substance are more likely to abuse other substances; for example, tobacco, cannabis, and alcohol abuse or dependence are highly comorbid with each other (13), as are cocaine, opioid, and nicotine dependence (14). This observation is in part explained by a common genetic predisposition leading to alternative manifestations of that predisposition (15). Therefore, the heritable trait is the use/dependence/abuse of alcohol, tobacco, and/or cannabis, with a heritability estimate of 60% for this phenotype (16). There is also evidence that additional genetic factors predispose to specific addictions to alcohol, tobacco, and cannabis, so future GWAS should be expected to identify several predispositional genes for alcohol, tobacco, and cannabis abuse, as well as several genes specific to each type of addiction (17).

SUD are also comorbid with psychiatric disorders such as mood, anxiety, and conduct disorders in particular (18). For example, individuals with SUD are 2–3 times more likely to also have depression or anxiety; conversely, alcohol-abuse disorders are more common in patients with mood disorders such as bipolar disorder or depression (18,19) (see chapters 9 and 14). It has been suggested that, as in the case of polysubstance comorbidity attributable to a common genetic mechanism, there is also a common genetic predisposition to both externalizing or behavioral disinhibition characteristics and SUD (6,20,21). Within this group as well, additional genetic factors may then predispose to specific addictions or behavioral disorders (1).

Some mental health conditions such as gambling, Internet addiction, sex addiction, and overeating are sometimes referred to as behavioral addictions. It is unknown whether these conditions should be studied under the umbrella of SUD. Of these, however, gambling has recently been classified as an addiction-related disorder in the *Diagnostic and Statistical Manual of Mental Disorders,* fifth edition (DSM-V) (22). Furthermore, the heritability of gambling is 35%–54% (23), indicating that a genetic component exists for this behavior. In addition, pathologic gambling has been found to be comorbid with SUD, with alcohol use disorders present in 73% of gamblers, and those with substance or alcohol dependence being almost three times more likely to have a gambling problem (24,25). Therefore, it has been suggested by some (22) that other behavioral addictions may also share genetic commonality with SUD, particularly since there are numerous similarities in terms of natural history, comorbidity, neurobiologic mechanisms, and so on, between behavioral addictions and SUD. Further study of those with behavioral and substance addictions may yield insights into relevant genetic pathways.

3.3 Gene classes

Despite some of these limitations noted earlier, there have been some interesting findings from genetic studies. What follows is not intended to be a comprehensive review, but only meant to highlight some of the recent findings. Several classes of genes have been identified (using the candidate gene approach, or GWAS) in the genetic etiology of SUD. One class is the dopamine system, which consists of receptors, transporters, and the enzymes involved in its metabolism (26) (see chapter 2). This system is also involved in the predisposition to psychiatric and psychotic disorders.

A second major gene class is the opioid system. There are four major subtypes of opioid receptors coded for by four distinct genes (OPRK1, OPRD1, OPRM1, and OPRL1) that are stimulated by the endogenous opioid peptides beta-endorphin (POMC), prodynomorphin (PDYN), enkaphalin (PENK), and orphanin/nociceptin (PNOC). These gene products (both receptors and opioid peptides) have been shown to interact with the dopaminergic system (27) and are implicated in the susceptibility to opioid, cocaine, alcohol, and methamphetamine addiction (28). A third class of relevant genes is the group regulating serotonin, which includes serotonin transporters and receptors. This class of genes is well known to be involved in the development of psychiatric and behavioral disorders, but only recently has been investigated as being involved in the etiology of SUD, particularly alcohol, nicotine, cocaine, and opioid dependence or abuse (29) (see chapters 7, 10, 11, and 16).

In addition, GWAS studies have identified close to 100 additional candidate genes that confer susceptibility to addiction, with many involved in cell adhesion (important for establishing and maintaining neural connections) (4,30) as well as genes that are primarily expressed in the brain, particularly the hippocampus and amygdala (31). Notably, recent studies have also identified candidate genes that are tightly linked to the various dopamine system genes, and that might also confer increased susceptibility to SUD. For example, ANKK1 (ankyrin repeat and kinase domain containing) is in a gene cluster with DRD2 (dopamine receptor D2), and it has been implicated as being involved in addictive disorders via its effect on signal transduction pathways (26).

3.4 Specific addictions

3.4.1 Alcohol

Studies on specific addictions have also found noteworthy results. Alcohol abuse or dependence has a significant genetic component, with heritabilities of approximately 50%–60% overall, but higher in females than in males (2,32) (see chapter 9). Using association studies, the alcohol dehydrogenase gene cluster had been found to be predispositional to alcohol dependence and aldehyde dehydrogenase 2 pathway protective. Both enzyme systems are in the same pathway that is involved in alcohol degradation (33). Other specific gene systems found to be involved are the glutamatergic system and the cholinergic system (34,35).

Using GWAS, other genes that predispose to the development of alcohol addiction have been identified, with many also predisposing to comorbidities. For example, several genes in the gamma-aminobutyric acid-ergic system also appear to predispose to the development of nicotine dependence (36); variants in cadherin 13 also appear to predispose to methamphetamine dependence (37). Astrotactin neuronal protein (ASTN1) is a gene associated with alcohol dependence that also has a role in glial-guided neuronal migration (38). This gene is interesting in that it is also implicated in autism, schizophrenia, bipolar disorder, and attention-defecit hyperactivity disorder (ADHD). Similarly, Wang et al. (39) found correlations between SNPs in C15orf53 and the number of alcohol-related symptoms (using the diagnostic criteria as defined by the DSM-IV), with a greater number of symptoms more likely to be associated with a greater likelihood of having a variant in this gene. Genetic variants in this gene are also thought to correlate with a predisposition to develop bipolar disorder, a condition that is comorbid with alcohol abuse (40).

An interesting approach to identifying alcohol dependence-related genes was that of Enoch et al. (41), who studied stress-related genes (i.e., those that mediate the response to stress) and found that certain polymorphisms were associated with an increased frequency of alcohol consumption secondary to stress. For example, carriers of a polymorphism in the PER1 (circadian rhythm gene period 1), which is activated by stress hormones, had a higher frequency of heavy drinking when also exposed to greater family adversity, thus demonstrating that response to environmental factors might also be under some genetic control.

3.4.2 Cannabis

Cannabis abuse/dependence is also markedly heritable, with a heritability of approximately 50% – it is more heritable in females than in males (2,42) (see chapter 8). Here again, studies are beginning to sort out the relevant genetic mechanisms that lead to cannabis dependence. For example, DRD2 and PENK are both expressed in the mesocorticolimbic system and certain polymorphisms are associated with a predisposition to cannabis dependence. Individuals with these polymorphisms in one or both genes are considered to have a high-risk genotype. One group found that individuals with the high-risk genotype who also had neuroticism were at a greater risk of developing cannabis dependence than those with the same genotype but no neuroticism. Specifically, if those with no neuroticism and the low-risk genotype had a baseline risk of 1, by comparison, those with either the low-risk genotype but presence of neuroticism or high-risk genotype with no neuroticism had an average relative risk of 2.1; those with both the high-risk genotype and presence of neuroticism had a relative risk of 8.8 (43).

3.4.3 Tobacco

Cigarette smoking initiation has a heritability that is estimated at 40% (see chapter 7). Quantity smoked is also genetically determined, with a heritability estimate of about 85% (44). Different genes are related to the various components of smoking behavior, with genes that code for cholinergic nicotine receptors (the primary sites of nicotine action) responsible for determining quantity, and in some instances, dependence. The activation of these receptors results in activation of the dopamine system in the mesoaccumbens, which in turn leads to behavioral reinforcement and addiction (45). Other smoking-related behaviors, however, are related to genes outside of this class; for example, variants in the brain-derived neurotrophic factor (BDNF) gene correlate to a predisposition to begin smoking in the first place (46).

Recently, Thakur et al. (47) demonstrated that a particular SNP in a noncoding RNA was significantly associated with both ADHD and difficulty with smoking cessation. Although it is fairly clear that those with ADHD are more likely to smoke (48), this particular study was noteworthy for demonstrating a link between a particular genetic variant and a specific component of smoking behavior. Recent studies have also found that variants in the cholinergic nicotine receptors are associated with other SUDs, such as cocaine, opioid, and alcohol dependence (49), indicating a broader role for some of these genes in determining vulnerability to develop SUDs.

3.4.4 Others

Addiction to cocaine is thought to be genetically related to marijuana dependence, but with a higher heritability, estimated at between 50% and 80% (2,50) (see chapter 11). Other heritabilities that have been identified include 30%–60% for heroin (2,51), for which the implied genes are those of the endogenous opioid pathway; and 40% for methamphetamine addiction, where variations in A2A adenosine receptor are suggested as the mechanism (52).

As outlined previuosly, studies such as GWAS are beginning to identify the genetic architecture of substance abuse disorders and some of their comorbidities, indicating that there is a complex interaction among genes for both generalized predisposition to SUD and psychiatric disorders as well as predisposition to specific addictions. The combination of these genes then determine the individual's phenotype.

Although significant advances have been made in our understanding of the genetic underpinnings of SUDs, there is a still the problem of what is called "missing heritability." This concept applies to the failure to identify a significant proportion of the genetic factors involved in causing the phenotype. For example, human height has a heritability of 80%, yet the identified genetic variants only account for 5% of the phenotypic variance (11). Several explanations have been proposed for this missing heritability, including epigenetic modification, epistasis (gene-gene interaction), rare genes with large effect, and undetected copy number variants.

3.5 Epigenetic effects

We are beginning to understand that epigenetic effects on gene expression (but not the gene sequence itself) (8) are contributory to the cause of SUD predispositions. Recent studies have found that exposure to various addictive substances cause changes in the chromatin structure of brain cells (8). For example, Martin et al. (53) injected rats with methamphetamine and found differences in the gene expression of histone acetyltransferase and deacetylase, both of which affect gene expression, especially in the nucleus accumbens. Romieu et al. (54) used histone deacetylase (HDAC) inhibitors (HDAC represses transcription so use of HDAC inhibitors would increase transcription of some genes) to decrease cocaine self-administration in rats.

There is also increasing evidence that at least some epigenetic modifications are heritable. For example, young mice exposed to stressful situations were more likely not only to exhibit depressive symptoms themselves but to also have offspring and grand-offspring with similar manifestations. Sperm of stressed males exhibited differences in DNA methylation (one means by which epigenetic modification occurs) so that expression levels of genes involved with stress response were altered. Similar changes in methylation were observed in brains of their offspring, suggesting that transmission of behavioral traits caused by postnatal exposure to stress could occur (55). For those interested in reading more about this topic, please see recent papers by Wong et al. (56), Maze and Nestler (57), and Robison and Nestler (58).

Prenatal exposure may also affect gene expression in the exposed fetus (see chapter 19). For example, DiNeiri et al. (59) found that maternal cannabis use led to decreased expression of dopamine receptor D2 (DRD2) in the fetal brain. Adults who had been prenatally exposed to cannabis also showed decreased levels of DRD2 mRNA, suggesting decreased transcription of the DRD2 gene. Studies in animals have shown that DRD2 dysregulation is implicated in increased addiction risk. Animal models with decreased DRD2 expression in the nucleus accumbens also had enhanced drug intake and, in humans, DRD2 variants are linked to an increased risk for certain types of addictions including alcohol, opiates, and stimulants (60). Therefore, those with prenatal exposure, particularly those with a genetic predisposition, might be particularly susceptible to development of a SUD.

The effect of gene-gene interaction (epistasis) also contributes to the missing heritability. Kumar et al. (61) showed that variants in OPRM1 or OPRK1 alone were not associated with a risk for alcoholism, but variants in both together conferred a two-fold increased risk. It is likely that in many cases of epistasis the relevant genes are in the same biologic pathway (62).

3.6 Complex diseases

As noted previously, complex diseases are thought to be caused by variation in predispositional genes, which are common in the general population, with each gene contributing a small effect. This is called the "common disease, common variant" hypothesis. Schorck et al. (63) discussed an alternative hypothesis, termed the "common disease, rare variant" hypothesis, which states that rare variants with great effect are causative of complex disorders. A recent demonstration of this hypothesis in a different complex trait, the predisposition to develop hypertriglyceridemia (HTG), was the finding that mutations in several rare HTG genes with major effects were found in individuals ascertained by the presence of HTG. In these patients, the rare variants were thought to be the major contributor to the genetic component of the phenotype (64). These rare variants would not have been expected to be detected on typical GWAS platforms. Although similar studies have not yet been published in SUD, it would not be surprising to find similar results. Of course, it must be remembered that both common variants with small effects and rare variants with large effects each play some role in the determination of the genetic component of the phenotype.

Finally, not all platforms are able to detect copy number variations (CNV), which are small deletions or duplications of genetic material. CNVs are likely to contribute to the cause of many complex disorders. Recently, Bae et al. (65) described the results of a study assessing the presence of CNVs in alcoholic patients and found some regions of interest, which the authors speculated may be related to the development of alcoholism. A similar approach was taken in autism with some success (66) in that a number of susceptibility loci were identified using this approach. It is entirely possible that a similar approach in other SUD will identify additional genetic causes.

3.7 Conclusion

So what is the relevance of identifying genetic causes, either structural or modifications? With knowledge of the pathophysiology that is gained by studying genetic variations and their relevance to SUD, potential treatments and clinical management protocols could be developed to improve success of intervention (67). Since epigenetic modifications are not changes of the genetic sequence, treatments that reverse abnormal modifications may be especially useful in treating this class of disorders. Exciting times are ahead in the area of research into the role of genetic influences on substance abuse disorders.

References

1. Merikangas KR, McClair VL. Epidemiology of substance abuse disorders. Hum Genet 2012; 131:779–89.
2. Swendsen J, Burstein M, Case B, Conway KP, Dierer L, He J, et al. Use and abuse of alcohol and illicit drugs in US adolescents. Arch Gen Psychiatry 2012;69:390–8.
3. Breslau N, Johnson EO, Hiripi E, Kessler R. Nicotine dependence in the United States: prevalence, trends, and smoking persistence. Arch Gen Psychiatry 2001;58:810–6.
4. Uhl GR, Drgon T, Johnson C, Li CY, Contoreggi C, Hess J, et al. Molecular genetics of addiction and related heritable phenotypes. Ann NY Acad Sci 2008;1141:318–81.
5. Merikangas KR, Dierker LC, Szatmari P. Psychopathology among offspring of parents with substance abuse and/or anxiety disorders: a high-risk study. J Child Psychol Psychiatry 1998;39: 711–20.
6. Hicks BM, Iacono WG, McGue M. Index of the transmissible common liability to addiction: heritability and prospective associations with substance abuse and related outcomes. Drug Alcohol Depend 2012;123S:S18–23.
7. Tsuang MT, Bar JL, Harley RM, Lyons MJ. The Harvard twin study of substance abuse: what we have learned. Harvard Rev Psychiatry 2001;9:267–79.
8. Epps C, Holt L. The genetic basis of addiction and relevant cellular mechanisms. Int Anesthesiol Clin 2011;49:3–14.
9. Agrawal A, Verweij KJH, Gillespie NA, Heath AC, Lessov-Schlaggar CN, Martin NG, et al. The genetics of addiction – a translational perspective. Trans Psychiatry 2012;2:e140; doi:10.1038/ tp.2012.54.
10. Bierut LJ. Genetic vulnerability and susceptibility to substance dependence. Neuron 2011;69 (4):618–27.
11. Manolio TA, Collins FS, Cox NJ, Goldstein DB, Hindorff LA, Hunter DJ, et al. Finding the missing heritability of complex diseases. Nature 2009;461:747–53.
12. Palmer RHC, McGeary JE, Francazio S, Raphael BJ, Lander AD, Heath AC, et al. The genetics of alcohol dependence: advancing towards systems-based approaches. Drug Alcohol Depend 2012;125:179–91.
13. Kapusta ND, Plener PL, Schmid R, Thau K, Walter H, Lesch OM. Multiple substance use among young males. Pharmacol Biochem Behav 2007;86:306–11.
14. McEachin RC, Sannareddy KS, Cavalcoli JD, Karnovsky A, Vink JM, Sartor MA. Convergence of genetic influences on comorbidity. BMC Bioinformatics 2012;13(suppl 2):S8.
15. Rhee SH, Hewitt JK, Young SE, Corley RP, Crowley TJ, Neale MC, et al. Comorbidity between alcohol dependence and illicit drug dependence in adolescents with antisocial behavior and matched controls. Drug Alcohol Depend 2006;84:85–92.
16. Palmer RHC, Button TM, Rhee SH, Corley RP, Young SE, Stallings MC, et al. Genetic etiology of the common liability to drug dependence: evidence of common and specific mechanisms for DSM-IV dependence symptoms. Drug Alcohol Depend 2012;123S:S24–32.
17. Haberstick BC, Zeiger JS, Corley RP, Hopfer CJ, Stallings MC, Rhee SH, et al. Common and drug-specific genetic influences on subjective effects to alcohol, tobacco, and marijuana use. Addiction 2011;106:215–24.

18. Grant BF, Stinson FS, Dawson DA, Chou SP, Dufour MC, Compton W, et al. Prevalence and co-occurrence of substance use disorders and independent mood and anxiety disorders: results from the National Epidemiologic Survey on Alcohol and Related Conditions. Arch Gen Psychiatry 2004;61:807–16.
19. Preisiq M, Fenton BT, Stevens DE, Merikangas KR. Familial relationship between mood disorders and alcoholism. Compr Psychiatry 2001;42:87–95.
20. Krueger RF, Hicks BM, Patrick CJ, Carlson SR, Iacono WG, McGue M. Etiologic connections among substance dependence, antisocial behavior, and personality: modeling the externalizing spectru. J Abnorm Psychol 2002;111:411–24.
21. Krueger RF, Markon KE. Reinterpreting comorbidity: a model-based approach to understanding and classifying psychopathology. Ann Rev Clin Psychol 2006;2:111–33.
22. Albayrak O, Wölfle SM, Hebebrand J. Does food addiction exist? A phenomenological discussion based on the psychiatric classification of substance-related disorders and addiction. Obes Facts 2012;5:165–79.
23. Eisen SA, Lin N, Lyons MJ, Scherrer JF, Griffith K, True WR, et al. Familial influences on gambling behavior: an analysis of 3359 twin pairs. Addiction 1998;93:1375–84.
24. Jazaeri SA, Habil MHB. Reviewing two types of addiction – pathological gambling and substance use. Indian J Psychol Med 2012;34:5–11.
25. Shek DTL, Chan EML, Wong RHY. Associations between pathological gambling and psychiatric comorbidity among help-seeking populations in Hong Kong. Scientific World Journal 2012; doi:10.1100/2012/571434.
26. Gorwood P, Le Strat Y, Ramoz N, Dubertret C, Moalic MG, Simonneau M. Genetics of dopamine receptors and drug addiction. Hum Genet 2012;131:803–22.
27. Kreek MJ, Levran O, Reed B, Schlussman SD, Zhou Y, Buterman ER. Opiate addiction and cocaine addiction: underlying molecular neurobiology and genetics. J Clin Invest 2012;122: 3387–93.
28. Levran O, Yuferov V, Kreek MJ. The genetics of the opioid system and specific drug addictions. Hum Genet 2012;131:823–42.
29. Meneses A, Liy-Salmeron G. Serotonin and emotion, learning, and memory. Rev Neurosci 2012; doi:10.1515/revneuro-2012–0060.
30. Liu QR, Drgon T, Johnson C, Walther D, Hess J, Uhl GR. Addiction molecular genetics: 639,401 SNP whole genome association identifies many "cell adhesion" genes. Am J Med Genet B 2006; 141B:918–25.
31. Johnson C, Drgon T, Liu QR, Zhang PW, Walther D, Li CY, et al. Genome wide association for substance dependence: convergent results from epidemiologic and research volunteer samples. BMC Med Genet 2008;9:113.
32. Gelernter J, Kranzler HR. Genetics of alcohol dependence. Hum Genet 2009;126:91–9.
33. Treutlein J, Rietschel M. Genome-wide association studies of alcohol dependence and substance use disorders. Curr Psychiatry Rep 2011;13:147–55.
34. Spanagel R. Alcoholism: a systems approach from molecular physiology to addictive behavior. Physiol Rev 2009;89:649–705.
35. Saccone SF, Hinrichs AL, Saccone NL, Chase GA, Convicka K, Madden PA, et al. Cholinergic nicotinic receptor genes implicated in a nicotine dependence association study targeting 348 candidate genes with 3713 SNPs. Hum Mol Genet 2007;16:36–49.
36. Cui WY, Seneviratne C, Gu J, Li MD. Genetics of GABAergic signaling in nicotine and alcohol dependence. Hum Genet 2012;131:843–55.
37. Uhl GR, Drgon T, Liu QR, Johnson C, Walther D, Komiyama T, et al. Genome-wide association for methamphetamine dependence: convergent results from 2 samples. Arch Gen Psychiatry 2008;65:345–55.

38. Hill SY, Weeks DE, Jones BL, Zezza N, Stiffler S. ASTN1 and alcohol dependence: family-based association analysis in multiplex alcohol dependence families. Am J Med Genet B 2012;159B: 445–55.
39. Wang JC, Foroud T, Hinrichs AL, Le NXH, Bertelsen S, Budde JP, et al. A genome-wide association study of alcohol-dependence symptom counts in extended pedigrees identifies C15orf53. Molecular Psychiatry 2012;doi:10.1038/mp/2012.143.
40. Sanchez-Pena JF, Alvarez-Cotoli P, Rodriguez-Solano JJ. Psychiatric disorders associated with alcoholism: 2 year follow-up of treatment. Actas Esp Psiquiatr 2012;40:129–35.
41. Enoch MA. The influence of gene-environment interactions on the development of alcoholism and drug dependence. Curr Psychiatry Rep 2012;14:140–55.
42. Agrawal A, Lynskey MT. Candidate genes for cannabis use disorders: findings, challenges and directions. Addiction 2009;104:518–32.
43. Jutras-Aswad D, Jacobs MM, Yiannoulos G, Roussos P, Bitsios P, Nomura Y, et al. Cannabis-dependence risk relates to synergism between neuroticism and proenkephalin SNPs associated with amygdala gene expression: case-control study. PLos ONE 2012;7:e39243.
44. Koopmans JR, Slutske WS, Heath AC, Neale MC, Boomsma DI. The genetics of smoking initiation and quantity smoked in Dutch adolescent and young adult twins. Behav Genet 1999; 29:383–93.
45. Saccone NL, Culverhouse RC, Schwantes-An TH, Cannon DS, Chen X, Cichon S, et al. Multiple independent loci at chromosome 15q25.1 affect smoking quantity: a meta-analysis and comparison with lung cancer and COPD. PLoS Genet 2010;6:e1001053.
46. Tobacco and Genetics Consortium. Genome-wide meta-analyses identify multiple loci associated with smoking behavior. Nat Genet 2010;42:441–7.
47. Thakur GA, Sengupta SM, Grizenko N, Choudhry Z, Joober R. Family-based association study of ADHD and genes increasing the risk for smoking behaviours. Arch Dis Child 2012;doi:10.1136/archdischild-2012–1882.
48. McClernon JF, Kollins SH. ADHD and smoking: from genes to brain to behavior. Ann NY Acad Sci 2008;1141:131–47.
49. Sherva R, Kranzler HR, Yu Y, Logue MW, Poling J, Arias AJ, et al. Variation in nicotinic acetylcholine receptor genes is associated with multiple substance dependence phenotypes. Neuropsychopharmacol 2010;35:1921–31.
50. Bevilacqua L, Goldman D. Genes and addictions. Clin Pharmacol Ther 2009;85:359–61.
51. Kendler KS, Jacobson KC, Prescott CA, Neale MC. Specificity of genetic and environmental risk factors for use and abuse/dependence of cannabis, cocaine, hallucinogens, sedatives, stimulants, and opiates in male twins. Am J Psychiatry 2003;160:687–95.
52. Kobayashi H, Ujike H, Iwata N, Inada T, Yamada M, Sekine Y, et al. The adenosine A2A receptor is associated with methamphetamine dependence/psychosis in the Japanese population. Behav Brain Funct 2010;6:50
53. Martin TA, Jayanthi S, McCoy MT, Brannock C, Ladenheim B, Garrett T, et al. Methamphetamine causes differential alterations in gene expression and patterns of histone acetylation/hypoacetylation in the rat nucleus accumbens. PLoS ONE 2012;7:e34236.
54. Romieu P, Deschatrettes E, Host L, Gobaille S, Sandner G, Zwiller J. The inhibition of histone deacetylases reduces the reinstatement of cocaine-seeking behavior in rats. Curr Neuropharmacol 2011;9:21–5.
55. Bohacek J, Gapp K, Saab BJ, Mansuy I. Transgenerational epigenetic effects on brain functions. Biol Psychiatr 2012;doi.org/10.1016/j.biopsych.2012.08.019.
56. Wong CCY, Mill J, Fernandes C. Drugs and addiction: an introduction to epigenetics. Addiction 2011;106:480–9.
57. Maze I, Nestler EJ. The epigenetic landscape of addiction. Ann NY Acad Sci 2011;1216:99–113.

58. Robison AJ, Nestler EJ. Transcriptional and epigenetic mechanisms of addiction. Nat Rev Neurosci 2012;12:623–37.
59. DiNieri JA, Wang X, Szutorisz H, Spano SM, Kaur J, Casaccia P, et al. Maternal cannabis use alters ventral striatal dopamine D2 gene regulation in the offspring. Biol Psychiatry 2011; 70:763–9.
60. LeFoll B, Gallo A, Le Strat Y, Lu L, Gorwood P. Genetics of dopamine receptors and drug addiction: a comprehensive review. Behav Pharmacol 2009;20:1–17.
61. Kumar D, Chakraborty J, Das S. Epistatic effects between variants of kappa-opioid receptor gene and A118G of mu-opioid receptor gene increase susceptibility to addiction in Indian population. Prog Neruopsychopharmacol Biol Psychiatry 2012;36:225–30.
62. Pandey A, Davis NA, White BC, Pajewski NM, Savitz J, Drevets WC, et al. Epistasis network centrality analysis yields pathway replication across two GWAS cohorts for bipolar disorder. Transl Psychiatry 2012;2:e154.
63. Schork NJ, Murray SS, Frazer KA, Topol EJ. Common vs. rare allele hypotheses for complex diseases. Curr Opin Genet Devel 2009;19:212–9.
64. Johansen CT, Wang J, Lanktree MB, Cao H, McIntyre AD, Ban MR, et al. Mutation skew in genes identified by genome-wide association study of hypertriglyceridemia. Nat Genet 2010;42:684–7.
65. Bae JS, Jung MH, Lee BC, Cheong HS, Park BL, Kim LH, et al. The genetic effect of copy number variations on the risk of alcoholism in a Korean population. Alcohol Clin Exp Res 2012;36:35–42.
66. Marshall CR, Scherer SW. Detection and characterization of copy number variation in autism spectrum disorder. In: Feuk L, ed. Genomic structural variants: Methods and protocols, methods in molecular biology. Volume 838. Springer Science and Business Media, LLC, 2012.
67. Lango H, Weedon MN. What will whole genome searches for susceptibility genes for common complex disease offer to clinical practice? J Intern Med 2008;263:16–27.

4 Essential diagnostic considerations

Helen D. Pratt and Sherry Pancost

Substance abuse disorders are one of the most commonly arising conditions among adolescents and young adults ages 13–22 years. In this chapter we review essential diagnostic issues that impact the identification and diagnosis the adolescent and young adult substance user and abuser. Adolescents and young adults across the developmental stages are exposed to substance use. Exposure to substances often begins during the middle school years (6th–8th grades, approximately ages 12–15 years). Research on validity and reliability of screening and diagnostic instruments with adolescents is limited. Most screening instruments are considered to be useful based on so-called expert opinion. Thirteen screening instruments were identified for use with adolescents and young adults. Five diagnostic instruments were identified for adolescents and young adults. Each of these instruments was listed in several empirical studies. Most offer free copies of their measurement instruments and instruction manuals on the Internet. One of the five diagnostic instruments offers free access on the Internet: Addiction Severity Baseline (ASI – B) and the Addiction Severity Index, 5th Edition. All adolescents should be routinely screened for substance use, abuse, and disorders beginning by the time they are ages 12–17 years. Young adults should be routinely screened for substance use, abuse, and dependence at all health visits.

4.1 Introduction

Substance abuse disorders are one of the most commonly arising conditions among adolescents and young adults ages 13–22 years (1,2). Experimenting by engaging in risk-taking behaviors during adolescence and young adulthood is considered normal behavior in the United States. Drug use during this developmental period (which includes refinement of functional skills, moving toward independence, and establishment of intimate relationships) is when these youth make lifestyle choices that will affect both their current and future health (2). Environmental factors such as family, peer group, school, and community characteristics also contribute to adolescents' health and risk behaviors. Adverse outcomes from these choices can cause significant morbidity and mortality as youth matriculate from childhood to adulthood (3).

All youth should be routinely screened for substance use, abuse, or dependence, especially if they present with the risk factors listed in table 4.1 (2,4,5). Screening for substance use/abuse or dependence allows organizations, clinicians, and physicians to identify adolescents with possible substance use problems and

Table 4.1: Risk factors for substance abuse in adolescents and young adults (2,4,5)

Individual Characteristic		
Personal Characteristics	**Personal Status**	
Behavior • High-risk life situations • Change in sleep patterns • Sexual promiscuity or other risky behavior • Increased oppositional behavior • Problem behaviors or discipline problems • Marked change in behavior or function • Deficits in self-regulation (poor behavioral control and poor emotional control)	**Educational Factor** • Dropped out of school • Special education students • Declining academic performance • Have a great number of unexcused school absences • Low academic achievement and/or academic aspirations	**Legal** • Entering into the child welfare system • Entering the juvenile detention system • Pending adjudication of a court case
Cognitive • Borderline intellectual functioning • Being diagnosed with mental retardation	**Special Circumstances** • Being a runaway • Homelessness	**Role within Family** • Serving as caretakers for ill or disabled parents or caregivers
Emotional • Very disruptive or persistent nightmares • Experiencing environmental distress • Marked change in mood • Significant losses • Traumatic events (such as exposure to an incident of violence, physical abuse, dating violence, parental violence, or a natural disaster) **Social Factors** • Peer use/abuse and attitude that substance use/abuse is "normal"	**Mental Health Status** • Untreated attention-deficit disorder (ADD) and attention-deficit hyperactivity disorder (ADHD), conduct disorder, oppositional defiant disorder, psychosis	**Health Status** • Prenatally exposed to drugs and alcohol Chronic recurrent or unexplained physical symptoms • Diagnosis or exacerbation of chronic medical conditions (such as HIV) • Presents at emergency medical services for trauma • Suddenly begin experiencing medical problems such as accidents, injury, • Or gastrointestinal disturbance
Family Factors • Parental history of substance use/abuse or mood disorders • Poor parental supervision and household disruption		
Environmental Factors • Living in a community with a high rate of poverty or violence • Living in a domestic violence shelter		

provide the option for further assessment. However, these professionals must remember that identification does not mean that the screened adolescents receive a diagnosis of a particular condition. Only mental health, substance abuse, or medical professionals (as determined by each state's licensing laws) are qualified to make a diagnosis.

Neither signs or symptoms of substance use/abuse or dependence nor screening tools provide sufficient information to reach a diagnosis (3,4). This chapter provides a review of essential diagnostic issues that can impact the accuracy and utility of information collected to identify and diagnose adolescents and young adult users and abusers of substances.

4.2 Review of the literature

The current authors conducted a review of assessments with attention to those that had (a) an empirical foundation and interview procedures – purposes, advantages, training required, and so on, and (b) included instruments for screening of general (overall) substance use/abuse versus substance-specific assessments. Diagnostic criteria and instruments were also reviewed. Two main databases were used to identify relevant articles.

- APA PsycNET® Platinum (PsycARTICLES, PsycEXTRA, and PsycINFO), membership required: https://my.apa.org/apa.
- EBSCOhost Connection (MEDLINE with Full Text, Cochrane Database of Systematic Reviews, and Psychology and Behavioral Sciences Collection), membership required: http://search.ebscohost.com.

4.3 Epidemiology

Adolescents and young adults across the developmental stages are exposed to substance use (see table 4.2) (1,2,5–8). Research supports that adolescents that develop substance use problems often have their first exposure to substances during their middle school years (6th–8th grades, approximately ages 12–15 years) and generally experiment as a result of peer pressure or imitation. This makes screening adolescents, starting at around age 12, important for treatment and prevention of long-term substance use problems. However, reports on pediatrician surveys have indicated that less than half of pediatricians reported screening for adolescent substance use/abuse (11). As opposed to adolescent substance use, young adult substance use is generally more about maintenance, continued, or increased use, which supports the need to continue routine screening into adulthood (12).

Table 4.2: Adolescent exposure to substances (1)

Tobacco Use
- 44.7% have smoked cigarettes.
- 10.3% of students had smoked a whole cigarette for the first time before age 13 years.
- 7.7% of students had used smokeless tobacco (e.g., chewing tobacco, snuff, or dip) on at least one day during the 30 days before the survey.

Alcohol Use
- 70.8% of students had taken at least one drink of alcohol on at least one day during their life (i.e., ever drank alcohol).

Marijuana Use
- 39.9% of students had used marijuana one or more times during their life (i.e., ever used marijuana).

Other Drug Use
- 6.8% of students had used any form of cocaine (e.g., powder, crack, or freebase) one or more times during their life (i.e., ever used cocaine).
- 11.4% of students had sniffed glue, breathed the contents of aerosol spray cans, or inhaled any paints or sprays to get high one or more times during their life (i.e., ever used inhalants).
- 2.9% of students had used heroin (also called "smack," "junk," or "China White") one or more times during their life (i.e., ever used heroin).
- 3.8% of students had used methamphetamines (also called "speed," "crystal," "crank," or "ice") one or more times during their life (i.e., ever used methamphetamines).
- 3.6% of students had taken steroid pills or shots without a doctor's prescription one or more times during their life (i.e., ever took steroids without a doctor's prescription).
- 20.7% of students had taken prescription drugs (e.g., Oxycontin, Percocet, Vicodin, codeine, Adderall, Ritalin, or Xanax) without a doctor's prescription one or more times during their life (i.e., ever took prescription drugs without a doctor's prescription).
- 2.3% of students had used a needle to inject any illegal drug into their body one or more times during their life (i.e., ever injected any illegal drug).
- 25.6% of students had been offered, sold, or given an illegal drug by someone on school property during the 12 months before the survey.

4.4 Empirical studies of assessment instruments

Few empirical studies comparing the efficacy, validity, and reliability of screening and diagnostic instruments exist for the adolescent population. One group of researchers did look at evidenced-based assessments in the pediatric clinical population. The study was focused on instruments that measured psychosocial adjustment and psychopathology in this group. Although the study did not specifically address substance use/abuse, it included the Minnesota Multiphasic Personality Inventory–A (MMPI-A) in their review because it was one of the measurement instruments used in the studies as a broad-band rating scale. Their examination of evidenced-based assessments (EBA) concluded that the MMPI-A is "well established" in the EBA classifications for 14–18-year-old adolescents (6–8). The MMPI was identified as having the similar impact for adults, which includes young adults (18–22 years) (6–8).

4.5 Comorbidity

Co-occurring substance use and mental health conditions are highly prevalent among adolescents and young adults who have either disorder (2,3,6). Current estimates place the prevalence of serious substance abuse and adolescent mental health conditions at around 2% and 5 %, respectively. The most prevalent mental health diagnoses that co-occur with substance use conditions are conduct disorder and mood disorders, followed by attention deficit hyperactivity disorder and anxiety disorders (6,9). Substance use/abuse or dependence is often comorbid with depression, other mental health disorders, and with adolescents who are also the victims of family discord (2–4). Clinicians should attempt to determine if the affective disorder or hallucinations are substance induced or simply comorbid (6,8).

4.6 Assessment

Two governmental reports on substance use/abuse recommend that organizations specializing, in whole or in part, in assessment and referral services for adolescents with substance use disorders must comply with federal confidentiality regulations (42 C.F.R. §2.12(e)) (see table 4.3 and table 4.4) (2,4,6). These regulations provide guidelines on confidentiality requirements, when confidentiality can be breached, who must obtain consent, who must provide consent, and who is able to receive confidential information about an adolescent (2,4,6).

Table 4.3: Attending to legal issues surrounding screening and assessment with adolescents (2, 4)

- Programs that specialize, in whole or in part, assessment and referral services for adolescents with substance use disorders must comply with the Federal confidentiality regulations (42 C.F.R. §2.12(e)).
- Information that is protected by Federal confidentiality regulations may always be disclosed after the adolescent has signed a proper consent form (parental consent must also be obtained in some states). The regulations also permit disclosure without the adolescent's consent in situations such as medical emergencies, child abuse reports, program evaluations, and communications among staff.
- Any disclosure made with written client consent must be accompanied by a written statement that the information disclosed is protected by Federal law and that the person receiving the information cannot make any further disclosure of such information unless permitted by the regulations (§2.32).
- When a program that screens, assesses, or treats adolescents asks a school, doctor, or parent to verify information it has obtained from the adolescent, it is making a client-identifying disclosure that the adolescent has sought its services. The Federal regulations generally prohibit this kind of disclosure unless the adolescent consents.
- Programs may not communicate with the parents of an adolescent unless they get the adolescent's written consent. The Federal regulations contain an exception permitting a program director to communicate with an adolescent's parents without his or her consent when the adolescent is applying for services.

(Continued)

Table 4.3: Attending to legal issues surrounding screening and assessment with adolescents (2, 4) (*Continued*)

- The organizational/program director believes that the adolescent, because of an extreme substance use disorder or a medical condition, does not have the capacity to decide rationally whether to consent to the notification of his or her guardians.
- The organizational/program director believes the disclosure is necessary to cope with a substantial threat to the life or well-being of the adolescent or someone else.
- Other exceptions to the Federal confidentiality rules prohibiting disclosure regarding adolescents seeking or receiving substance use disorder services are:
  - Information that does not reveal the client as having a substance use disorder
  - Information ordered by the court after a hearing
  - Medical emergencies
  - Information regarding crimes on program premises or against program personnel
  - Information shared with an outside agency that provides service
  - Information discussed among people within the program
  - Information disclosed to researchers, auditors, and evaluators with appropriate Institutional Review Board review and approval to ensure the protection of program participants

Table 4.4: Substance Abuse and Mental Health Services Administration (SAMHSA) recommends (2,4,6)

- First, do no harm.
- Abide by the legal requirements of Federal, state, and local governments (see Table 3).
  - Be clear on the legalities required in your state regarding:
    a) The age of consent for adolescents and
    b) When to obtain written, informed consent from the legal guardian.
- Confidentiality must be ensured.
- Use a scientifically sound screening process.
- Screening instruments must be valid and reliable.
- Screening and evaluation instruments must be developmentally, age, gender, and racially/ethnically, culturally, and linguistically appropriate for the adolescent, his or her family, and communities.
- All screeners and evaluators should be qualified and appropriately trained.
- Safeguard the screening information and ensure its appropriate use.
- Identifying possible problems should never be used to make a diagnosis or to label an adolescent or young adult.
- Provide a contact name for someone who can answer questions and make a copy of the screening tool available to the legal guardians. This approach often puts parental concerns about the process to rest.
- Your organization should require active consent: a child or adolescent is not screened unless the legal guardian has signed a consent form and returned it to the organization. SAMHSA advises against using passive consent: parents are informed of the screening, and unless they indicate that they want to opt their adolescent out of the program, the child will be screened. Blanket consents given should not be used as a substitute for a signed parental consent form to administer a mental health or substance use/abuse screening tool.
- In emergency situations involving mental health or substance use problems, a youth's identification, assessment, and treatment may take place without obtaining parental consent. However, consent should be obtained as soon as possible during or after a screening.

Clinicians must be careful when gathering an adolescent's personal data from other organizations. Asking a school, doctor, or parent to verify information obtained from the adolescent is making a client-identifying disclosure that the adolescent has sought services. The Federal regulations generally prohibit this kind of disclosure unless the adolescent consents (2,4). Confidentially for young adults are the same for any adult using mental health services and are being assessed at schools and colleges. Regulations are enumerated in the policies and procedures of all agencies, community mental health boards, schools, and colleges. Clinicians and staff who screen for substance use/abuse should know those policies governing patient/client/student rights.

4.7 Screening

The purpose of screening is to identify adolescents and young adults who need a more comprehensive assessment for substance use disorders. Screening does so by uncovering "red flags," or indicators of serious substance-related problems (2,10,11). As such, it covers the general areas in a young person's life that pertain to substance use without making an involved diagnosis.

Selection of screening and assessment instruments for use with adolescents and young adults should be guided by several factors (see table 4.5): (a) reliability and validity of the tool, (b) its appropriateness to an adolescent population, (c) the type of settings in which the instrument was developed, and (d) the intended purpose of the instrument (2,4,10,11).

Screening and assessment should cover multiple domains pertaining to the individual, including his or her environment, and the process should involve more than one method and source of data collection (4). The screening process should last no more than 30 minutes, although a process time of 10–15 minutes would be better. The instrument should be simple enough that a wide range of health professionals can administer it (2). Several researchers and governmental agencies publish screening instruments with at least limited empirical support or have been used by "experts" and are considered to be useful in community and clinical settings (2,4,8,7,10).

Screening for substance use/abuse as a routine matter of providing comprehensive health care would improve the chances for detecting adolescents at earlier stages of substance use/abuse and allow for early intervention. This is especially important when working with at-risk youth (see table 4.2) (1,2,5,8).

In order to improve the opportunities to screen adolescent and young adults for substance use/abuse, a wide range of professionals should be trained to screen adolescents and young adults for mental health and substance use/abuse issues; for example, health service providers, other professionals who work with adolescents and at-risk youth, street youth workers, and community organizations (e.g., school

Table 4.5: Purpose of conducting comprehensive post-screening assessment of substance use/abuse (2,4,10,11)

1. To accurately identify those youth who need treatment.
2. To further evaluate if a substance use disorder exists.
3. To determine the severity of use/abuse.
4. To determine if a substance use disorder exists based on formal criteria (e.g., DSM-IV, ICD-10).
5. To permit the evaluator to learn more about the nature, correlates, and consequences of the adolescent's or young adult's substance-using behavior.
6. To ensure that additional related problems not flagged in the screening process are identified (e.g., problems in medical status, psychological status, nutrition, social functioning, family relations, educational performance, delinquent behavior).
7. To examine the extent to which the youth's family is able and prepared to be involved in comprehensive assessment and possible subsequent interventions.
8. To identify specific strengths of the adolescent or young adult (e.g., coping skills) that can be used in developing an appropriate treatment plan.
9. To provide a diagnosis that drives treatment.
10. To develop a written report that:
    a. Identifies the severity of the substance use disorder
    b. Identifies factors that contribute to or are related to the substance use disorder
    c. Identifies a corrective plan of action to address these problem areas
    d. Details an interim plan to ensure that the treatment plan is implemented and monitored to its conclusion
    e. Makes recommendations for referral to agencies or services
    f. Describes how resources and services of multiple agencies can best be coordinated and integrated

The assessment should be conducted in an office or other site that is comfortable, private, and secure.

staff, teachers, school counselors, college staff in student services, health care delivery systems, the judiciary staff, juvenile justice workers, probation officers, vocational rehabilitation staff, and religious organization staff). Thus, many health and judicial professionals should have screening expertise, especially pediatric, family medicine, and internal medicine physicians, as they are most likely to be the first professionals an adolescent has contact with after engaging in substance use (2,4). College professors and student services staff are often the first to detect young adults who are struggling with substance use/abuse issues (skipping classes, getting in fights, being physically harmed by peers, being arrested, etc.).

Parents/guardians are no longer present on a daily basis to guide and protect the young adults; these young people are often experiencing an environment where they are living more independently for the first time. Screening instruments can play an important role; they are often a first step in the evaluation process and can be used as time savers, as a method for identifying youth who are in trouble, or as a preventative assessment tool.

The best method for organizational staff, college staff, and those who are not mental health or substance abuse professionals to quickly identify adolescents and young adults with substance use problems is to use an appropriate and well-tested screening tool that includes items identifying high-risk conditions (2,4). For young persons at high risk for a substance use disorder, a negative screening result should be followed up with a reevaluation, perhaps after six months (1,2,4). If a tool's predictive effectiveness has not been fully researched for an organization's target population, the findings may not be as reliable (9).

All assessment instruments should be selected on the basis of their purpose, content, administration requirements, time required for completion, training needed by the assessor, how the instrument can be obtained, its cost, and persons to contact for further guidance. The two most important criteria in the evaluation of any measurement instrument are reliability and validity (4).

The majority of screening instruments are self-report instruments. The adolescent or young adult is given a list of questions and asked to provide a response. Self-report instruments do present a problem with respect to whether the answers provided by the adolescent or young adult are a true reflection of actual level of use, either as a result of underreporting or overreporting (10). It is important not to use these screens as the sole means of identifying substance use/abuse because research shows that such reports only have fair validity (2). Few clinicians actually observe the signs and symptoms of substance use/abuse/dependence. That information is often collected from self-reports, family reports, police reports, or staff/care-provider reports. Therefore, this data may not be accurate and use may look different for youth at different stages of development or ages (2,4,11). One study that examined self-report data offered that such measures should be routinely combined with biochemical laboratory tests (10).

Screening tools are the best brief method available for personnel who are not mental health or substance abuse professionals to identify children and adolescents at risk of mental health and substance use problems, even though no screening tool is correct all of the time (2). Screening instruments for this chapter were selected based on our review. Our findings indicate that they have either data supporting validity and reliability or are recommended by professional organizations based on so-called expert opinion. The screening and diagnostic instruments selected are shown in table 4.6 (11–27).

If a screening instrument reveals that a youth is using/abusing substances or is at high risk for developing dependency, the screening must be followed by notifying the youth and if under the age of 18 his or her parents, guardians, or the entity with legal custody as allowable by confidentiality requirements. For adolescents and young adults, the clinician must explain the results to the patient and involved parties and offer referrals for an appropriate, in-depth assessment conducted by trained personnel who have the ability to provide the adolescent and his or her family or support persons with links to appropriate services and supports (2,4).

The SAMHSA-HRSA Center for Integrated Health Solutions (CIHS) has developed a comprehensive set of procedures that outlines the process of identifying and

Table 4.6: Screening instruments for detecting substance use or abuse and identifying adolescents and young adults in need of further assessment (11–27)

Screening Instruments	Description	Population	Assessment Format	Who Can Administer	Website and Other Information
Alcohol Use Disorders Identification Test (AUDIT and AUDIT-C)	Alcohol screen for hazardous or harmful alcohol consumption in the past year	Adults	• AUDIT 10-item multiple choice questionnaire • AUDIT-C 3-item multiple choice questionnaire • Self-report • Can be given as pen-and-paper or computerized format	• Health professionals or paraprofessionals. • Training required for administration.	• Cost: None • http://whqlibdoc.who.int/hq/2001/who_msd_msb_01.6a.pdf
Alcohol Dependence Scale (ADS)	Screens for alcohol use, including compulsion to drink, inability to control drinking, withdrawal symptoms, alcohol tolerance, and alcohol-seeking behaviors	Adults, although can be used with adolescents	• 25 items • Can be given in a computerized format, pen-and-paper format, or as an interview • Up to 10 minute administration time	• Health professionals or paraprofessionals. • No special training is required to administer.	• Cost: $15.00 for kit with users guide and questionnaires • http://pubs.niaaa.nih.gov/publications/AssessingAlcohol/InstrumentPDFs/10_ADS.pdf
CAGE	Screen for alcohol use disorders	Adolescents and adults	• 4 questions • Can be given as an interview or self-report	• Health professionals or paraprofessionals. • No special training is required to administer.	• Cost: None • http://www.hopkinsmedicine.org/johns_hopkins_healthcare/downloads/CAGE%20Substance%20Screening%20Tool.pdf

CAGE AID	Brief screen for alcohol and/or drug use	Adolescents and adults	• 5 items • Can be given as an interview or self-report	• Health professionals or paraprofessionals. • No special training is required to administer.	• Cost: None • http://www.integration.samhsa.gov/images/res/CAGEAID.pdf
CRAFFT	Screen for alcohol and other drug use disorders	Designed for persons under the age of 21	• 6 items • Brief interview format	• Health professionals or paraprofessionals. • No special training is required to administer.	• Cost: None • http://www.drtepp.com/pdf/substance_abuse.pdf
Drug Abuse Screening Test (DAST)	Screen for a person's overall view of drug use and a gauge of drug-use intensity	Adolescents and adults	• 28 questions • Self-report or interview format	• Health professionals or paraprofessionals. • No special training is required to administer.	• Cost: None • Has two alternate forms, a 10-item version and a 20-item version • http://www.suboxone.com/hcp/quality_patient_care/pdfs/15_Drug_Abuse_Screening_Test_-_DAST_10.pdf
NIDAMED Drug-Use Screening Tool	Screens for drug, alcohol, and tobacco use	Adolescents and adults	• 4 questions • Can be administered as a self-report, pen-and-pencil, interview, or computerized	• Health professionals or paraprofessionals. • No special training is required to administer.	• http://www.drugabuse.gov/nmassist/
Personal Experience Screening	Screens for chemical dependency	Adolescents ages 12–18 years	• 10 questions • Self-report	• Health professionals and clinicians.	• Cost: $75.00 per kit (25 administrations) • http://portal.wpspublish.com/portal/page?_pageid=53,69732&_dad=portal&_schema=PORTAL

(*Continued*)

Table 4.6: Screening instruments for detecting substance use or abuse and identifying adolescents and young adults in need of further assessment (11–27) (*Continued*)

Screening Instruments	Description	Population	Assessment Format	Who Can Administer	Website and Other Information
Questionnaire (PESQ)				Training required for administration.	
Personal Experience Screening Questionnaire for Adults (PESQ-A)	Screens for chemical dependency	Adults	• 10 questions • Self-report	• Health professionals and clinicians. Training required for administration.	• Cost: $75.00 per kit (25 administrations) • http://portal.wpspublish.com/portal/page?_pageid=53,70480&_dad=portal&_schema=PORTAL
Personal Experience Inventory (PEI)	Screen for substance use problems, psychosocial problems, and personal risk factors	Adolescents ages 12–18 years	• 276 items • Self-report, pen-and-pencil, or computerized administration	• Health professionals and clinicians. Training required for administration.	• Cost: $285.00 for 12 mail-in answer sheets • http://pubs.niaaa.nih.gov/publications/AssessingAlcohol/InstrumentPDFs/48_PEI.pdf
Problem-Oriented Screening Instrument for Teenagers (POSIT)	Screen for problem substance use and nine other functional areas	Adolescents	• 139 yes/no questions • Self-report, pen-and-paper administration	• Health professionals or paraprofessionals. No special training is required to administer.	• Cost: None • http://www.emcdda.europa.eu/attachements.cfm/att_4444_EN_tposit.pdf
Substance Abuse Subtle Screening Inventory (SASSI-3)	Screens for substance dependence and identifies high or low probability of dependence	Adults	• 62 true/false questions • Self-report, pen-and paper	Professional who has a degree from an accredited 4-year college or university in psychology, counseling, or a closely related field *plus*	• Cost: Starting at $125.00 (SASSI-3 Manual, SASSI-3 User's Guide, scoring key, and 25 paper tests and profiles) • http://www4.parinc.com/Products/Product.aspx?ProductID=SASSI-3# • Audio version of questionnaire available

				satisfactory completion of coursework in test interpretation, psychometrics and measurement theory, educational statistics, or a closely related area; *or* license or certification from an agency that requires appropriate training and experience in the ethical and competent use of psychological tests.	
Substance Abuse Subtle Screening Inventory–Adolescent (SASSI-A2)	Screens for substance dependence and identifies high or low probability of dependence	Adolescents	• 72 true/false questions • Self-report, pen-and-paper	Professional with a degree from an accredited 4-year college or university in psychology, counseling, or a closely related field *plus* satisfactory completion of coursework in test interpretation, psychometrics and measurement theory, educational statistics,	• Cost: Starting at $125.00 (SASSI-A2 Manual, SASSI-A2 User's Guide, scoring key, and 25 paper tests and profiles) • http://www4.parinc.com/Products/Product.aspx?ProductID=SASSI-A2 • Audio version of questionnaire available

(*Continued*)

Table 4.6: Screening instruments for detecting substance use or abuse and identifying adolescents and young adults in need of further assessment (11–27) (*Continued*)

Screening Instruments	Description	Population	Assessment Format	Who Can Administer	Website and Other Information
				or a closely related area; *or* license or certification from an agency that requires appropriate training and experience in the ethical and competent use of psychological tests.	
Addiction Severity Baseline (ASI-B) and Addiction Severity Index–5th Edition	Used to diagnose substance abuse severity and addresses seven lifestyle areas	Adults	One-hour interview, pen-and-paper, or computerized questionnaire	Health professionals or paraprofessionals. Training required for administration.	• Cost: None • http://adai.washington.edu/instruments/pdf/Addiction_Severity_Index_Baseline_Followup_4.pdf • The Addiction Severity Follow-Up (ASI-F) takes approximately 15 minutes and measures the individual's progress and changing needs
Composit International Diagnostic Interview Substance Abuse Module (CIDI-SAM)	Assessment used for the diagnosis of substance abuse disorders	Adults	• Up to 45 minutes to complete • Can be administered as pen-and-paper or computerized assessment	Health professionals or paraprofessionals. Training required for administration.	• Cost: $35.00 pen-and-paper; $500.00 computerized • https://zork.wustl.edu/nida/study_descriptions/study_11/sam_entire.pdf
Minnesota Multiphasic	Measure of adolescent psychopathology, has	Adolescents	• 478 true/false items	Expertise in test interpretation, or a	

Personality Inventory–Adolscent (MMPI-A)	three scales to measure substance abuse problems: MacAndrew Alcoholism Scale–Revised (MAC-R), Addiction Acknowledgement Scale (AAS), and Addiction Potential Scale (APS)		• Paper-and-pencil, CD, or computer administration	doctorate degree in psychology, education, or closely related field with formal training in the ethical administration, scoring, and interpretation of clinical assessments related to the intended use of the assessment.	• Cost: variable – contact publisher • http://psychcorp.pearsonassessments.com/HAIWEB/Cultures/en-us/Productdetail.htm?Pid=PAg522
Minnesota Multiphasic Personality Inventory, 2nd Edition (MMPI-2)	Used to assist with the diagnosis of mental disorders and the selection of appropriate treatment methods, has three scales relevant to assessing individuals who may use substances: MacAndrew Alcoholism Scale–Revised (MAC-R), Alcohol/Drug Problem Proneness scale (PRO), and the Alcohol/Drug Problem	Adults	• 567 true/false items • Paper-and-pencil, CD, or computer administration	Expertise in test interpretation or a doctorate degree in psychology, education, or closely related field with formal training in the ethical administration, scoring, and interpretation of clinical assessments related to the intended use of the assessment.	• Cost: variable – contact publisher • http://psychcorp.pearsonassessments.com/HAIWEB/Cultures/en-us/Productdetail.htm?Pid=MMPI-2&Mode=summary

(Continued)

Table 4.6: Screening instruments for detecting substance use or abuse and identifying adolescents and young adults in need of further assessment (11–27) (*Continued*)

Screening Instruments	Description	Population	Assessment Format	Who Can Administer	Website and Other Information
	Acknowledgement scale (ACK)				
Personality Assessment Inventory (PAI)	Assesses psychopathological syndromes and provides information relevant for clinical diagnosis, treatment planning, and screening for psychopathology; has two scales relevant to assessing individuals who may use substances: Alcohol Problems (ALC) and Drug Problems (DRG)	Adult	• 334 items • Self-report, pen-and-paper or audio administration	Advanced professional degree that provides appropriate training in the administration and interpretation of psychological tests; *or* license or certification from an agency that requires appropriate training and experience in the ethical and competent use of psychological tests	• Cost: variable – contact publisher • Sample report: http://www.psychassessments.com.au/products/184/prod184_report1.pdf

working with a patient that is likely to have alcohol or drug problems. This set of procedures, the Screening, Brief Intervention, and Referral to Treatment (SBIRT), is designed to be brief enough to be able to be used in any setting where a high-risk person presents (i.e., hospital, college health center, primary care physician's office, and so on). The first step of the procedure involves screening for alcohol/drug problems with a validated brief questionnaire, such as the Substance Abuse Subtle Screening Inventory (SASSI-3) or Substance Abuse Subtle Screening Inventory – Adolescent (SASSI-A2), the NIDAMED (National Institute on Drug Abuse: Medical and Health Professionals) Drug Use Screening Tool, Personal Experience Screening Questionnaire (PESQ) or Personal Experience Screening Questionnaire – Adults (PESQ-A), Personal Experience Inventory (PEI), or the Problem-Oriented Screening Instrument for Teenagers (POSIT) (briefly described in table 4.6) (11–27). Once screened, a trained professional provides a personalized and brief intervention (of 5–10 minutes) and discusses alcohol and drug-use issues with the person who may be at risk. The last step involves making a referral to treatment if warranted. In most cases Medicare, Medicaid, and commercial insurance will pay for this service (28).

4.8 Diagnosis

Once the screening process is complete and youths needing further evaluation are identified, a comprehensive psychosocial and medical history should be conducted (see table 4.7) (1,2,4). Mental health professionals can use this system to diagnose substance use disorders in terms of the following categories: acute intoxication, abuse, dependence, withdrawal, delirium, and other disorders. In contrast to screening, diagnosis typically involves a broader evaluation of signs, symptoms, family and individual medical and psychosocial history, as well as laboratory data as these relate to the patient's illness. The purpose of diagnosis is to provide the clinician with a logical basis for planning treatment and estimating prognosis (10).

Physicians primarily use two major classification systems for billing purposes: the *International Classification of Diseases*, 10th Revision (ICD-10) and the *Diagnostic and Statistical Manual for Primary Care* (DSM-PC), where as mental health professionals use the following two diagnostic classification systems: ICD-10 and *Diagnostic and Statistical Manual of Mental Disorders*, Fourth Edition, Text Revision (DSM-IV-TR) (28–30). A major diagnostic category that has received increasing attention in research and clinical practice is "substance abuse" in contrast to dependence (28,30).

DSM-IV-TR offers that substance-related disorders include using drugs (drug of abuse, medication, toxin exposure). The DSM-IV-TR offers substance use disorders (dependence and abuse) and substance-induced disorders (intoxication, withdrawal, delirium, persisting dementia, persisting amnesic, psychotic, mood disorder, anxiety disorder, sexual dysfunction, sleep disorders) (28). The reader is referred to

Table 4.7: Components of a psychosocial history designed to obtain an accurate picture of the adolescent's problems (2)

Identifying the following:
1. Individual History a. Strengths and deficits: self-esteem, coping skills, religiosity, access to resources, coping skills, and motivation for treatment. b. Resources: peer, family, other community supports. c. Is homelessness or is a runaway. d. Issues regarding the youth's history of child abuse or neglect, involvement with the child welfare agency, and foster care placements are also key considerations. e. History of substances use over the counter and prescription drugs (including, length of use, pattern of use, and mode of ingestion). f. Medical history: previous illnesses, infectious diseases, medical trauma, pregnancies, and sexually transmitted diseases. g. Mental health history: assessments, diagnoses (focus on depression, diagnoses of conduct disorders [CDD], attention deficit disorders, oppositional defiance and conduct disorders [ODD], anxiety disorders, disability status, and treatment status for each diagnosis). h. Findings of most recent physical examination (including evidence of cutting, tattoos, picking, piercings, and self-injurious behavior). i. Sexual history, including sexual orientation, sexual abuse, and HIV risk behavior status (e.g., does he or she inject drugs, practice unsafe sex?). j. Developmental history. k. History of trauma such as exposure to domestic violence, being a victim of neglect, physical or sexual abuse. l. Safety status (presence/absence of current threats to safety [e.g., pressure from gang members to participate in drug trafficking]). m. History of and presence of suicidal ideation attempts, or plans (collect onset, frequency, duration, exact nature of attempts, and plans). Determine if the adolescent or young adult has a plan to commit suicide and has access to tools to carry out the plan. n. History of and presence of homicidal ideation attempts, or plans (collect onset, frequency, duration, exact nature of attempts, and plans). Determine if the adolescent or young adult has a plan to commit homicide and has access to tools to carry out the plan. Get the name and contact information of the person he or she targets and follow "Duty to Warn" laws in your state. o. Leisure activities, including recreational activities, hobbies, interests, and any aspirations associated with them. p. School history (this is college history for young adults), including academic performance and behavior, learning-related problems, extracurricular activities, and attendance problems. Has the child been assessed with a learning disability, or perhaps received special education services at some time in his or her educational career? q. Vocational history, including paid and volunteer work. r. Peer relationships, interpersonal skills, gang involvement, and neighborhood environment. s. Juvenile justice involvement and delinquency, including types and incidence of behavior and attitudes toward that behavior. This is legal history and involvement with the police for young adults. 2. Family History a. Including the parent's and/or guardian's history of substance use, mental and physical health problems, chronic illnesses, incarceration or illegal activity, child management concerns, and

(*Continued*)

Table 4.7: Components of a psychosocial history designed to obtain an accurate picture of the adolescent's problems (2) (*Continued*)

the family's cultural, linguistic racial/ethnic, and degree of acculturation. When working with young adults ask for a contact person for whom they will give you/your organization consent and sign a release of information in case of an emergency. Spell those conditions out in writing. This is especially critical when working with homicidal and suicidal individuals.
b. Socioeconomic status of family: Include descriptions of the home environment that includes whether the family lives in substandard housing, are homelessness, or live in shelters.
c. The family's strengths should also be noted because they will be important in intervention efforts.
d. Are the families basic needs being met?
3. Social service agency program involvement, child welfare involvement (number and duration of foster home placements), and residential treatment.

Adapted by the authors from their clinical practice in which they use a diagnostic interview form.

pages 191–295 of the DSM-IV-TR for detailed descriptions of these disorders and diagnostic criteria (28). In the latest version of the DSM (DSM-IV-TR), substance abuse is defined as a maladaptive pattern of alcohol or drug use leading to clinically significant impairment or distress (28). In the ICD-10 the term *harmful* use refers to a pattern of using one or more psychoactive substances that causes damage to health (30). The following represents the types of substance abuse listed in the previous texts (28,31):

1. *Salience.* Salience means that drinking or drug use is given a higher priority than other activities in spite of its negative consequences.
2. *Impaired control.* The main characteristic of impaired control is the lack of success in limiting the amount or frequency of substance use.
3. *Tolerance.* Tolerance is a decrease in response to a psychoactive substance that occurs with continued use.
4. *Withdrawal signs and symptoms.* A withdrawal state is a group of symptoms occurring after cessation of substance use.
5. *Other features of dependence.* To be labeled as substance dependent, symptoms must have persisted for at least one month or must have occurred repeatedly (two or more times) over a longer period of time (28,31).

4.9 Biochemical testing

A variety of drug-testing products are available to test for the presence of substances in a patient's body, including breath and saliva tests for alcohol, a multidrug panel hair test, and a variety of laboratory and instant urine tests. Pediatricians should advise parents of the limitations and potential risks associated with home drug-testing products (32).

4.10 Discussion

When assessing family members, certain principles should be kept in mind:

- Adolescents may define family in nontraditional ways. Treatment providers should allow adolescents to identify and acknowledge the people they would describe as "family," even though they may not live with the adolescent.
- The law and society may define family in ways that differ from the actual experiences of substance-abusing youth.
- Cultural and ethnic differences in family structures should be respected (2,4).

After the information from the different sources (interview, observation, specialized testing) has been assembled, the assessor writes a report of what he or she has learned about the patient in terms that can be understood by all concerned, including the patient. The receiving clinician who writes the report should also include information that helps the receiving clinician, guardians, and the adolescent understand (a) the way the adolescent processes information most effectively and how this will affect treatment, and (b) how the adolescent's past experiences will affect her or his reaction to certain treatment interventions. The report should also include (a) specific treatment and placement recommendations as well as justifications, (b) counselor recommendations, and (c) a plan for recidivism. Clinicians should also make sure that both guardians and the adolescent, or the young adult, understand that treatment is a slow laborious process that generally does not produce large effects on substance-abuse-related outcomes. The clinician also needs to help them remember that individual outcomes vary widely within different types of treatments. Finally, warn them that no one treatment approach is effective for all youth (34).

References

1. Centers for Disease Control and Prevention. Youth risk behavior surveillance – United States, 2011. MMWR 2012;61(No. 4): 1–168. Accessed 2012 Aug 24. URL: http://www.cdc.gov/healthyyouth/yrbs/pdf/us_overview_yrbs.pdf http://www.cdc.gov/mmwr/pdf/ss/ss6104.pdf http://brightfutures.aap.org/pdfs/Preventive%20Services%20PDFs/Screening.PDF
2. Substance Abuse and Mental Health Services Administration. (2011). Identifying mental health and substance use problems of children and adolescents: A guide for Child-serving organizations (HHS Publication No. SMA 12–4670). Rockville, MD: Author. Accessed 2012 Aug 31. URL: http://www.samhsa.gov/children/508compliant_Identifying_MH_and_SU_Problems_1-30-2012.pdf
3. Perepletchikova F, Krystal JH, Kaufman J. Practitioner review: adolescent alcohol use disorders: assessment and treatment issues. J Child Psychol Psychiatry 2008;49(11):1131–54.
4. Center for Substance Abuse Treatment (CSAT). Screening and assessing adolescents for substance use disorders. Treatment improvement protocol (TIP) Series, No. 31. Rockville MD: Substance Abuse and Mental Health Services Administration (US); 1999. Accessed 2012 Aug 24. URL: http://store.samhsa.gov/product/TIP-31-Screening-and-Assessing-Adolescents-for-Substance-Use-Disorders/SMA09-4079

5. Wills TA, Walker C, Mendoza D, Ainette MG. Behavioral and emotional self-control: Relations to substance use in samples of middle and high school students. Am Psychol Assoc 2006;20(3): 265–78.
6. Preda A. Depression and mania in substance-induced mood disorders. Medscape references drugs, disease, procedures 2012. Accessed 2012 Aug 30. URL: http://emedicine.medscape.com/article/286885-overview
7. Knight J, Roberts T, Gabrielli J, Van Hook, S. Adolescent alcohol and substance use and abuse. In: Tanski S, Garfunkel LC, Duncan PM, Weitzman M, eds. Pediatrics performing preventive services: A bright futures handbook, 3rd ed. Elk Grove Village, IL: American Academy of Pediatrics, 2010. Accessed 2012 Aug 28. URL: http://brightfutures.aap.org/continuing_education.html
8. Holmbeck GN, et al. Evidence-based assessment in pediatric psychology: measures of psychosocial adjustment and psychopathology. J Pediatr Psychol 2008;33(9):958–80.
9. Chi FW, Sterling S, Weisner C. Adolescents with co-occurring substance use and mental conditions in a private managed care health plan: prevalence, patient characteristics and treatment initiation and engagement. Am J Addict 2006;15:67–79.
10. Williams RJ, Nowatzki N. Validity of adolescent self-report of substance use. Misuse 2005;40: 299–311.
11. Wintres KC and Kaminer YK. Screening and assessing adolescent substance use disorders in clinical populations. J Am Acad Child Adolesc Psychiatry 2008;47:740–4.
12. Bovasso GB, Alterman AI, Cacciola JS, and Cook TG. Predictive validity of the addiction severity scale index's composite scores in the assessment of 2-year outcomes in a methadone maintenance population. Psychol Addict Behav 2001;15:171–6.
13. Freimuth M. Another missed opportunity? Recognition of alcohol use problems by mental health providers. Psychother Theor Res 2008;45:405–9.
14. Butcher JN, Miller KB. Assessment of substance abuse in psychotherapy clients: the effectiveness of the MMPI-2 substance abuse scales. Psychol Assessment 1999;11:101–7.
15. Fals-Stewart W. The ability of individuals with psychoactive substance use disorders to escape detection by the personality assessment inventory. Psychol Assess 1996;8:60–8.
16. Gallucci NT. On the identification of patterns of substance abuse with the MMPI-A. Psychol Assess 1997;9:224–32.
17. Winters KC, Leitten W. Brief intervention for drug-abusing adolescents in a school setting. Psychol Addict Behav 2007;21:249–54.
18. Carpenter KM, Hasin DS. Reasons for drinking alcohol: relationships with DSM-IV alcohol diagnoses and alcohol consumption in a community sample. Psychol Addict Behav 1998;12:168–84.
19. Myerholtz LE, Rosenburg H. Screening dui offenders for alcohol problems: psychometric assessment of substance abuse subtle screening inventory. Psychol Addict Behav 1997;11:155–65.
20. Carey KB, Teitelbaum LM. Goals and methods of alcohol assessment. Prof Psychol-Res Pr 1996;27:460–6.
21. Andrews JA, Tildesley E, Hops H, Li F. The influence of peers on young adult substance use. Health Psychol 2002;21:349–57.
22. Winters KC, Remafedi G, Chan BY. Assessing drug abuse among gay-bisexual young men. Psychol Addict Behav;10:228–36.
23. Kogan SM, Lou Z, McBride Murry V, Brody GH. Risk and protective factors for substance use among African American high school dropouts. Psychol Addict Behav 2005;19:382–91.
24. Winters KC, Latimer WW, Stinchfield RD, Egan E. Measuring adolescent drug abuse and psychosocial factors in four ethnic groups of drug-abusing boys. Exp Clin Psychopharm 2004; 12:227–36.
25. Borsari B, Neal DJ, Collins SE, Carey KB. Differential utility of three indexes of risky drinking for predicting alcohol problems in college students. Psychol Addict Behav 2001;15:321–4.

26. Curry J, et al. Onset of alcohol or substance use disorders following treatment for adolescent depression. J Consult Clin Psych 2012;80:299–12.
27. SAMHSA-HRSA Center for Integrated Health Solutions. Screening, brief intervention, and referral to treatment (SBIRT). Accessed 01 Sept 2012. URL: http://www.integration.samhsa.gov/about-us
28. American Psychiatric Association (APA). Diagnostic and statistical manual of mental disorders, 4th ed. Washington, DC: APA, 1994:191–295.
29. Wolrich ML, Felice MF, Drotar D, eds. The classification of child and adolescent mental diagnoses in primary care. Diagnostic and statistical manual for primary care (DSM-PC). Child and adolescent Version. Elk Grove Villiage, IL: American Academy of Pediatrics, 1996.
30. World Health Organization (WHO). The ICD-10 classification of mental and behavioural disorders: Clinical descriptions and diagnostic guidelines, 2nd ed. Geneva: WHO, 2004.
31. Carson-DeWitt R, ed. Diagnosis of drug abuse: Diagnostic criteria. encyclopedia of drugs, alcohol, and addictive behavior. eNotes.com 2001. Accessed on 2012 Aug 12. URL: http://www.enotes.com/diagnosis-drug-abuse-diagnostic-criteria-reference/diagnosis-drug-abuse-diagnostic-criteria
32. Levy S, Van Hookand S, Knight J. A review of internet-based home drug-testing products for parents. Pediatrics 2004;113:720–6.
33. Waldron HB, Turner CW. Evidence-based psychosocial treatments for adolescent substance abuse. J Clin Child Adoles Psychol 2008;37(1):238–61.

Section II: **Treatment**

5 Psychosocial treatments for substance use disorders

Ahsan Nazeer and Michael R. Liepman

Millions of adolescents all over the world meet one or more of the criteria of substance use disorders (SUDs) set forth in the *Diagnostic and Statistical Manual of Mental Disorders*, fourth edition (*DSM-IV*). For various reasons, only a small percentage of these adolescents seek professional care for the treatment of these disorders. During the past 30 years, numerous psychosocial treatments have been developed and validated. This chapter is a brief review of the empirically validated treatments in this category.

5.1 Introduction

Psychosocial treatment of SUDs is a broad term that includes numerous nonpharmacological modalities with the goal to achieve and sustain abstinence, or change patterns of use to avoid harm, and improve function. The long-term goal of maintaining abstinence lies at the heart of many effective SUD treatment programs and psychosocial interventions are considered to be the key for success in achieving this goal. Implementation of these interventions may differ; efficacy usually is influenced by patient characteristics, nature of drugs involved, types of pharmacological interventions that are being applied, psychiatric comorbidities, and psychosocial stressors that may be unique to a particular individual. Despite the individualized nature of these programs, the long-term goals of making positive lifestyle changes and maintaining a drug-free lifestyle or a life free of drug-related harm are critical, common elements of these modalities.

Failure to engage adolescents in effective treatment for SUDs is the principal reason for adult SUDs since most substance use behavior begins during childhood and adolescence. While experimentation with getting high via drug use typically begins in the pediatric population, those who find this practice most captivating will progress over time into chronic substance dependence; their choice of drug may morph over time, but their entire life existence is infused with drug use as a major goal. Demonstrating the chronicity is the extent to which many require multiple SUD treatments and the number of consequences that must accumulate before they achieve recovery, if they ever do. As is said in jest, "The monkey is off my back, but the organ grinder is still in town."

Behavioral therapies have long been known to be an effective treatment option for common psychiatric disorders. By the mid-1980s, behavioral treatments for SUDs were available, but there was significant pessimism regarding their effectiveness. It was not until the 1990s that the National Institute on Drug Abuse started supporting research and implementation of these approaches in community settings. In the following chapter, we will briefly review the following psychosocial treatments: motivational treatments, contingency management (CM) approaches, cognitive behavioral therapies (CBTs), and couple and family interventions.

A 2008 meta-analysis reviewing the efficacy of psychosocial treatments for SUDs found a moderate effect size in general, but with greater efficacy when applied to cannabis use than with polysubstance dependence. The largest effect size was achieved by CM treatments followed by relapse prevention (RP) and CBT (1).

5.2 Motivational treatments

Motivational treatments are aimed at helping individuals to take action and to make a change with the long-term goal of abstinence from drugs. This process of change occurs in individualized talk-therapy sessions between the therapist and patient. Change is characterized by moving through the stages of precontemplation (denial), contemplation (ambivalence), preparation, action, maintenance, and termination (2). On the basis of this process, Miller and Rollnick have developed a counseling style (motivational interviewing [MI]) that is designed to reduce ambivalence (move past contemplation) and to promote change (3). It is important to understand that individuals may cycle through these stages of readiness to change numerous times before solidifying a recovery-oriented new lifestyle. It is possible to use this approach to motivate change leading to total abstinence or to harm reduction by using substances in a manner that leads to no harm or less harm.

5.2.1 Precontemplation stage

Precontemplation is the initial stage that signifies resistance to change. In this stage, individuals are not ready to make a change in their life and are not consciously aware of their mistakes and the consequences of their behaviors. They may project their troubles onto those around them (e.g., their parents, the police, and teachers) who seem intolerant of their substance use. The pros of continuing the behavior that troubles those around them far outweigh the cons, and the cons of change far outweigh the pros of the changes others want them to make. Seen as rebelliousness by outsiders and autonomy by the youth with the problem, the youth will deny the relationship between the problem behavior and the consequences that have occurred and the risk of future consequences that adults who care about him/her may anticipate.

The therapist must remain neutral in motivational enhancement therapy, avoiding confrontation, and trying to understand the world from the patient's point of view. The therapist provides feedback and explores the patient's perspective. She/he discusses the patient's hopes, raises consciousness about connections between choices made and consequences of those choices, and highlights the discrepancy between actions and goals. At times, involving families during this phase further helps the patient to connect the drug use behaviors with identifiable consequences, as insightful family members will supply more examples of consequences and risky behaviors than the youth may offer.

Adolescents with SUDs tend to have fewer consequences than adults simply because they have been abusing drugs for a shorter time. In addition, cognitive impairment may cause the adolescent to forget what may have happened during an episode of intoxication or have virtually no insight (4). Minimization of the severity of consequences or risks, blaming others for being caught, and comparing self to others are common defenses that youth use to convince themselves not to worry about what is happening during precontemplation.

5.2.2 Contemplation stage

The contemplation stage follows precontemplation and is characterized by an individual who is considering making a change in the future. The patient begins to become aware of the addictive behavior and its causal relationship to consequences. However, the patient also values certain positive aspects of the substance use (e.g., relief of social anxiety, fitting in with peers, and improving performance), and reluctance to lose these stands in the way of committing to change. Without effective support, some individuals procrastinate about deciding to change, which can lead to chronicity of the disorder and accumulation of more consequences. Adolescents are particularly prone to rebellion against adults, so confrontational approaches are more likely to promote defensive resistance than MI or motivational enhancement therapy.

During this phase, by examining pros and cons of continued substance use and of recovery, the therapist helps the patient to resolve ambivalence. Whereas during contemplation the decisional balance between pros and cons in fairly even, this will need to shift toward greater pros and fewer cons related to recovery and greater cons and fewer pros related to continued use before any effective change will occur. Shifts in the opposite direction will lead to a return to precontemplation, relapse or continuing substance abuse, and dropping out of treatment. During this stage, the therapist does not advise or seek action, patiently waiting until the patient is ready for change. Listening for change talk is key to moving on to the next stage. When the patient expresses a genuine desire to change, the therapist flags this statement and explores what that might look like in terms of new behaviors including better decision making and participation in treatment and recovery support activities (3).

The desire to control the continued use of drugs in such a manner as to avoid harm is common among persons suffering from SUDs, especially adolescents. There is published research that documents a small number of alcoholics who have successfully morphed their pattern of drinking to avoid further harm (5,6). However, this work was done on adults. Also, long-term follow-up data are scant. There has been much controversy over whether abstinence is a healthier outcome than controlled use of substances (7). Attempts to train alcoholic adults to control their drinking showed some promising results in the short run, but evidence from longer-term follow-up raises questions about whether this can realistically be accomplished for most patients.

Those with dependence may do better when things in their environment are going well, but they may resume former heavier drinking patterns when under stress (8). Furthermore, what seems like "normal drinking" to the alcoholic may be much in excess of what others would consider safe. However, abstinence as a goal for teens, especially from drugs that are socially accepted (such as alcohol and cannabis) and prescribed medications (such as opioids, anxiolytics, and stimulants) may be unacceptable. While the brain reward center is a single entity, triggered by a wide variety of addictive drugs, it makes sense to recommend staying away from all drugs that can trigger a relapse of addictive behavior (see chapter 2). However, the research on outcome of controlled use has not been done on teen drug users, so extrapolating from studies on dependent adult alcoholics may not be scientifically valid.

In the individual work with a teen, the therapist looks at the goals of the use of intoxicants. If such goals are relief of unpleasant feelings (e.g., anxiety, depression, pain, and boredom), these might need to be addressed before the patient would consider giving up substance use (see chapter 14). If social pressure to join in with others who are also abusing substances is the main goal, changing with whom one associates may be critical in the change process; this may be difficult depending on various factors including where one lives and goes to school, and substance use patterns among relatives. Adolescents usually have little influence over these matters other than choices of friends. A realistic understanding of the process of one's substance use behavior, including the frequency and dose of typical drug consumption, may be necessary to tackle the fantasy of becoming a nonproblem substance user.

5.2.3 Preparation stage

The preparation stage is significant for the individual's intentions to take action in the near future. Individuals usually craft a plan of action in this stage, and they work actively to get ready to execute that plan. During this stage, the therapist clarifies the patient's specific, realistic goals of behavior change and guides the process of discovery of a plan of action that is most likely to succeed. In this stage, it is appropriate to make arrangements, assemble a supportive team, and counsel family members to curtail expressions of negativity in exchange for recovery supportive expressions.

5.2.4 Action stage

Action is the stage during which the individual makes specific changes in behavior. Complete abstinence from some psychoactive drugs may be attempted by some, while others may attempt to control the dose, setting, or frequency of drug use. Entry into a formal substance abuse treatment program frequently is necessary to guide and support change. Peer interactional group therapy for adolescents who are working on recovery may be counterproductive if the therapist is unable to curb cross talk between group members, within or outside of group sessions; this problem glorifies drug use or suggests additional drugs to try. Dishion and colleagues reported on two experimental studies that demonstrated increased substance use and deviant behavior among low-risk youth who participated with high-risk youth in therapy groups (9). However, others have shown that structured CBT groups do not lead to this effect (10,11). It is likely that the therapist direction plays an important role in whether the group achieves constructive or destructive results.

The contagion effect also can occur at 12-step meetings in the community where there are no controls over what participants do or say to one another; indeed, not everyone in attendance may be there for the purpose of recovery. The recovering members in attendance with the longest sobriety are likely to try to quash that kind of activity. In 12-step groups other than Alateen, the group's senior members are likely to be fairly young with shorter sobriety histories. There is evidence for better outcomes when either CBT done in groups or a structured family therapy is used.

During the action stage, the therapist avoids passive and nondirective therapy and is more actively engaged in behavior change-oriented treatments. Specific suggestions are given that include facilitating participation in self-help group meetings such as young people's Alcoholics Anonymous (AA) or Narcotics Anonymous (NA) or alternatives, changing the peer group, trying alternative recreational activities, or dealing with underlying emotional problems. Help to identify craving and cues that trigger the urge to use and strategies to cope with urges are important elements of treatment.

Processing examples of craving and successful or unsuccessful attempts to avert relapses is critical. It is important to encourage brutal honesty in treatment sessions so guilt and shame do not promote concealing these important slips from the therapist that reveal gaps in the armor that is being built to prevent slips in the future. Frequent drug testing (saliva and urine) when properly done is critical in detecting slips and making it clear to the patient that lying to the therapist will not be effective; in outpatient settings, missed visits may be in part motivated by a desire to conceal slips and dodge shame.

Some patients may benefit from participation in self-help groups. In large cities, there are many options, but in rural communities and smaller towns there may not be any appropriate self-help groups for adolescents. Young people's groups may exist on college campuses or be associated with adolescent treatment programs. Online recovery-oriented chat rooms exist that may be helpful, but parental oversight might be in order given the lack of professional oversight that exists. In cases where an adolescent patient needs to discuss conflict with this parent, another surrogate adult might be identified to monitor the utilization of such chat rooms. AA and NA have a strong focus on spiritual investment mentioning faith in "God" or a "higher power" in the literature and steps. Many interpret this as pushing religion on them; those with objections to religion may find themselves distracted from the healing elements of these groups. There are other programs that provide alternatives in which faith or religion is not promoted as an element in the recovery process; these include SMART Recovery, Secular Organization for Sobriety (SOS), Women for Sobriety, Rational Recovery, and Moderation Management (12).

CBT is the mainstay during the action stage. RP treatment is a variant of CBT that is aimed at maintaining sobriety. After the initial period of sobriety, patients are taught to identify high-risk situations including drug paraphernalia, peers who use drugs, and stressful life situations that may trigger urges to use called cravings. While usually transient, coping strategies such as distraction, disclosing the urge to a support person, or just waiting until it passes are usually effective. These strategies also are recommended at 12-step groups. "Slips" are identified and are processed in the treatment sessions as "learning experiences." Efforts are made to differentiate these brief incidents from complete loss of control or "relapses."

Numerous studies have shown the effectiveness of MI in the management of drug use, whereas others have failed to show consistent results with this modality (13,14,15). In a recent 2011 Cochrane review, authors reviewed 59 randomized clinical trials of 13,342 participants using or abusing drugs. Results were categorized into four different groups, and MI was compared to "no treatment control," "treatment as usual," "assessment and feedback," and "other active intervention." These results were also compared for their efficacy immediately after the intervention and after short-, medium-, and long-term follow-up intervals. When compared with "no treatment," MI showed significant postintervention effect, weaker short- and medium-term effect, and nonsignificant long-term effect. MI also fared better than the comparison group "assessment and feedback" for medium-term efficacy. There was no significant difference among the outcomes when the MI was compared with "treatment as usual" and "other active treatment" for any of the follow-ups. The authors concluded that MI is effective for the management of substance abuse in comparison to no treatment (16).

5.2.5 Maintenance stage

The maintenance stage is characterized by the patient's and therapist's work to prevent relapse. Reflecting the chronic, relapsing clinical course of this disorder, this stage requires prolonged effort, and patients may remain in this stage from months to years before relapsing. Most patients are not ready for the sustained effort that is needed to maintain sobriety and are particularly prone to relapse during times of emotional distress. Adolescents typically have strong denial that persistent abstinence is necessary; rather, they tend to believe that all they need to do is to stay out of trouble for a while until people forget about what brought their behavior under adult scrutiny. It is easy for them to find peers who are still consuming alcohol, tobacco, or other drugs and who would be happy to have them join in. Also, the adolescent fantasy of omnipotence makes it easy to believe that the rules of nature and laws of the community do not really apply to them. Those who are required to be monitored by a juvenile drug court or by parents are likely to cheat to test the monitoring process.

5.2.6 Contemplation of relapse

If the commitment to recovery begins to erode, the adolescent may enter a contemplation of relapse stage. Much like the contemplation of recovery stage, where the pros and cons of changing, and of not changing, are of approximately equal strength, ambivalence tends to paralyze decision making. If the supports and coping tools are properly utilized, the youth may avoid relapse. If a slip occurs, quick reconsideration may result in resumption of maintenance of recovery. On the other hand, the pros-and-cons impasse may be overturned by impulsivity, peer pressure, or a desire to relieve dysphoria with a full relapse resulting (relapse action); in this case, the next stage is maintenance of relapse, which is equivalent to precontemplation. There may be a significant delay before enough harm has accrued that the youth can be engaged in recovery efforts again.

5.3 CM and community reinforcement approaches (CRAs)

5.3.1 CM

CM therapies are based on learning and operant conditioning theories. These theories are based on the principle that negative or positive consequences to a behavior can increase or decrease the target behavior, which in turn can lead to a desired outcome. Within this model, it is conceptualized that drug use and the associated lifestyle provides constant reinforcement to the user. In CM, the patient's environment is gradually reorganized, and drug reinforcements are systematically replaced with alternative neutral reinforcing activities. Using coupons for the exchange of goods or vouchers contingent upon negative urine drug screens (UDSs) is an example of alternate reinforcement. Aversive consequences including forfeiting the available incentives or loss of certain privileges are usually considered in the face of continued drug use.

Voucher-based CM has shown success in individuals with cocaine use. These are usually 12-week programs that need a signed contract with the individual at the start of the program. Vouchers are contingent upon providing negative UDSs; also, subsequent vouchers incrementally increase in their dollar value as the number of consecutive negative UDSs increases. A bonus is provided after three consecutive negative UDSs in order to continue reinforcing continuous abstinence. A positive UDS in this ongoing process resets the voucher value back to the initial amount as a punishment. Like other behavioral interventions, these interventions are directed to a single behavior; the promptness of the rewards or negative consequences can lead to a stronger treatment effect.

These approaches have good empirical support and have been known to be an effective management strategy from studies conducted as early as the 1970s. In one study, alcoholic human volunteers were placed in residential facilities where they were allowed to purchase and consume ethanol at will. Numerous consequences to this behavior were applied with the goal to modify ethanol self-administration. Researchers noted an increase in abstinence when the volunteers were provided with monetary reinforcements and were given access to alternate reinforcements. Abstinence also increased when the amount of work required to access alcohol was increased and when periods of isolation were imposed (17). There is also a significant body of evidence from methadone clinics that supports the notion that positive consequences (rewards) are more effective in maintaining these patients in treatment and managing long-term abstinence than negative consequences (18).

5.3.2 CRA

CRA provides a way to achieve abstinence by using the contingencies that are present in the individual's natural environment. This approach is different than the voucher- and coupon-based programs that are systematically put in place for the explicit reason to get a negative UDS specimen. Comprehensive treatment programs usually involve both strategies in which individuals gradually phase from voucher-based programs that provide initial abstinence to more naturalistic resources in their community to maintain long-term abstinence.

In CRA, patients learn to recognize the antecedents and consequences of their behavior. Ongoing counseling is provided to help them change their daily activities as well as their social contacts and to pursue a healthier lifestyle. Individual therapy sessions focus on changing attitudes and learning skills such as anger management, problem solving, and assertiveness (being a good team member). Counselors gradually help the users to get their reinforcements from alternate recreational or other activities that do not rely on drugs to have fun. This goal also can be achieved by participation in self-help groups including AA or NA. This phase usually lasts for 24 weeks (assuming that they stay more or less engaged and abstinent during this interval) after which patients are encouraged to be in contact with the counselors on a monthly basis for brief therapy sessions.

Researchers have found an important relationship between the length of time spent in the program and the treatment outcomes including longer abstinence and decreased legal troubles (19). These data are consistent across studies targeting adult and adolescent populations. In the Drug Abuse Treatment Outcome Study (DATOS), 10,000 users from 96 programs were evaluated for long-term outcomes. This study supported the relationship between the previous two variables and identified a minimum threshold of 90 days for the treatment to be effective on a longer-term basis (20). The adolescent DATOS study (DATOS-A) also found that adolescents who stayed in the outpatient programs for more than 90 days or in inpatient programs for more than 21 days had better abstinence outcomes than others (21).

5.4 Cognitive behavioral approaches

CBT including RP is based on learning theory including classical and operant conditioning. Therapists conceptualize drug use as a learned behavior that is associated over time with certain internal or external stimuli. Some of these include cues that remind one to self-administer drugs such as being offered some drug; encountering drug paraphernalia or something that resembles the same, such as a sweetener packet resembling a bag of heroin; stressful life experiences; or exposure to certain situations including drinking at parties. These triggers are called antecedents to use; exposure to these triggers causes an urge to use a particular drug. Drug use following these cues usually leads to desired rewarding effects such as "feeling high" or "becoming relaxed"; these are positive consequences or rewards that further consolidate this behavior. Behavioral treatment is based on the following: (1) detailed analysis of the target behavior including identification of antecedents and consequences, (2) skills training, and (3) RP.

As with any other behavioral treatment, the CBT model relies on the individual's motivation to change the existing behavior and to replace it with a new healthy behavior. This change happens on a continuum as the individual goes through the process of precontemplation, contemplation, preparation, action, and maintenance. Counselors also understand that motivation is more dynamic than static and numerous factors influence this state at a given time. Dissatisfaction with the old behaviors increases motivation to change them and to replace them with new behaviors.

Change in life including job requirements and newly diagnosed medical or psychiatric comorbidities further affect this dissatisfaction.

Adolescents typically have less insight into the situation; denial and their limited sense of future can make it difficult for them to realize the extent to which their drug use behavior is harming them and how it will progress and damage their future potential. Also, many of their peers, especially those they have been hanging out with, are drug users too; thus, they believe that drug use is the norm. This is reinforced if others in their family and surroundings (e.g., older siblings, parents, other relatives, neighbors, and celebrities) also use drugs. They are much less likely to be exposed to recovering former drug users or sensible people who have chosen not to become drug involved. So, while authority figures may be telling them to stop using, their peers may be saying the opposite, giving them mixed community reinforcements.

This makes treatment difficulty in an open society where deviance is accepted or at least tolerated. This may explain why one of the most effective treatment settings for adolescents is an isolated, longer-term residential facility where for an extended interval, the peer group is made up of other recovering teens, and where access to drugs is extremely difficult and would lead to likely detection and expulsion from the program. Other highly effective treatment programs take place in outpatient settings where either family or drug court probation officers closely monitor teens' choices and promptly apply consequences.

5.4.1 Functional analysis

Analysis of the target behavior, also called functional analysis, is the next step in this process of change. According to classical conditioning, neutral stimuli can become associated with cravings and with drug use. These are usually neutral triggers that in a nonuser do not elicit these responses. In users, certain environments, people or inner emotions can lead to drug use. If these triggers occur in close proximity to the drug self-administration behavior, gradually they become paired with each other, and as a result, a previous neutral stimulus now becomes a trigger for drug use. In operant conditioning, rewarding consequences of drug use lead to a higher likelihood of future drug use.

Structured and nonstructured interviews can be conducted to identify the patterns of use, triggers, and consequences. These triggers are then organized in a hierarchical pattern according to their frequency of occurrence and the strength of association with the target behavior. Numerous behavioral strategies and techniques have been derived from the previously discussed theories. In cue exposure, an individual is exposed to the stimulus that is most closely associated with drug use. Users are then repeatedly exposed to those stimuli without being permitted to self-administer the drug. The model of extinction is applied in this strategy with a goal to disrupt the cycle of antecedent leading to drug self-administration behavior. For example, if one repeatedly holds a cigarette pack in one's hands but does not take a cigarette out and light or puff on it, eventually the connection between encountering a pack of cigarettes in a store will be less compelling. Pharmacological treatments such as nicotine replacements or varenicline and bupropion reduce the craving and reinforcement from smoking leading to extinction of smoking behavior (see chapters 2 and 7).

5.4.2 Drug refusal skills

After the functional analysis of the behavior, the main thrust of CBT is to teach necessary drug refusal skills. Behavioral theorists believe that after motivation, specific sets of skills are needed in order to learn and sustain new behavior. Numerous factors threaten long-term abstinence including cravings, withdrawal symptoms, and social stressors. During the initial few attempts to quit drug use, most users lack necessary skills to deal with day-to-day stressors. Skill training is helpful in preventing these limitations and barriers that prevent abstinence. There are numerous manual-based approaches that teach necessary skills that are known to be absent in drug-using individuals. These skills are as follows:

- Anger management
- Relaxation training to combat stress
- Using assertiveness with people in place of passivity or aggressiveness
- Drug refusal to respond to invitations from peers and ask them to stop inviting
- Handling criticism and compliments gracefully without becoming upset
- Expressing feelings and emotions in intimate relationships
- Managing negative thoughts (e.g., resentments and negative self-talk)
- Selecting and engaging in pleasant nondrug activities to maintain a balance in daily life
- Decision-making training to foresee the consequences of the decisions
- Problem solving (i.e., identification of the problem, reviewing alternative solutions, and choosing the best possible solution among these options)
- Expanding the social network to include peers who do not use drugs and diminishing exposure to peers who do (22)

5.4.3 RP

RP applies the CBT skills learned to the challenges of the maintenance stage. RP treatment is based on the assumption that an individual's ability to maintain abstinence is directly related to his/her ability to successfully negotiate stressful situations without relying on drug use. Counselors help the individuals to identify high-risk situations such as mood dysregulations, medical care, and social situations with drug-using peers promoting the use of abusable drugs. Specific areas of problems are evaluated in depth, and a plan of coping strategies is crafted for each of these situations.

It is important to note that most of these situations are identical to the ones for which they have already received skills training. Thus, decision making and interpersonal skills that they have learned in the past are helpful for individuals to make rational decisions and to avoid risky situations and encounters. In this model, "slips" are considered part of the treatment process in which the motivational aspects of the individual are reevaluated, the situation that led to the slip is analyzed, and strategies are discussed to prevent complete relapse. If a slip occurred for which the patient had strategies that were not used, the reason they were not applied must be determined. If a slip occurred for a novel situation that was not anticipated before, a new set of strategies must be created (23).

5.5 Family interventions

Adolescent substance abuse has always been considered as a multidimensional problem with impaired interactions among individuals, family, and society. Family interventions have been the mainstay of successful substance abuse treatment in adolescents. SUDs cause significant morbidity in the family system. Research has shown that genetic factors inherited from biological family members determine about half of the cause of substance abuse by adolescents, while the environment explains the other half (see chapter 3). The environment may be more responsible for determining which drugs are tried based on ease of access and whether a youth will experiment with drugs. On the other hand, genetic factors may be responsible for how a person reacts to particular drugs and may be influential in creating needs in the teen that can be fulfilled by use of a specific drug (e.g., attention-deficit/hyperactivity disorder and stimulants, anxiety and alcohol, and pain and opioids). In addition to genetic factors, having drug-abusing parents can result in the following:

- Role models for drug use
- Access to drugs in the home
- Tolerance of or lack of parental concern about youth drug use
- Frightening traumatic life experiences associated with accidents; domestic violence; child abuse or neglect; or early loss of parents through death, incarceration, or divorce
- Poverty, deprivation, or failure to be properly evaluated and treated for medical/psychiatric problems
- Exposure to unsavory characters without parental protection

It has been shown that these hereditary factors and environmental experiences increase the incidence of SUDs and add comorbidities that must be addressed in treatment for recovery to be achieved (24).

During the treatment process, families can be engaged in managing resistance and denial as well as identifying the early signs of recovery or relapse. However, families also have denial and resistance, so it is important to address their clinical needs as well. Family psychoeducation and support groups, such as Al-Anon or Families Anonymous, frequently are helpful.

5.5.1 Multidimensional family therapy (MDFT)

MDFT is an intervention that focuses on identifying and changing adolescents' behaviors within the context of family interactions as well as within the family relations with the broader community. It is not unusual for youths with SUDs to have families that are more critical, are emotionally unavailable, only respond to negative behaviors, have inconsistent rules, and display a high level of conflict. In MDFT, therapists serve as an advocate for the youth and the family with the school, other community resources, and the legal system. Sessions may be conducted in the office or at the family's home with individual sessions with the youth with each of the family members.

During the initial phase of treatment, therapists work with the adolescents to engage them in therapy, to break through resistance, and to establish a positive patient-therapist alliance.

Factors that are evaluated include pattern of drug use, personality style, quality of relationship with the parents, and their interactions with the broader group. As the treatment progresses, the family is gradually integrated into the sessions, and the emphasis is placed on reducing conflict and emotional detachment between the patient and the family. Therapists also seek collaboration between the family and the other community resources including the school and legal systems that are important in the adolescent's life.

Families are provided help with housing, transportation, and medical care in an effort to engage them fully in the treatment plan and to work with the adolescent closely. In a recent study, 11- to 15-year-old Hispanic and African American youth were randomly assigned to MDFT or group-based CBT for 12–16 weeks (25). Outcomes were assessed during the treatment, at the end of treatment, and then 6 and 12 months after termination. Adolescents in the MDFT showed more robust and longer-lasting abstinence than those in group therapy (54% as compared to 13%). Researchers also noticed a decrease in frequency of drug use and in delinquent behaviors.

There are other models of family therapy that are effective with adolescents (26). Family involvement, if accomplished in a positive manner, can bring efficacy as high as 80%–85%. In contrast, individual therapy approaches are more prone to relapse.

In addition, a perverse process has been observed in which another family member becomes sick with an SUD following onset of remission in the original chemically dependent family member. This may be avoided by treating the entire family. It is believed that substance use in some way may incur benefits to the family as a whole, despite its negative effects on the family. This becomes a challenge for the therapist to discover what advantage this is and to find another alternative (27).

5.6 Conclusion

During the past three decades, psychosocial treatments for SUDs have undergone substantial growth as scientific scrutiny of outcomes has generated new therapies that have been validated. Adolescents with SUDs present a challenge in the degree of their denial, the influence of acceptance from peers, and resistance to authority in their quest for autonomy. Family approaches, motivational enhancement therapies, and CBTs have shown the best efficacies for this group.

References

1. Dutra L, Stathopoulou G, Basden SL, Leyro TM, Powers MB, Otto MW. A meta-analytic review of psychosocial interventions for substance use disorders. Am J Psychiatry 2008;165:179–87.
2. Prochaska JO, DiClemente CC, Norcross JC. In search of how people change: Applications to addictive behaviors. Am Psychol 1992;47:1102–14.
3. Miller WR, Rollnick S. Motivational interviewing: Preparing people for change, 2nd ed. New York: Guilford, 2002.
4. Morrison MA. White rabbit: A doctor's own story of addiction, survival and recovery. New York: Berkley, 1981.
5. Vaillant GE. The natural history of alcoholism revisited. Cambridge, MA: Harvard University Press, 1995.
6. Sobell MB, Sobell LC. Controlled drinking after 25 years. Addiction 1995;90:1149–53.
7. Glatt MM. Controlled drinking after a third of a century. Addiction 1995;90:1157–60.
8. Sobell MB, Sobell LC, eds. Review of moderation as a goal or outcome of treatment for alcohol problems: A dialogue. New York: Haworth Press, 1987.
9. Dishion TJ, McCord J, Poulin F. When interventions harm: Peer groups and problem behavior. Am Psychol 1999;54:755–64.
10. Weiss RD, Jaffee WB, de Menil VP, Cogley CB. Group therapy for substance use disorders: What do we know? Harv Rev Psych 2004;12:339–50.
11. Burleson JA, Kaminer Y, Dennis ML. Absence of iatrogenic or contagion effects in adolescent group therapy: Findings from the Cannabis Youth Treatment (CYT) Study. Am J Addict 2006;15 (Suppl 1):s4–15.
12. Galanter M, Egelko S, Edwards H. Rational recovery: Alternative to AA for addiction? Am J Drug Alc Abuse 1993;19:499–510.
13. Dunn C, Deroo L, Rivara FP. The use of brief interventions adapted from motivational interviewing across behavioral domains: A systematic review. Addiction 2001;96:1725–42.
14. Burke BL, Arkowitz H, Menchola M. The efficacy of motivational interviewing: A meta-analysis of controlled clinical trials. J Consult Clin Psychol 2003;71:843–61.

15. Miller WR, Yahne CE, Tonigan JS. Motivational interviewing in drug abuse services: A randomized trial. J Consult Clin Psychol 2003;71:754–63.
16. Smedslund G, Berg RC, Hammerstrom KT, Steiro A, Leiknes KA, Dahl HM, et al. Motivational interviewing for substance abuse. Cochrane Database Syst Rev 2011;5:1–128.
17. Bigelow GE, Griffiths RR, Liebson IA. Experimental models for the modification of human drug self-administration: Methodological developments in the study of ethanol self-administration by alcoholics. Fed Proc 1975;34:1785–92.
18. Kidorf M, Stitzer ML. Contingent use of take-homes and split dosing to reduce illicit drug use of methadone patients. Behav Ther 1996;27:41–51.
19. Simpson DD. Treatment for drug abuse: Follow-up outcomes and length of time spent. Arch Gen Psychiatry 1981;38:875–80.
20. Simpson DD, Joe GW, Broome KM, Hiller ML, Knight K, Rowan-Szal GA. Program diversity and treatment retention rates in the Drug Abuse Treatment Outcome Study (DATOS). Psychol Addict Behav 1997;11:279–93.
21. Hser YI, Grella CE, Hubbard RL, Hsieh SC, Fletcher BW, Brown BS, et al. An evaluation of drug treatments for adolescents in four U.S. cities. Arch Gen Psychiatry 2001;58:689–95.
22. Monti PM, Kadden R, Rohsenow DJ, Cooney N, Abrams D. Treating alcohol dependence: A coping skills training guide, 2nd ed. New York: Guilford, 2002.
23. Marlatt GA, Donovan DM, eds. Relapse prevention: Maintenance strategies in the treatment of addictive behaviors, 2nd ed. New York: Guilford, 2005.
24. Liepman MR, Calles JL Jr, Kizilbash L, Nazeer A, Sheikh S. Genetic and non-genetic factors influencing substance use by adolescents. Adol Med 2002;13:375–401.
25. Liddle HA, Rowe CL, Dakof GA, Henderson CE, Greenbaum PE. Multidimensional family therapy for young adolescent substance abuse: Twelve-month outcomes of a randomized controlled trial. J Consult Clin Psychol 2009;77(1):12–25.
26. Liepman MR, Parran TV, Farkas K, Lagos-Saez M. Family involvement in addiction, treatment and recovery. In: Ries RK, Fiellin DA, Miller SC, Saitz R, eds. Principles of addiction medicine, 4th ed. Baltimore: Lippincott Williams Wilkins, 2009:857–67.
27. Liepman MR, Flachier R, Tareen RS. Family behavior loop mapping: A technique to analyze the grip addictive disorders have on families and to help them to recover. Alcohol Treatment Quart 2008;26(1/2):59–80.

6 General pharmacotherapy principles

Gabriel Kaplan

It has been known for a long time that substances such as alcohol and opioids can be abused; ancient documents even warned about the dangers of intoxication. In this book, you will find many chapters that examine the treatment strategies appropriate for specific substance use disorders (SUDs) and review the role of pharmacological agents for each disorder. It is unlikely that many primary care practitioners will prescribe these types of medicines; however, patients returning to the primary care clinician for ongoing medical care may be on them for long periods of time, and therefore, it is important that primary care clinicians gain familiarity with these agents. This chapter outlines general principles that should be followed to determine if pharmacotherapy is appropriate for adolescents and young adults with substance abuse disorders.

6.1 Introduction

Substances that can be abused such as alcohol and opioids have been available for thousands of years (1,2); ancient documents even warned about the dangers of intoxication (3). While the link between the ingestion of certain substances and the resulting socially unacceptable behaviors was established early on in civilization, effective treatments have only recently become widely available.

Many chapters in this book (particularly chapters 7–12) examine the treatment strategies appropriate for specific SUDs and review the role of pharmacological agents for each disorder. Although it is unlikely that many primary practitioners will prescribe these types of medicines, patients returning to the clinician for ongoing medical care may be on them for long periods of time (see chapter 13). Therefore, it is important that clinicians gain familiarity with these agents. This chapter outlines general principles that should be followed to determine if pharmacotherapy is appropriate for adolescents and young adults with substance abuse disorders. Other chapters in this book focus on specific SUDs and provide more detailed information.

6.2 Evaluation for pharmacotherapy

The American Psychiatric Association (APA) and the American Academy of Child and Adolescent Psychiatry have published comprehensive evaluation and treatment guidelines for SUDs (4,5). Experts from both professional associations agree that, for most patients, there is strong evidence regarding the benefits of psychosocial treatments. These are covered in detail in other sections of this book including chapters 5 and 15. While psychosocial treatments are effective, current pharmacotherapy options are also recommended for a more selected population of patients and during certain clinical stages of specific disorders. For adolescents, there is less available evidence of effectiveness because of concerns regarding the risk/benefit ratio of medications in youth, lack of approval by the U.S. Food and Drug Administration (FDA), and little published data regarding younger subjects (6).

As delineated in other sections of this volume, the *Diagnostic and Statistical Manual of Mental Disorders*, fourth edition, text revision (7), classifies substance-related diagnoses into two groups: (1) substance-induced disorders (SIDs) including intoxication and withdrawal, which consist of physical and psychological symptoms that result from acute exposure to, or interruption of, a particular substance; and (2) SUDs, which encompass abuse and dependence, as well as chronic behavioral patterns causing significant detrimental functional impact.

The goals of SUD treatment include the achievement of abstinence or reduction in the use and effects of substances, reduction in the frequency and severity of relapse to substance use, and improvement in psychological and social functioning (4). The APA presents six categories of pharmacological treatments: (1) medications to treat intoxication and withdrawal states, (2) medications to decrease the reinforcing effects of abused substances, (3) agonist maintenance therapies, (4) antagonist therapies, (5) abstinence-promoting and relapse prevention therapies, and (6) medications to treat comorbid psychiatric conditions (4). The table 6.1 lists available treatment agents according to specific SUDs.

The decision to recommend pharmacotherapy is considered in the context of a treatment plan approach that takes into account multiple factors such as the clinical stage of the disorder (withdrawal vs. maintenance), failure or success of previous treatments, level of care required (outpatient vs. inpatient), overall medical health, presence of comorbid psychiatric features, and patient motivation, to name a few. The process leading to determining if medications are appropriate starts with obtaining a comprehensive psychiatric evaluation, which should include the following: (1) history of (a) current and previous substance use and any medical or legal sequelae, (b) general medical and psychiatric problems, (c) psychiatric treatments and outcomes, and (d) family as well as social focusing on substance abuse; (2) mental status; and (3) laboratory work such as blood and urine for toxicology as well as other assessments to rule out co-occurring pathology such as tuberculosis and HIV/AIDS. With adolescents in particular, it is very important to obtain permission to contact family/significant others to validate the extent of abuse and for additional information. A completed evaluation will yield a case formulation that lists the specific diagnosis(es), determines the level of acuity, and recommends an initial level of care with precise treatment options.

The American Society of Addiction Medicine (8) publishes universally accepted and extremely detailed criteria to assess the most appropriate level of care placement for patients seeking treatment. In general, these available multiple levels to manage SUDs can be classified in order of complexity and acuity as follows:

Table 6.1: Medications for the treatment of SUDs

	FDA approved (18 years and older unless otherwise noted)			Not FDA approved
	Intoxication	Withdrawal	Maintenance	
Alcohol (see chapter 9)	Acute medically supportive measures	Chlordiazepoxide (6 years and older)	Acamprosate, disulfiram, naltrexone	Topiramate
Opioids (see chapter 10)	Naloxone (any age)	Methadone, buprenorphine (16 years and older)	Methadone, buprenorphine (16 years and older), naltrexone	Clonidine, trazodone, benzodiazepines
Tobacco (see chapters 7 and 16)	None	5 Nicotine replacement therapy (NRT) formulations	5 NRT formulations, bupropion, varenicline	Nortriptyline, clonidine
Cocaine, stimulants (see chapters 11 and 16)	Acute medically supportive measures	None	None	Topiramate, disulfiram, modafinil, stimulants
Marijuana (see chapters 8 and 16)	None			N-acetylcysteine, buspirone, nabilone
Benzodiazepines (see chapter 10)	Flumazenil	None	None	Benzodiazepines

(1) inpatient medical complex settings for acute withdrawal, (2) inpatient detoxification units, (3) inpatient or residential rehabilitation units, (4) day hospital rehabilitation and/or detoxification programs, (5) intensive outpatient rehabilitation programs, and (6) aftercare/outpatient settings. Because of the chronic and recurring nature of SUDs, it is common for patients to receive treatment at almost all levels of care along this continuum at some point during the course of illness.

6.3 When is pharmacotherapy appropriate?

Various agents have been approved by the FDA for treating tobacco, alcohol, and opioid SUDs (see chapters 7, 9, 10, and 16). Pharmacotherapy treatment for other SUDs remains on an "off-label" status, although agents are routinely used given that the devastation of poor-outcome SUDs tilts the benefit/risk ratio in favor of trying less well-researched but generally considered safe medications (see table 6.1). Treatment for SIDs is more likely to be conducted in a hospital or rehabilitation setting and, in severe cases, may require intensive medical interventions (e.g., intubation, intravenous formulations, and continuous monitoring of vital signs) in order to quickly reverse the symptoms of intoxication and prevent or ameliorate withdrawal. Therefore, pharmacotherapy is considered routine in most instances of withdrawal.

By definition, detoxification also requires the administration of a pharmacological agent(s). In contrast, maintenance treatments for SUDs attempt to improve maladaptive patterns where the use of biological agents may be a helpful adjunct within the context of a comprehensive array of modalities (e.g., group or supportive psychotherapy) (6). After completion of detoxification of alcohol and opioids, physicians may recommend rehabilitation programs without medication or programs that combine psychotherapeutic/12-step strategies with pharmacotherapy.

Despite recent advances in the understanding of the neurobiology of addiction (see chapter 2) that point to the potentially beneficial impact of pharmacotherapy on outcomes, the field of substance abuse rehabilitation was somewhat slow to embrace pharmacotherapy. This is because abstinence had been the ultimate goal of treatment. In a world where no medications were available to improve outcomes, it was logical to pursue abstinence as the ideal status. Research over the past few years, however, has shown that medications actually do improve outcomes in terms of treatment retention and reduced substance use (9). Even very traditional longstanding abstinence model facilities have started offering pharmacotherapy (10). The availability of newer alcohol treatment agents such as acamprosate and naltrexone (intramuscular) has additionally improved patient access to medical therapies (see chapter 9). Furthermore, with the FDA approval of buprenorphine in 2002 for use in private clinician offices, the maintenance treatment for opioids became more widely available and unlinked from the long-stigmatized methadone clinics (see chapter 10).

The APA guidelines (4) favor the use of pharmacological agents as part of a comprehensive multimodal treatment plan, as follows: (1) For tobacco (chapters 7 and 16), agents are recommended for individuals who wish to stop smoking and have not achieved cessation without pharmacological agents or who prefer to use such agents. (2) For alcohol (chapter 9), agents for treating dependency have well-established efficacy and moderate effectiveness. (3) For cocaine (chapter 11), pharmacological treatment is not ordinarily indicated as an initial approach; however, for individuals who fail to respond to psychosocial treatment alone, some off-label medications may be promising. (4) For opioids (chapter 10), maintenance treatment with methadone or buprenorphine is appropriate for patients with a prolonged history (>1 year) of dependence. No pharmacological treatment can be recommended for marijuana at this time (see chapters 8 and 16).

6.4 Conclusion

The field of pharmacotherapy for the treatment of SUDs is in its infancy, but as discussed elsewhere in this volume, it shows great promise. Even the evidence available today makes a strong case for recommending medications for alcohol, tobacco, and opioid dependence. Wider dissemination among the public and professionals of information regarding pharmacotherapy's beneficial effects on SUD outcomes is necessary to improve patient access to effective care in the continuing fight against substance abuse disorder – the number one public health challenge in the United States and around the globe.

References

1. World's earliest wine. Accessed December 20, 2012. URL: www.archaeology.org/9609/newsbriefs/wine.html
2. van Reel JM, Gerrits MAFM, Vanderschuren LJMJ. Opioids, reward and addiction: An encounter of biology, psychology, and medicine. Pharmacol Rev 1999;51(2):341–96.
3. Mendelbaum D. Wine and culture. Accessed December 20, 2012. URL: http://escholarship.org/uc/item/66m323jv
4. American Psychiatric Association. Practice guideline for the treatment of patients with substance use disorders, 2nd ed. In: American Psychiatric Association practice guidelines for the treatment of psychiatric disorders: Compendium 2006. Arlington, VA: American Psychiatric Association, 2006.
5. Bukstein O, Bernet W, Arnold V, Beitchman J, Shaw J, Benson RS, et al. Work group on quality issues: Practice parameter for the assessment and treatment of children and adolescents with substance use disorders. J Am Acad Child Adolesc Psychiatry 2005;44:609–21.
6. Kaplan G, Ivanov I. Pharmacological management of substance abuse disorders. Pediatr Clin North Am 2011;58:243–58.
7. American Psychiatric Association. Diagnostic and statistical manual of mental disorders, 4th ed., text rev. Washington, DC: APA, 2000.
8. Mee-Lee D, Shulman GD, Fishman M, eds. ASAM patient placement criteria for the treatment of substance-related disorders, 2nd ed., rev. Philadelphia, PA: Lippincott Williams Wilkins, 2001.
9. Mattick RP, Breen C, Kimber J, Davoli M. Methadone maintenance therapy versus no opioid replacement therapy for opioid dependence. Cochrane Database Syst Rev 2009;8:CD002209.
10. Hazelden introduces anti-addiction medications into recovery for first time. Accessed December 20, 2012. URL: http://healthland.time.com/2012/11/05/hazelden-introduces-antiaddiction-medications-in-recovery-for-first-time/#ixzz2Fu5S7hrG

7 Use of pharmacological agents for smoking cessation

Dilip R. Patel and Danielle Hirsch

Tobacco use has been clearly demonstrated to have negative health consequences. Smoking cigarettes is the predominant method of tobacco use. The tar contained within cigarettes and other similar products is also harmful. Other tarless tobacco-containing products do exist but carry no significantly decreased risk. While nicotine is considered to be principally responsible for tobacco addiction, other chemicals in the cigarette smoke including acetaldehyde may contribute to the addictive properties of tobacco products. The adverse health consequences of tobacco use have been well documented. Studies have shown that a combined behavioral and pharmacological approach is more effective in smoking cessation than either approach alone. Pharmacotherapy can achieve 50% reduction in smoking. With pharmacotherapy, the estimated 6-month abstinence rate is about 20%, whereas it is about 10% without pharmacotherapy. The first line of drugs for smoking cessation includes varenicline, bupropion sustained release (SR), and nicotine replacement drugs, which are approved for use in adults. Data are insufficient to recommend their use in adolescents. This article reviews the pharmacological agents used for smoking cessation.

7.1 Introduction

The tobacco plant is native to South America, Mexico, and the West Indies (1). The American Indians used various forms of tobacco for its medicinal properties for hundreds of years before the discovery by Christopher Columbus of the New World (1). The common tobacco, *Nicotiana tabacum*, is named after Jean Nicot, the French ambassador to Lisbon, who is believed to have sent its seeds to Catherine de Medicis, the queen consort and regent of France in 1566 (1). Nicotine was first extracted in its crude form in 1571 and its purified form in 1928, and it was synthesized in a laboratory in 1904 (1). Over the decades, the causative role of smoking and other forms of tobacco use in cancer has been well established. This article reviews the health effects of smoking and pharmacological agents used for smoking cessation in adolescents and young adults.

7.2 Epidemiology

Cigarette smoking is the most popular method of using tobacco; other forms of smoking and tobacco use are summarized in table 7.1 (2–4). Worldwide, tobacco use causes more than 5 million deaths per year, and if the current trends in use

Table 7.1: Main forms of tobacco used

Cigarettes	Cigarette brands are categorize based on their tar content: • Ultralight, 1–6 mg tar • Light, 6–15 mg tar • Full flavor, > 15 mg tar Of all cigarettes sold in the United States, 84% are either light or ultralight. Low-yield cigarettes and cigarette-like products are examples of a classification of products referred to as "potentially reduced-exposure products" (PREPs).
Cigars	Cigars contain the same toxic and carcinogenic compounds found in cigarettes. The three major types of cigars sold in the United States are large cigars, cigarillos, and little cigars.
Bidis	Bidis are small, thin hand-rolled cigarettes imported to the United States primarily from India and other Southeast Asian countries. They consist of tobacco wrapped in a tendu or temburni leaf (plants native to Asia) and may be secured with a colorful string at one or both ends. They have higher concentrations of nicotine, tar, and carbon monoxide than conventional cigarettes sold in the United States.
Kreteks	Kreteks (clove cigarettes), imported from Indonesia, typically contain a mixture consisting of tobacco, cloves, and other additives. Kreteks deliver more nicotine, carbon monoxide, and tar than conventional cigarettes.
Smokeless tobacco	Chewing tobacco comes in the form of loose leaf, plug, or twist. Snuff is finely ground tobacco that can be dry, moist, or in sachets (tea bag–like pouches). Although some forms of snuff can be used by sniffing or inhaling into the nose, most smokeless tobacco users place the product in their cheek or between their gum and cheek. Users then suck on the tobacco and spit out the tobacco juices, which is why smokeless tobacco is often referred to as spit or spitting tobacco.
Betel quid with tobacco (Gutka)	Gutka (*ghutka* or *gutkha*) is a dry, relatively nonperishable commercial preparation that consists of betel leaf (*Piper betle*), tobacco, areca nut (*Areca catechu*), catechu (extract of the *Acacia catechu* tree), and slaked lime (calcium hydroxide). Gutka is available in sachets and tins. It is consumed by placing a pinch of the mixture in the mouth between the gum and cheek and gently sucking and chewing. The excess saliva produced by chewing may be swallowed or spit out. *Gutka* is primarily consumed in the Indian subcontinent (India, Pakistan, and Bangladesh). In the Indian subcontinent, nonperishable, commercially manufactured preparations of betel quid without tobacco are known as *pan masala*, and freshly prepared betel quid (with or without tobacco) is known as *pan*.

Based on data from: Centers for Disease Control and Prevention. Smoking and tobacco use: Fact sheets. Available at http://www.cdc.gov/tobacco/data_statistics/fact_sheets. Accessed August 11, 2009.

of tobacco continue, it will cause 8 million deaths per year by 2030 (5). Cigarette smoking is the leading preventable cause of death in the United States, responsible for about 1 in 5 or a half-million deaths every year (4). Exposure to environmental tobacco smoke results in an estimated 49,000 deaths every year (2). Smoking and use of other forms of tobacco by youth is of particular significance, with 60% of new smokers being under the age of 18 when they first smoked a cigarette.

In 2007, more than 3 million American adolescents (aged 12–17 years) reported using a tobacco product in the month prior to the survey (2). Tobacco use by adolescents is influenced by multiple psychosocial and biological factors that increase adolescents' vulnerability for nicotine use (2,6,7). Studies show that adolescents are more sensitive to the reinforcing effects of nicotine and other chemicals found in cigarettes, further increasing their susceptibility to tobacco addiction. Intermittent smoking, such as over the weekends or at parties, has also been shown to result in tobacco addiction in adolescents. Tobacco use, especially of the smokeless forms, is of special concern in athletes (8–17).

7.3 Chemistry and pharmacology

Approximately 4,000 chemicals are found in the smoke of tobacco products, of which nicotine is primarily responsible for tobacco addiction (2,6,7). The chemistry and neuropharmacology of nicotine has been extensively studied (18–21). Other main constituents of smoke that result in adverse health consequences include ammonia, benzene, carbon monoxide, cyanide, formaldehyde, acetaldehyde, phenols, and tar. Approximately 90% of the constituents of the smoke are in the form of vaporized chemicals, while the rest are in the particulate form (2,4,22).

Cigarettes are categorized (see table 7.1) based on their tar content (total particulate matter in smoke, excluding water and alkaloid compounds), which is measured using a standardized protocol on a smoking machine (2,3,4). In filtered cigarettes (99% of cigarettes currently on the market), the filter vents dilute the smoke with air, reducing standard yields of tar, nicotine, and carbon monoxide. Many smokers block the vents or compensate with increased inhalations when smoking low-yield cigarettes. By doing so, they typically get as much tar and nicotine from cigarettes with low-yield ratings as those with higher yields. On average, a cigarette contains between 13 mg and 19 mg of nicotine, and smoking of one cigarette typically delivers 1–2 mg of nicotine (2,6,7). The nicotine content of tobacco smoke is 1%–2%, and each inhalation delivers approximately 0.05–0.15 mg (2,7).

Smoke is produced by incomplete combustion of tobacco. The fate of the cigarette smoke is depicted in figure 7.1 (22). Mainstream smoke – the smoke inhaled by the smoker directly through the mouthpiece of the cigarette – constitutes approximately 45% of the total smoke; whereas, side stream smoke, which is the smoke emitted by smoldering tobacco between puffs and the smoke diffusing through

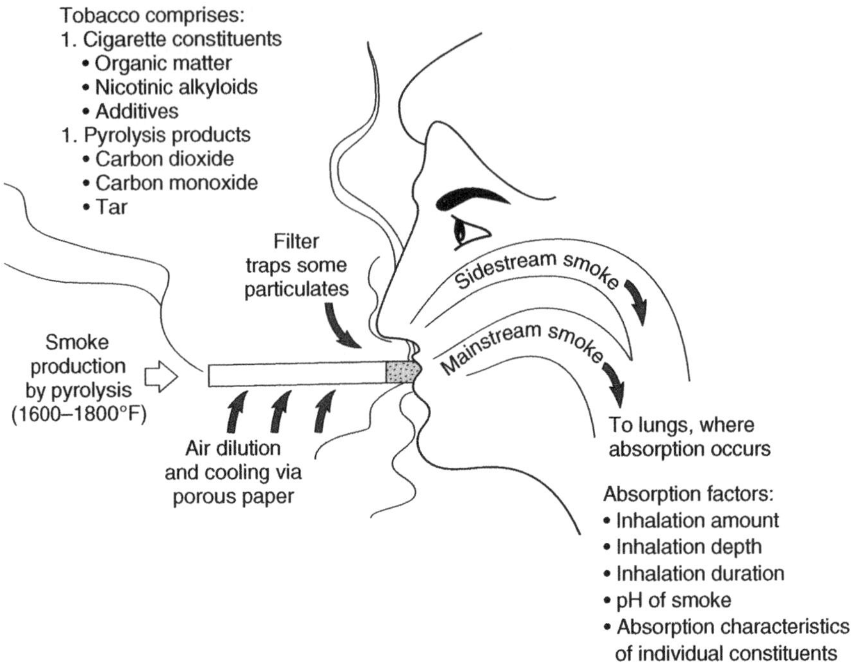

Figure 7.1: Fate of cigarette smoke (From U.S. Department of Health and Human Services. The health consequences of smoking – Nicotine addiction: A report of the surgeon general. Washington, DC: DHHS, 1988)

the lit cigarette paper and escaping from the burning cone during smoking, constitutes 55% of the total smoke (22).

Nicotine, whose chemical structure resembles that of the neurotransmitter acetylcholine, acts on stereospecific nicotinic cholinergic receptors (nAChRs) in the brain and other organs (7,21). The chemical structure and metabolic pathway of nicotine is depicted in figure 7.2. It also has direct and indirect effects on the neuroendocrine system.

The initial phase of stimulation of the central nervous system (CNS) by nicotine is typically followed by a phase of CNS depression (7,20). The action of nicotine on nAChRs stimulates the release of various neurotransmitters and hormones including acetylcholine, norepinephrine, dopamine, vasopressin, serotonin, and beta-endorphins (2,6,7,19). Research shows that smoking is associated with a marked decrease in monoamine oxidase (MAO) levels in the brain (7). It is postulated that this decrease in MAO is caused by chemicals in the smoke other than nicotine. Decreased levels of MAO-A and MAO-B in the brain result in a higher level of dopamine. The action of nicotine on the CNS increases alertness, improves memory, improves concentration, and decreases anxiety. The pharmacokinetic properties of nicotine are summarized in table 7.2 (2,4,7,8,21).

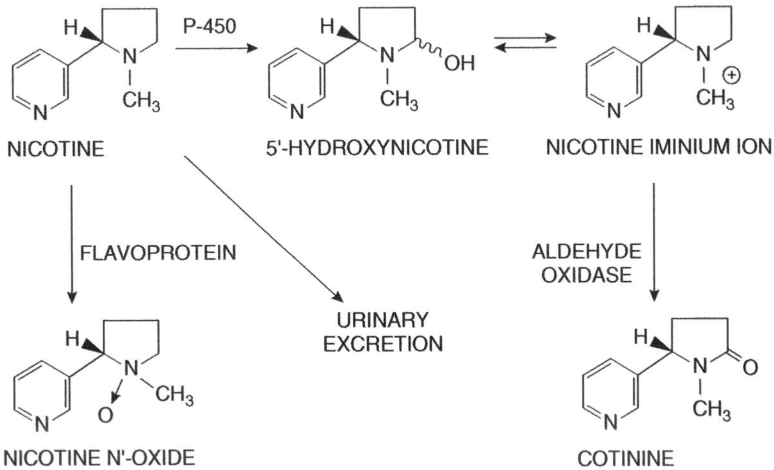

Figure 7.2: Chemical structure and metabolic pathway of nicotine (From U.S. Department of Health and Human Services. The health consequences of smoking – Nicotine addiction: A report of the surgeon general. Washington, DC: DHHS, 1988)

Table 7.2: Pharmacokinetics of nicotine (2,4,7,8,21)

Absorption	• 10%–50% of available nicotine is absorbed during puffing, and 80% during deep inhalation. • Readily and completely absorbed via mucous membranes and skin.
Distribution	• Readily distributed in all body tissues. • Reaches the brain within 10 sec. • Acute spike in arterial nicotine level occurs. • Steady-state volume of distribution is approximately 2.6 times the body weight in kilograms.
Metabolism	• 80% is metabolized in the liver to cotinine by enzyme CYP2A6 (and to a lesser extent by CYP2B6 and CYP2E1). • The rest is metabolized in the lungs and kidneys.
Elimination	• Average elimination half-life is 2 h. • Average elimination half-life of nicotine metabolite cotinine is 16 h. • Cotinine is not detectable in urine after complete abstinence of 1 week. • Unaltered nicotine and its metabolites are excreted by the kidneys.

7.4 Effects on health

The wide-ranging adverse effects of tobacco use have been well established and well documented (2,4,6,22–28). The numerous health consequences of smoking are summarized in table 7.3. Nicotine activates reward pathways in the brain that regulate feelings of pleasure (7). These effects of nicotine are mediated by dopamine. Nicotine

Table 7.3: Adverse health effects of smoking and tobacco use

Disease	
Cancer	• Bladder cancer • Cervical cancer • Esophageal cancer • Kidney cancer • Laryngeal cancer • Leukemia • Lung cancer • Oral cancer • Pancreatic cancer • Stomach cancer
Cardiovascular diseases	• Abdominal aortic aneurysm • Acute and episodic increase in blood pressure • Acute increase in peripheral vascular resistance and blood pressure • Atherosclerosis • Cerebrovascular disease • Coronary heart disease • Decreased coronary blood flow (due to constriction of coronary arteries) • Decreased oxygen carrying capacity of the hemoglobin • Hypertension • Increased baseline heart rate • Increased oxygen demands of the myocardium (due to increased heart rate and blood pressure) • Increased risk for thromboembolism • Increased risk of ventricular arrhythmias and sudden death (due to increased platelet adhesiveness, releasing catecholamines causing acute thrombosis and promoting ventricular arrhythmias) • Peripheral vascular disease
Respiratory diseases	• Bronchiolitis • Bronchitis • Chronic cough • Chronic obstructive pulmonary disease • Decreased forced expiratory volume (FEV1) • Decreased peak expiratory flow rate (PEFR) • Development and exacerbation of asthma • Dyspnea • Eosinophilic granuloma • Halitosis • Hoarseness • Idiopathic pulmonary fibrosis • Impaired lung growth

(*Continued*)

Table 7.3: Adverse health effects of smoking and tobacco use (*Continued*)

Disease	
	• Impaired respiratory immunity • Increased respiratory allergies • Interstitial lung disease • Laryngitis • Otitis media and middle ear effusions • Pneumonia • Pulmonary hemorrhage • Pulmonary hypertension • Rhinitis • Sinusitis • Snoring • Spontaneous pneumothorax • Upper respiratory infections
Reproductive effects	• Fertility • Fetal death and stillbirths • Low birth weight • Pregnancy complications • Premature menopause
Musculoskeletal	• Decreased bone mineral density • Increased risk for fractures • Increased spinal disk disease
Gastrointestinal	• Decreased appetite • Gastroesophageal reflux disease • Impaired glucose tolerance • Increase insulin resistance • Peptic ulcer disease
Mental health and psychosocial	• Addiction • Anxiety, palpitations, tremors • Nervousness, depression • Tolerance and dependence • Withdrawal symptoms
Effects on offspring of maternal smoking during pregnancy	• Certain childhood cancers • Increased cotinine in breastfed infants if mother smokes • Increased incidence of conduct disorders • Increased probability of female children to be smokers • Low birth weight • Miscarriage • Prematurity • Sudden infant death syndrome
Specific effects of smokeless tobacco use	• Excess salivation • Gingivitis, gingival recession • Halitosis

(*Continued*)

Table 7.3: Adverse health effects of smoking and tobacco use (*Continued*)

Disease	
	• Leukoplakia • Oropharyngeal cancers • Periodontal disease • Staining of teeth
Other effects	• Altered lipid profile • Altered metabolism of therapeutic drugs • Anorexia and weight loss • Cataracts • Decreased exercise performance • Diminished health status/increased morbidity • Esophagitis • Gastroesophageal reflux disease • Hip fractures • Low bone density • Macular degeneration • Nicotine addiction (tolerance, dependence, withdrawal symptoms) • Osteoporosis • Peptic ulcer disease • Spinal disk disease

Sources: U.S. Department of Health, Education, and Welfare 1964, 1967, 1979; U.S. Department of Health and Human Services 1980, 1982, 1983, 1984, 1989, 1990, 1994, 2001. Data from: (1) U.S. Department of Health and Human Services. The health consequences of smoking – Nicotine addiction: A report of the surgeon general. Washington, DC: DHHS, 1988. (2) U.S. Department of Health and Human Services. The health consequences of smoking: A report of the surgeon general. Atlanta, GA: U.S. Department of Health and Human Services, CDC, National Center for Chronic Disease Prevention and Health Promotion, Office of Smoking and Health, 2004. Available at http://www.cdc,gov/tobacco/data_statistics/sgr_2004/index.htm. Accessed August 11, 2009.

increases levels of dopamine mainly by its action on the mesolimbic dopamine system (7,21). Chronic use of nicotine results in an increase in the number of nicotine receptors in the brain (6,7,19). Consequently, more nicotine is required to achieve the desired effect, eventually resulting in tolerance and dependence. Regular tobacco use results in nicotine accumulation in the body, exposing the user to the effects of nicotine throughout a 24-hour period. Nicotine levels in the brain and the associated feelings of pleasure and reward peak within 10 seconds of inhalation (2,4,7).

However, the acute effects of nicotine dissipate rapidly. This causes the smoker to continue to smoke to maintain the effects of the nicotine and prevent withdrawal symptoms. The significant neurochemical changes in the brain that result from chronic nicotine use make it very difficult for the smoker to quit. Animal studies have shown that acetaldehyde, a chemical found in tobacco smoke, dramatically increases the reinforcing properties of nicotine and may also contribute to tobacco addiction (2,4,7). Adolescent animals show far more sensitivity to this reinforcing effect, suggesting increased vulnerability of adolescents to tobacco addiction.

Abrupt cessation of smoking results in withdrawal symptoms primarily due to decreased nicotine levels. Symptoms of nicotine withdrawal include irritability, craving, depression, anxiety, cognitive and attention deficit, sleep disturbances, and increased appetite (6,22). The withdrawal symptoms, in most cases, begin within a few hours after the last cigarette, peak within the first few days of smoking cessation, and usually subside within a few weeks. In some cases, however the symptoms may persist for months (4,6).

7.5 Behavioral approaches to smoking cessation

Behavioral treatment is integral to smoking cessation – studies have shown that a combination of behavioral and pharmacological treatment is more effective than either approach alone (3,29–32). In addition to the neurochemical effects of nicotine, behavioral factors also affect the severity of withdrawal symptoms. For some people, the feel, smell, and sight of a cigarette and the ritual of obtaining, handling, lighting, and smoking a cigarette are all associated with the pleasurable effects of smoking. Consequently, this can worsen withdrawal symptoms or cravings. Behavioral therapies can help smokers identify environmental triggers of craving so that they can employ strategies to prevent or circumvent these symptoms and urges.

7.6 Pharmacological agents

Factors that should to be considered when prescribing pharmacological agents for smoking cessation are summarized in table 7.4 (3). Patients who smoke may be on therapeutic drugs for other chronic diseases. The effective dosages of these therapeutic drugs reflect the adjustments made because of concomitant exposure to nicotine. With smoking cessation and elimination of nicotine from the body, a new state of metabolic homeostasis will result that may necessitate adjusting the dosage of therapeutic drugs (3).

Tobacco dependence should be considered a chronic disease, and as such, its management requires ongoing patient education, counseling, and use of medications as indicated (3). Relapses are common during smoking cessation, and patients require long-term monitoring and treatment. Long-term pharmacotherapy, combination therapy, and reuse of drugs previously used (recycling) should be considered in relapse prevention and treatment. In some patients who are not able to quit completely, pharmacotherapy has been used to reduce smoking, with some achieving

Table 7.4: Factors to be considered in the use of smoking cessation drugs

Practical considerations	Health insurance coverage, out-of-pocket costs, likelihood of adherence, dentures when considering the gums, or dermatitis when considering the patch.
Patient's prior experience with a medication	Prior successful experience (sustained abstinence with the medication) suggests that the medication may be helpful to the patient in a subsequent quit attempt, especially if the patient found the medication to be tolerable and or easy to use. However, it is difficult to draw firm conclusions from prior failure with a medication.
Heavy users or smokers	The higher-dose preparations of nicotine gum, patch, and lozenge have been shown to be effective in highly dependent smokers. Combination nicotine replacement therapy (NRT) may be particularly effective in suppressing tobacco withdrawal symptoms. NRT combinations are especially helpful for highly dependent smokers or those with a history of severe withdrawal.
Light users or smokers	Cessation medications are generally not beneficial to light smokers. If NRT is used with light smokers, consider reducing the dose of the medication. No adjustments are necessary when using bupropion sustained release (SR) or varenicline.
Gender	NRT can be effective with both sexes; however, evidence is mixed as to whether NRT is less effective in women than men. This may encourage the clinician to consider use of another type of medication with women, such as bupropion SR or varenicline.
Weight gain concern	Bupropion SR and NRTs, in particular 4 mg nicotine gum and 4 mg nicotine lozenge, delay – but do not prevent – weight gain.
Depression	Bupropion SR and nortriptyline appear to be effective, but nicotine replacement medications also appear to help individuals with a history of depression.
History of cardiovascular disease	The nicotine patch has been demonstrated safe for patients with a history of cardiovascular disease.
Long-term use	Long-term use is helpful with smokers who report persistent withdrawal symptoms during the course of medications, who have relapsed in the past after stopping medication, or who desire long-term therapy. A minority of individuals who successfully quit smoking use ad libitum NRT medications (gum, nasal spray, inhaler) long term. The use of these medications for up to 6 months does not present a known health risk, and developing dependence on medications is uncommon. The FDA has approved the use of bupropion SR, varenicline, and some NRT medications for 6-month use.
Combination therapy	Combining the nicotine patch long term (> 14 weeks) with nicotine gum or nicotine nasal spray, the nicotine patch with the nicotine inhaler, or the nicotine patch with bupropion SR increases long-term abstinence rates relative to placebo treatments. Combining varenicline with NRT agents has been associated with higher rates of side effects (e.g., nausea, headaches).

Modified from: Fiore MC, Jaen CR, Baker TB, Bailey WC, Benowitz N, Curry SJ, et al. Treating tobacco use and dependence 2008 update: Clinical practice guideline. Rockville, MD: U.S. Department of Health and Human Services, Public Health Service, May 2008.

a 50% reduction in smoking (3,7). With pharmacotherapy, the estimated 6-month abstinence rate is about 20%, compared to approximately 10% without pharmacotherapy (3,6,7). All pharmacological agents have been shown to be effective in smoking cessation with odds ratios between two and four when compared to placebo treatment (3,6). Absolute smoking cessation rates vary depending on the particular pharmacological agent used and the intensity of concomitant counseling; rates vary in range from 5% to 35% (3,6,7).

The first line drugs for smoking cessation approved by the U.S. Food and Drug Administration (FDA) are varenicline, bupropion SR, and nicotine replacement drugs (3,33–44) (see chapter 16). These drugs are approved by the FDA for use in adults. Data are insufficient to assess their efficacy in adolescents (3). Pharmacotherapy has not been shown to be effective in light smokers and in those who use smokeless tobacco.

7.6.1 Varenicline

Varenicline acts by selective binding at $\alpha 4\beta 2$ neuronal nicotinic acetylcholine receptors, which results in agonist activity, while simultaneously preventing nicotine binding to $\alpha 4\beta 2$ receptors (7,39–41). The FDA recommendation for varenicline product label includes a warning that serious neuropsychiatric symptoms have been reported in patients being treated with this drug. It is not uncommon for patients to experience feelings of depression, anxiety, irritability, and sleep disturbances during smoking cessation. Although some of these symptoms may be associated with nicotine withdrawal, symptoms have occurred in patients who continued to smoke. Patients on varenicline should be monitored for agitation, depressed mood, and changes in behavior that are not typical for the patient. The patient also must be assessed for suicidal ideation or suicidal behavior. Varenicline is reported to be well tolerated for up to 1 year and may reduce the incidence of relapse (41). Prescribing information for varenicline is summarized in table 7.5.

Table 7.5: Varenicline^{Rx}

Product	Chantix (Pfizer Inc., New York, NY) • 0.5 mg, 1 mg tablet
Precautions	• Pregnancy • May worsen preexisting psychiatric illness. • Dosage adjustment required in patients with kidney disease (creatinine clearance < 30 mL/min) or who are on dialysis. • WARNING: Can cause depressed mood, agitation, change in behavior, suicidal ideation, suicide. Reported in patients attempting to quit smoking while using varenicline. Monitor closely.

(*Continued*)

Table 7.5: Varenicline[Rx] (*Continued*)

Dosage	Recommended: 1-week titration: Days 1–3: 0.5 mg tablet daily Days 4–7: 0.5 mg tablet BID (AM and HS) Days 8+: 1 mg tablet BID (AM and HS) • Set quit date. • Start 1 week before quit date. • Take after eating and with a full glass of water. • Nausea is dose related; if persistent and troubling, consider dose reduction. Duration: 12 weeks; if successful after 12 weeks, an additional 12 weeks is recommended for increased likelihood of long-term abstinence.
Side effects	• Dose-dependent nausea (most common) • Insomnia • Abnormal dreams • Headache • Dyspepsia • Constipation • Flatulence • Vomiting
Advantages	• Provides nicotine effects to reduce withdrawal symptoms and cravings. • Blocks the nicotine effects from smoking and reduces reward of smoking. • May be used in those with cardiovascular disease. • No clinically meaningful drug interactions. • Found to be more effective than bupropion SR.
Disadvantages	• Not studied in combination with other therapies. • Nausea associated with higher doses may be bothersome. • Does not reduce weight gain. • May cause impaired ability to drive or operate heavy machinery. • May cause neuropsychiatric symptoms including behavioral changes, agitation, depressed mood, suicidal ideation, and suicidal behavior.

7.6.2 Bupropion SR

The proposed mechanisms of action of bupropion SR include blockade of neuronal reuptake of dopamine and norepinephrine (42). Similar to varenicline, bupropion SR also carries an FDA warning for neuropsychiatric adverse events. Bupropion SR is also antidepressant, and like other antidepressant drugs, it carries a warning for increased risk of suicidal ideation. Patients on bupropion should therefore be closely monitored for emerging neuropsychiatric symptoms and signs of suicidal ideation. Prescribing information for bupropion SR for smoking cessation is summarized in table 7.6.

Table 7.6: Bupropion SR^{Rx}

Product	Zyban (GlaxoSmithKline plc, Brentford, London, England, UK), Generic • 150 mg sustained-release tablet
Contraindications	• History of seizure disorder • History of stroke • History of brain tumor, brain surgery, or serious closed-head injury • Eating disorders • Those taking another form of bupropion • Monoamine oxidase inhibitor therapy within previous 14 d • Abrupt discontinuation of alcohol or benzodiazepines at same time
Precautions	• Pregnancy • Concomitant therapy with medications known to lower the seizure threshold.
Dosage	150 mg PO q AM × 3 d, then increase to 150 mg PO BID • Treatment should be initiated while patient is still smoking. • Set quit date 1–2 weeks after initiation. • DO NOT exceed 300 mg/d. • Allow at least 8 h between doses. • Avoid bedtime dosing to minimize insomnia. • Can be used safely with NRT. • If progression toward abstinence unsuccessful by week 7, discontinue. Duration: 8–12 weeks, maintenance up to 6 months
Side effects	• Insomnia most common (35%–40%) • Dry mouth • Nervousness • Agitation • Anxiety • Weight loss • Constipation • Seizures (risk is 1/1,000)
Advantages	• Bupropion can be safely used with NRT. • Bupropion may be beneficial in patients with depression. • No tapering required.
Disadvantages	• Seizure risk is increased. • May increase the risk of suicidal thinking in patients who have depression.

7.6.3 Nicotine replacement therapies

Nicotine replacement therapy (NRT) drugs reduce craving and withdrawal symptoms by partially replacing lost nicotine intake. The main characteristics and prescribing information of available NRT products are summarized in tables 7.7 through Table 7.11 (3,29,33–35,43,44).

Table 7.7: Transdermal preparations[OTC/Rx]

Products		Nicotrol Patch (McNeil Consumer Healthcare, Fort Washington, PA) • 5 mg • 10 mg, 15 mg (16 h)	Nicoderm CQ (Sanofi-Aventis S.A., Paris, France); Generic nicotine patch • 7 mg • 14 mg, 21 mg (24 h)
Dosage	> 10 cigarettes/d	• 15 mg/d × 6 weeks • 10 mg/d × 2 weeks • 5 mg/d × 2 weeks	• 21 mg/d × 6 weeks • 14 mg/d × 2 weeks • 7 mg/d × 2 weeks
	≤ 10 cigarettes/d	• 10 mg/d × 6 weeks • 5 mg/d × 2 weeks	• 14 mg/d × 6 weeks • 7 mg/d × 2 weeks If < 100 lb. or cardiovascular disease: • 14 mg/d × 4–6 weeks • 7 mg/d × 2–4 weeks
Comments[a]		• Remove before bedtime. • Nicotine released over 16 h.	• May wear patch for 24 h. • Remove at bedtime if patient experiences sleep disturbances.
Contraindications		• Pregnancy • Recent (2 or fewer weeks postmyocardial infarction) • Unstable angina pectoris • Serious underlying arrhythmias	
Side effects		• Local skin reactions: erythema, pruritis, burning • Headache • Sleep disturbances: insomnia, vivid dreams	
Advantages		• Provides consistent nicotine levels over 16–24 h. • Easy to use and conceal. • Fewer adherence issues. • Available without prescription.	
Disadvantages		• Patients cannot titrate the dose. • Allergic reactions to adhesive. • Patients with certain skin conditions cannot use patch. • Patch may contain aluminum.	

[a]Patch should be applied in the morning when patient wakes on the quit day. Apply on relatively hairless areas between the neck and waist.

Table 7.8: Gum[OTC]

Product	Nicorette (GlaxoSmithKline plc, Brentford, London, England, UK), Nicorette DS (GlaxoSmithKline plc, Brentford, London, England, UK), Generic • 2 mg, 4 mg; regular, mint, orange
Contraindications	• Pregnancy • Recent (≤ 2 weeks) myocardial infarction • Serious underlying arrhythmias • Serious or worsening angina pectoris • Temporomandibular joint disease

(*Continued*)

Table 7.8: Gum^{OTC} (*Continued*)

Dosage	≥ 25 cigarettes/d: 4 mg < 25 cigarettes/d: 2 mg Weeks 1–6: 1 piece q 1–2 h Weeks 2–4: 1 piece q 2–4 h Weeks 10–12: 1 piece q 4–8 h • Chew each piece slowly until peppery or flavored taste emerges. • Park between cheek and gum when tingling sensation appears. • Resume chewing when tingle fades. • Repeat chew/park steps until most of the nicotine is gone (taste or tingle does not return; generally 30 min). • Park in different areas of mouth. • No food or beverages 15 min before or during use (acidic beverages reduce buccal absorption). • If there are strong or frequent cravings, may use a second piece within the hour. Max: 24 pieces/d Duration: up to 12 weeks
Side effects	• Mouth soreness • Throat irritation • Jaw pain • Hiccups • Dyspepsia • Hypersalivation • Flatulence • Nausea and vomiting • Unpleasant taste • Lightheadedness
Advantages	• Might satisfy oral cravings. • May delay weight gain. • Patients can titrate therapy to manage withdrawal symptoms. • Available over the counter.
Disadvantages	• Gum chewing may not be socially acceptable. • Difficult to use with dentures. • May cause loosening of dental fillings. • Patients must use proper chewing technique to minimize adverse effects.

Table 7.9: Lozenge^{OTC}

Product	Commit (GlaxoSmithKline plc, Brentford, London, England, UK) • 2 mg, 4 mg
Contraindications	• Pregnancy • Recent (≤ 2 weeks) myocardial infarction • Serious underlying arrhythmias • Serious or worsening angina pectoris

(*Continued*)

Table 7.9: Lozenge^{OTC} (*Continued*)

Dosage	First cigarette ≤ 30 min after waking up: 4 mg First cigarette > 30 min after waking up: 2 mg Weeks 1–6: 1 lozenge q 1–2 h; minimum 9/ d Weeks 7–9: 1 lozenge q 2–4 h Weeks 10–12: 1 lozenge q 4–8 h • Allow lozenge to dissolve slowly (20–30 min). • Nicotine release may cause a warm or tingling sensation. • Do not chew or swallow the lozenge. • Rotate the lozenge to different areas of the mouth. • No food or beverages 15 min before, during, or after use. • Do not use more than 1 lozenge at a time. Max: 5 lozenges every 6 h; 20 lozenges/d Duration: up to 12 weeks
Adverse events	• Nausea • Hiccups • Cough • Heartburn • Headache
Advantages	• Might satisfy oral cravings. • May delay weight gain. • Patients can titrate therapy to manage withdrawal symptoms. • Provides ~25% more nicotine than gum. • Available over the counter.
Disadvantages	• Gastrointestinal side effects might be bothersome. • Contains phenylalanine.

Table 7.10: Nasal spray^{Rx}

Product	Nicotrol NS (Pfizer Inc., New York, NY) • Metered spray (0.5 mg nicotine/actuation) aqueous nicotine
Contraindications	• Pregnancy • Recent (≤ 2 weeks) myocardial infarction • Serious underlying arrhythmias • Serious or worsening angina pectoris
Dosage	1–2 doses/h (8–40 doses/d) One dose: 2 sprays (one in each nostril); each spray delivers 0.5 mg of nicotine to the nasal mucosa. • Patients should not sniff, swallow, or inhale through the nose as the spray is administered. • For best results, initially use at least 8 doses/d. • DO NOT exceed 5 doses/h and 40 doses/d. • Gradually decrease usage. Duration (maximal): 3 months

(*Continued*)

Table 7.10: Nasal spray^{Rx} (*Continued*)

Side effects	• Nasal and throat irritation (hot, peppery, or burning sensation) • Transient change in sense of smell and taste • Rhinitis • Tearing • Sneezing • Cough • Headache • Nausea
Advantages	• Patients can easily titrate therapy to rapidly manage withdrawal symptoms. • Fastest-acting nicotine product.
Disadvantages	• Nasal/throat irritation may be bothersome. • Dependence can result. • Patients must wait 5 minutes before driving or operating heavy machinery. • Patients with chronic nasal disorders (allergy, rhinitis, nasal polyps, or sinusitis) or severe reactive airway disease should NOT use the spray. • No optimal tapering schedule. • Prescription only.

Table 7.11: Oral inhaler^{Rx}

Product	Nicotrol Inhaler (Pfizer Inc., New York, NY) • 10 mg cartridge delivers 4 mg of inhaled nicotine vapor
Contraindications	• Pregnancy • Recent (≤ 2 weeks) myocardial infarction • Serious underlying arrhythmias • Serious or worsening angina pectoris
Dosage	6–16 cartridges/d; individualize dosing • Initially, use at least 6 cartridges/d for first 3–6 weeks. • Best effects with continuous puffing for 20 min. • Nicotine in cartridge is depleted after 20 min of active puffing (oral inhalation). • Patients should inhale deeply into back of throat or puff in short breaths. • Open cartridge retains potency for 24 h. • Each cartridge delivers 4 mg of nicotine over 80 inhalations. • Avoid eating or drinking for 15 min before and after use (acidic beverages reduce absorption). Duration: Treat for 3 months, and then taper over next 3 months.
Adverse events	• Mouth and throat irritation (40%) • Unpleasant taste • Cough (32%) • Rhinitis (23%) • Dyspepsia • Headache

(*Continued*)

Table 7.11: Oral inhaler^{Rx} (*Continued*)

Advantages	• Patients can easily titrate therapy to rapidly manage withdrawal symptoms. • The inhaler mimics hand-to-mouth ritual of smoking.
Disadvantages	• Initial throat or mouth irritation can be bothersome. • Dependence can occur. • Cold temperatures (< 60°F) reduce amount of nicotine delivered. • Avoid hot environments (> 77°F), and protect from light. • Patients with underlying bronchospastic disease must use with caution. • No definitive tapering schedule. • Prescription only.

7.6.4 Second-line medications

Clonidine and nortriptyline are second-line medications used for smoking cessation (3,45). Although second-line medications have been shown to be effective in treating tobacco dependence, their use is limited mainly because of a less favorable side-effect profile when compared to the first-line medications. Second-line medications are not approved by the FDA specifically for use in smoking cessation (3). Second-line medications should be considered for use on a case-by-case basis after first-line medications (either alone or in combination) have been used without success or are contraindicated (3).

Clonidine is contraindicated in pregnant women and in those who engage in potentially hazardous activities. The most common side effects of clonidine include dry mouth (40%), drowsiness (33%), dizziness (16%), sedation (10%), and constipation (10%) (3). Because its abrupt discontinuation can result in severe rebound hypertension, clonidine should be tapered. Clonidine is available as 0.1 mg, 0.2 mg, and 0.3 mg scored tablets and 0.1 mg/24 h, 0.2 mg/24 h, and 0.3 mg/24 h transdermal patches. The usual dosage is 0.2 mg–0.6 mg per day in divided doses. (3,45). A specific dosage of clonidine for smoking cessation has not been established.

Nortriptyline is a tricyclic antidepressant and therefore carries an FDA warning about increased suicide risk (3). The most serious side effects of nortriptyline are arrhythmias and impairment of myocardial contractility. More common and less serious side effects include sedation, dry mouth, blurred vision, urinary retention, lightheadedness, and shaky hands (3). Nortriptyline is available as 10 mg, 25 mg, 50 mg, and 75 mg capsules and 10 mg/5 mL liquid. The dosage of nortriptyline in smoking cessation studies ranges between 25 mg per day and 100 mg per day (3,45,46). Therapeutic drug level and cardiovascular monitoring, including electrocardiogram, is recommended.

7.6.5 Vaccine

Some of the latest research for smoking cessation is coming in the form of a vaccine. The principal behind this idea is that after the vaccine enters the systemic circulation, a substantial proportion of nicotine can bind with antibodies and then once bound can no longer cross the blood-brain barrier (47). The pathophysiological mechanism underlying the addictive properties of smoking is due to the impact nicotine has on locomotion, cognition, affect, pain sensitivity, arousal, and most importantly, the reward stimuli in the brain. In regular smokers, studies have shown an almost complete saturation of the receptors, which may serve to prevent occurrences of withdrawal symptoms. Thus, further developments in pharmacotherapy for smoking cessation should focus on reducing the rewarding effects of smoking – hence, the development of vaccinations. Basically, an immunogenic substrate that causes T- and B-cell activation leads to the formation of specific antibodies that bind to a drug and thus disable that drug from crossing the blood-brain barrier. This idea was first tested in an animal model of heroin addiction, and what the five reports of phase I and II trials have shown is that therapeutic antibody levels are only established several weeks after the first vaccine injection (47,48).

Vaccination for the treatment of nicotine or even other substances of abuse has various attractive features. However, efficacy of vaccination is largely related to subjects achieving the highest serum antibody concentration. Immunization can be achieved in two ways: actively through vaccination or passively via administering a drug-specific monoclonal antibody. Clinical trials have focused on vaccination because of the safety profile, low cost, and long duration of action (48). Passive immunization achieves higher serum antibody concentrations but is more costly than vaccines. Vaccination, although promising, is still at a very experimental stage and not currently available as a treatment option.

7.6.6 E-cigarettes

As of this writing, electronic cigarettes (e-cigarettes) were marketed legally in the United Sates without any clinical trials (49,50). E-cigarettes are battery-operated devices that contain a cartridge that is generally filled with nicotine, flavor, and other chemicals (49). They do not burn tobacco; thus they do not emit smoke. The nicotine contained in the refill bottles can contain more than 500 mg, which is approximately 10 times the lethal dose. E-cigarettes promise to reduce toxins in the mainstream and secondhand smoke, as well as help smokers quit (49).The FDA and other health agencies are concerned about the marketing to the public about e-cigarettes because it can promote nicotine addiction, delay or derail serious quit attempts, and even encourage youth to try them (49). The chemical propylene glycol is what is used to make the "vapor" emitted from e-cigarettes, and this chemical has the potential to generate acute and chronic respiratory effects, as well as reduced lung function with increased proximity and cumulative exposure (49). The U.S. surgeon general has made statements repeatedly that there is no safe level of exposure to tobacco smoke; however, no clear-cut scientific research is available on the safety of the vapor from e-cigarettes. Despite this lack of research, the sales of e-cigarettes continue to increase.

7.7 Conclusion

Tobacco use remains a great public health concern, especially in adolescents. The significant health hazards of smoking and other forms of tobacco use are well documented. Smoking can also adversely affect exercise and sports performance. Tobacco addiction is primarily caused by nicotine, though other chemicals contained within tobacco products are now believed to play a secondary role in addiction. A combined behavioral and pharmacological approach has been found to be more effective for smoking cessation than either approach used alone. A range of pharmacological agents and behavioral therapies are available for smoking cessation. Varenicline, bupropion SR, and NRTs are recommended as first-line drugs for smoking cessation. In selected cases, the first-line drugs may also be used in combination with each other to improve outcomes. Treatment interventions have been shown to double the rate of smoking cessation when compared to quit attempts without intervention. Tobacco dependence should be considered a chronic disease with anticipated relapses requiring long-term monitoring and treatment.

Acknowledgments

Adapted with permission from Patel DR, Feucht C, Reid L, Patel ND. Pharmacological agents for smoking cessation: A clinical review. Clin Pharmacol Adv Applications 2010;2:17–29. The authors thank Kim Douglas for assistance with the preparation of this manuscript. Data in table 7.5 to table 7.11 are derived with permission from (1) Fiore MC, Jaen CR, Baker TB, et al. Treating tobacco use and dependence 2008 update: Clinical practice guideline. Rockville, MD: U.S. Department of Health and Human Services, Public Health Service, May 2008; (2) Food and Drug Administration product information available at http://www.fda.gov; and (3) drug manufacturer product labels available at manufacturer websites, including the following: Chantix (http://www.accessdata.fda.gov/drugsatfda_docs/label/2008/021928s007lbl.pdf), Zyban (http://www.fda.gov/Safety/MedWatch/SafetyInformation/ucm176815.htm), Nicotrol inhaler (http://media.pfizer.com/files/products/uspi_nicotrol_inhaler.pdf), Nicotrol NS (http://media.pfizer.com/files/products/uspi_nicotrol.pdf), Nicoderm CQ (http://www.nicodermcq.com/), Commit (http://www.commitlozenge.com/), and Nicorette (http://www.nicorette.com/).

References

1. Britannica.com (Encyclopaedia Britannica). Accessed December 10, 2012. URL: http://www.britannica.com
2. Centers for Disease Control and Prevention. Smoking and tobacco use: Fact sheets. Accessed December 10, 2012. URL: http://www.cdc.gov/tobacco/data_statistics/fact_sheets
3. Fiore MC, Jaen CR, Baker TB, Bailey WC, Benowitz N, Curry SJ, et al. Treating tobacco use and dependence 2008 update: Clinical practice guideline. Rockville, MD: U.S. Department Health Human Services, 2008.
4. U.S. Department of Health and Human Services. National Institute on Drug Abuse. Research Report Series: Tobacco addiction. Accessed December 10, 2012. URL: http://www.nida.hih.gove/reserachreports/nicotine/nicotine.html
5. World Health Organization. WHO report on the global tobacco epidemic, 2008. Geneva: WHO, 2008.
6. Hatsukami DK, Stead LF, Gupta PC. Tobacco addiction. Lancet 2008;371(9629):2027–38.
7. Benowitz NL. Pharmacology of nicotine: Addiction, smoking-induced disease, and therapeutics. Annu Rev Pharmacol Toxicol 2009;49:57–71.
8. Walsh MM, Ellison J, Hilton JF, Chesney M, Ernster VL. Spit (smokeless) tobacco use by high school baseball athletes in California. Tob Control 2009;9(Suppl 2):32–9.
9. Melnick MJ, Miller KE, Sabo DF, Farrell MP, Barnes GM. Tobacco use among high school athletes and nonatheletes: Results of the 1997 Youth Risk Behavior Survey. Adolescence 2001;36(144): 727–47.
10. Green GA, Uryasz FD, Petr TA, Bray CD. NCAA study of substance use and abuse habits of college student-athletes. Clin J Sport Med 2001;11(1):51–6.
11. Alaranta A, Alaranta H, Patja K, Palmu P, Prättälä R, Martelin T, et al. Snuff use and smoking in Finnish Olympic athletes. Int J Sports Med 2006;27(7):581–6.
12. Peretti-Watel P, Guagliardo V, Verger P, Pruvost J, Mignon P, Obadia Y. Sporting activity and drug use: Alcohol, cigarette and cannabis use among elite student athletes. Addiction 2003;98(9): 1249–56.
13. Walsh MM, Hilton JF, Ernster VL, Masouredis CM, Grady DG. Prevalence, patterns, and correlates of spit tobacco use in a college athlete population. Addict Behav 1994;19(4):411–27.
14. Davis TC, Arnold C, Nandy I, Bocchini JA, Gottlieb A, George RB, et al. Tobacco use among male high school athletes. J Adolesc Health 1997;21(2):97–101.
15. Epps RP, Lynn WR, Manley MW. Tobacco, youth, and sports. Adolesc Med 1998;9(3):483–90.
16. Rainey CJ, McKeown RE, Sargent RG, Valois RF. Patterns of tobacco and alcohol use among sedentary, exercising, nonathletic, and athletic youth. J Sch Health 1996;66(1):27–32.
17. Yusko DA, Buckman JF, White HR, Pandina RJ. Alcohol, tobacco, illicit drugs, and performance enhancers: A comparison of use by college student athletes and nonathletes. J Am Coll Health 2008;57(3):281–90.
18. Fletcher PJ, Lê AD, Higgins GA. Serotonin receptors as potential targets for modulation of nicotine use and dependence. Prog Brain Res 2008;172:361–83.
19. Gamberino WC, Gold MS. Neurobiology of tobacco smoking and other addictive disorders. Psychiatr Clin North Am 1999;22:301.
20. Rose JE. Disrupting nicotine reinforcement: From cigarette to brain. Ann NY Acad Sci 2008; 1141:233–56.
21. Taylor P. Agents acting at the neuromuscular junction and autonomic ganglia. In: Hardman JG, Limbird LE. Goodman and Gilman's pharmacologic basis of therapeutics, 9th ed. New York: McGraw-Hill, 1996:177–98.
22. U.S. Department of Health and Human Services. The health consequences of smoking – Nicotine addiction: A report of the surgeon general. Washington, DC: DHHS, 1988.

23. Aubry M, Wright JL, Myers JL. The pathology of smoking-related diseases. Clin Chest Med 2000; 21:11.
24. Fiore MC, Piaseck TH, Baker LJ, Decren SM. Cigarette smoking: The leading preventable cause of pulmonary disease. In: Bone RC, ed. Pulmonary and critical care medicine. St. Louis, IL: Mosby, 1998.
25. Patel DR, Homnick DN. Pulmonary effects of smoking. Adolesc Med 2000;11:547–65.
26. Sethi JM, Rochester CL. Smoking and chronic obstructive pulmonary disease. Clin Chest Med 2000;21:67.
27. U.S. Department of Health and Human Services. The health consequences of smoking: A report of the surgeon general. Atlanta, GA: U.S. Department Health Human Services, CDC, National Center for Chronic Disease Prevention and Health Promotion, Office of Smoking and Health, 2004. Accessed December 10, 2012. URL: http://www.cdc.gov/tobacco/data_statistics/sgr/sgr_2004/index.htm
28. U.S. Department of Health and Human Services. The health benefits of smoking cessation: A report of the surgeon general. Washington, DC: DHHS, 1990.
29. Burke MV, Ebbert JO, Hays JT. Treatment of tobacco dependence. Mayo Clin Proc 2008;83 (4):479–83.
30. Lemmens V, Oenema A, Knut IK, Brug J. Effectiveness of smoking cessation interventions among adults: A systematic review of reviews. Eur J Cancer Prev 2008;17(6):535–44.
31. Patel DR, Greydanus DE. Office interventions for adolescent smokers. Adolesc Med 2000;11: 577–88.
32. Shah SD, Wilken LA, Winkler SR, Lin SJ. Systematic review and meta-analysis of combination therapy for smoking cessation. J Am Pharm Assoc 2008;48(5):659–65.
33. Carrozzi L, Pistelli F, Viegi G. Pharmacotherapy for smoking cessation. Ther Adv Respir Dis 2008;2(5):301–17.
34. Eisenberg MJ, Filion KB, Yavin D, Bélisle P, Mottillo S, Joseph L, et al. Pharmacotherapies for smoking cessation: A meta-analysis of randomized controlled trials. CMAJ 2008;179(2):135–44. Erratum in: CMAJ 2008;179(8):802.
35. Fant RV, Buchhalter AR, Buchman AC, Henningfield JE. Pharmacotherapy for tobacco dependence. Handb Exp Pharmacol 2009;192:487–510.
36. The Medical Letter: Drugs for tobacco dependence. Treatment guidelines. Medical Letter 2008; 6(73):61–6.
37. Hajeck P, Stead LF, West R, Jarvis M, Lancaster T. Relapse prevention interventions for smoking cessation. Cochrane Database Syst Rev 2009(1):CD003999.
38. Galanti LM. Tobacco smoking cessation management: Integrating varenicline in current practice. Vasc Health Risk Manage 2008;4(4):837–45.
39. Garrison GD, Dugan SE. Varenicline: A first-line treatment option of smoking cessation. Clin Ther 2009;31(3):463–91.
40. Hays JT, Ebbert JO. Varenicline for tobacco dependence. New Engl J Med 2008;359(19):2018–24.
41. Lee JH, Jones PG, Bybee K, O'Keefe JH. A longer course of varenicline therapy improves smoking cessation rates. Prev Cardiol 2008;11(4):210–14.
42. Paterson NE. Behavioural and pharmacological mechanisms of bupropion's anti-smoking effects: Recent preclinical and clinical insights. Eur J Pharmacol 2009;603(1–3):1–11.
43. Walsh RA. Over-the-counter nicotine replacement therapy: A methodological review of the evidence supporting its effectiveness. Drug Alcohol Rev 2008;27(5):529–47.
44. Amodei N, Lamb RJ. Over-the-counter nicotine replacement therapy: Can its impact on smoking cessation be enhanced? Psychol Addict Behav 2008;22(4):472–85.
45. Stahl SM. Essential psychopharmacology: A prescriber's guide. New York: Cambridge University Press, 2006:53–8, 353–60.

46. Hughes JR, Stead LF, Lancaster T. Antidepressants for smoking cessation. Cochrane Database Syst Rev 2007;24(1):CD0000311.
47. Raupach T, Hoogsteder PH, Onno van Schayck CP. Nicotine vaccines to assist with smoking cessation, current status of research. Drugs 2012;5(72):e1–16.
48. Cornish KE, Harris AC, LeSage MG, Keyler DE, Brroughs D, Earley C, et al. Combined active and passive immunization against nicotine: Minimizing monoclonal antibody requirements using a target antibody concentration strategy. Int Immunopharmacol 2011;11(11):1809.
49. Riker CA, Darville LK, Hahn EJ. E-cigarettes: Promise or peril? Nurs Clin North Am 2012;47(2):315.
50. McNeil JJ, Piccenna L, Ioannides-Demos LL. Smoking cessation-recent advances. Cardiovascular Drugs Ther 2010;24(4):359.

8 Marijuana: Current concepts and conundrums

Donald E. Greydanus, Elizabeth K. Hawver, and Megan M. Greydanus

Marijuana (cannabis) remains a controversial drug in the 21st century. This chapter considers current research on the use of *Cannabis sativa* and its constituents such as the cannabinoids. Topics reviewed include prevalence of cannabis use, other drugs consumed with pot, the endocannabinoid system, use of medicinal marijuana, medical adverse effects of cannabis, and psychiatric adverse effects of cannabis use. Treatment of cannabis withdrawal and dependence is difficult and remains mainly based on psychological therapy; current research on pharmacological management of problems related to cannabis consumption is also considered. The potential role of specific cannabinoids for medical benefit will be revealed as the 21st century progresses. However, potential dangerous adverse effects from smoking marijuana are well known and should be clearly taught to a public often confused by a media-driven, though false, message and promise of benign pot consumption. Caveat emptor!

8.1 Introduction

A number of chemicals are inhaled for the development of euphoria, including cannabis (marijuana), methamphetamine, heroin, crack cocaine, phencyclidine (PCP), and nitrites (amyl and butyl) (1). Marijuana (cannabis, pot) has been known to *Homo sapiens* for thousands of years, and concern has been raised over the past two centuries regarding its potential adverse effects – leading to various laws in the United States and other countries to control its production and use (2) (see chapter 1). The psychoactive chemical delta-9-tetrahydrocannabinol (THC) was isolated in the mid-1960s, while other aspects of the endocannabinoid system (cannabinoid receptors [CB1R and CB2R] and key endogenous cannabinoids [2-arachidonoyl glycerol and anandamide]) were identified more than 20 years later. Though use of phytocannabinoids is being increasingly linked to improvement of some health conditions, frequent users of cannabis are at increased risk for adverse effects, which can lead to additional health problems (3). Research is identifying components of cannabis that are not psychoactive and may become established parts of the pharmacopoeia as the 21st century continues.

8.1.1 *Cannabis sativa* plant

The products of cannabis are made from the easily grown hemp plant, *C. sativa*, and the psychoactive ingredient, THC, has been at the heart of the complex cannabis controversy in this and the past century (see chapter 19). The euphoria can last minutes to hours. The enzyme, Δ1-tetrahydrocannabinolic acid synthase, catalyzes the oxidative cyclization of cannabigerolic acid into Δ1-tetra-hydrocannabinolic acid, which is the precursor of THC (4). This enzyme controls the psychoactivity of *C. sativa* (4) due to THC, which is present in the dried leaves, seeds, stems, flowers (sensimilla), and oil of *C. sativa* (5). The pot of the 1960s and 1970s contained 1%–2% THC, while the Hawaiian sensimilla product was 3%; this is in contrast to current versions with much a higher THC percentage as measured by the Potency Monitoring Project and other research (5,6). A recent survey in Japan revealed an average potency of 11.2% with a maximum potency of 22.6% (7). High-potency cannabis is referred to as "skunk."

Cannabis remains a popular global drug that is easily obtained around the world. Movements are increasing to legalize this drug because of the research noting positive medical benefits as well as the intense euphoria it produces along with a popular though false impression that this is a "safe" drug (8,9). Cannabis remains a controversial drug because its illegal status places it in conflict with the popular notion that pot is a harmless chemical – a notion made fashionable or trendy by many media and Hollywood personalities who may promote its use to enhance their joie de vive. Such promotions seem to be effective as noted by the popularity of this illicit drug. However, marijuana (cannabis) has been prohibited in the United States since the 1937 Marijuana Tax Act and is classified by the U.S. Drug Enforcement Agency as an illegal Schedule I drug. Some states in the United States have legalized small amounts of cannabis that a person can carry without forensic consequences.

8.1.2 Prevalence

Prevalence data for cannabis can be determined in various ways such as self-report data, wastewater (sewage) analysis, and sales of cigarette paper (10,11). Research notes that marijuana is the most commonly used illicit drug on earth (12,13). The most frequently used substances among American adolescents are tobacco, alcohol, and marijuana. Marijuana ("weed, pot, hash, BC Bud, Ganja, grass, smoke, doobs," others) is an illicit Schedule I drug that constitutes about three-fourths of the illegal drug utilization in the United States (14–16).

Many studies have been done to confirm the high use of cannabis among adolescents and young adults of the world (see chapter 16). The 2007 European School Survey Project on Alcohol and Other Drugs (ESPAD) reported that lifetime use of cannabis among students in Europe ranged from 3% in Armenia to 45% in the Czech Republic with an average of 19% among 35 countries (see table 8.1). One-third of Canadian university students use cannabis (17).

Table 8.1: Lifetime use of marijuana: 2007 ESPAD*

Armenia: 3%	Italy: 23%
Austria: 17%	Latvia: 18%
Belgium (Flanders): 24%	Lithuania: 18%
Bulgaria: 22%	Malta: 13%
Croatia: 18%	Monaco: 28%
Cyrus: 5%	Netherlands: 28%
Czech Republic: 45%	Norway: 6%
Estonia: 26%	Poland: 16%
Faroe Islands: 6%	Portugal: 13%
Finland: 8%	Romania: 4%
France: 31%	Russia: 19%
Germany: 20%	Slovak Republic: 32%
Greece: 6%	Slovenia: 22%
Hungary: 13%	Sweden: 7%
Iceland: 9%	Switzerland: 33%
Ireland: 20%	Ukraine: 14%
Isle of Man: 34%	United Kingdom: 29%
AVERAGE: 19%	

*Hibell B, Guttormsson U, Ahlström S, Balakireva O, Bjarnason T, Kokkevi A, et al. ESPAD (The European School Survey Project on Alcohol and Other Drugs) report 2007: Substance use among students in 35 European countries. Stockholm: Swedish Council Information Alcohol Other Drugs, 2009.

The U.S. Centers for Disease Control and Prevention Youth Risk Behavioral Surveillance reported a lifetime use (once or more times) among U.S. high school students of 31.3% in 1991 that increased to 47.2% in 1999 and was 36.8% in 2009 (18). Use of marijuana by U.S. high schools students that occurred 30 days before the survey ranged from 14.7% in 1991 to 26.7% in 1999 and 20.8% in 2009. Other studies note marijuana use by adolescents that ranges from 28% in New York City versus 38% across the United States (19). Prevalence of cannabis use disorders has increased in veterans in the United States and is higher in states that allow cannabis for medical purposes (20).

8.1.2.1 Consumption of cannabis (marijuana)

Marijuana is typically smoked as a joint but can be taken orally in various foods, teas, or capsules, which may be used as "medicinal" marijuana. It can be prepared in food for oral consumption, as in brownies, cookies, or spaghetti. Various kinds of oral consumption are found in different countries. For example, in eastern Iran, there is a special solid "pie" called Majoon Birjandi, which is consumed by adolescents to reach a cannabis-induced euphoria (21).

The marijuana (bhang) cigarette is rolled from the *C. sativa* plant (upper leaves, tops, and stems) that is cut and dried. Hashish refers to dried exudate that comes from the top and underside of the plant leaves, while concentrated hashish distillate is called hashish oil. Sensimilla is another potent marijuana product that is made from the seedless female flower of the cannabis plant. The "typical" marijuana cigarette includes about 20 mg of THC, which is produced from a gram of *C. sativa* leaves and buds; however, much variation in potency can be found (vida supra). THC can be found in the body for up to 2 weeks after use of a single pot cigarette. A blunt is a cigarette or cigar form made from tobacco and filled with marijuana in a process called boosting; this can be used to boost the effects of other drugs such as alcohol (22).

8.1.2.2 Cannabis and other drug use

Pot is often combined with consumption of alcohol or diazepam, which increases the sedative effects of cannabis. Addition of various other drugs enhances the euphoric effects. For example, marijuana is often mixed with various drugs such as nicotine, cocaine, opioids, or hallucinogens (as LSD [lysergic acid diethylamide]). It is also mixed with drugs such as PCP, in which the joint is dipped (hand rolled) into PCP dissolved in an organic solvent (such as formaldehyde); after drying, it is smoked – called "water, wet, or Sherms." Such additions add to the complications of pot use. Other additives include glutethimide and methaqualone, which have been popularized in the past. Persons abusing marijuana who also take disulfiram due to alcohol abuse can develop increased psychoactive effects of cannabis due to THC blockage by the disulfiram (23).

Cannabis users also smoke tobacco, and research notes that this occurs for a variety of reasons, including shared genetic factors, the similar cue of smoking for both, and withdrawal symptoms that are seen to some extent in both (24). One study of 467 adults who regularly smoked both cannabis and tobacco noted that one-third started with cannabis first, nearly half initiated tobacco before cannabis, and most cannabis smokers who stopped tobacco did so after taking up regular cannabis consumption (25).

As noted, those who consume marijuana also tend to use other drugs, and it may serve as a gateway drug from early experimentation in adolescence to other drug use (26,27). For example, two different studies report that 45% of college students who illegally used prescription drugs also abused marijuana, while 24% to 57% also abused alcohol (28). Cannabis initiation usually follows alcohol use, though cannabis use can start before alcohol use and African Americans (vs. European Americans) have an increased risk for this cannabis-first trend (29). Other research notes increased risk for cannabis-related problems in African American females versus European Americans (29). Some research identifies declining socioeconomic position from childhood to adulthood as a risk factor for cannabis as well as tobacco consumption (30).

Some researchers report that patients seen in a pain clinic are at increased risk for use of marijuana; for example, one study of these patients with 21,746 urine specimens found 13.0% incidence of urine with cannabis (tetrahydrocannabinol); also, 4.6% were positive for cocaine, and 1.07% were positive for methamphetamine. (31). A case-crossover research design study noted that cannabis was a trigger for onset of cocaine use even when genetic influences and various environmental conditions were held constant (32).

8.1.2.3 Cannabinoids

C. sativa contains more than 60 cannabinoids as well as more than 400 other chemicals including benzopyrene, a known carcinogen. Table 8.2 lists some of the known cannabinoids (33). The cannabinoids of the *C. sativa* plant include cannabidiol (CBD), cannabigerol (CBG), and cannabinol, which, in contrast to THC, are not psychoactive. CBD may activate central nervous system (CNS) limbic and paralimbic regions, which can reduce autonomic arousal and feelings of anxiety; this is in contrast to THC, which can be anxiogenic (34) (see chapter 19). CBG is found in higher concentrations in hemp and has been used to lower intraocular pressure.

Other research also notes that THC and CBD influence different CNS regions and thus have different effects on cannabis users (35). In addition to anxiolytic effects, CBD has been shown to have antiemetic, anti-inflammatory, and antipsychotic effects (36). There is no effect on vital signs (i.e., blood pressure, pulse, body temperature), gastrointestinal transit, or psychological functioning. Doses up to 1,500 mg per day as well as chronic use of CBD have been reported as being well tolerated by humans (36). There can be hepatic drug metabolism inhibition, reduced activities of some drug transporters (i.e., p-glycoprotein), and lowered capacity of fertilization (36).

Euphoria is produced from effects of this lipophilic drug on cannabinoid receptors (ECS: endogenous cannabinoid system CB1R and CB2R) in the mesocortical and limbic systems; THC also affects the striatum and lateral prefrontal cortex.

Table 8.2: Types of cannabinoids

Endogenous cannabinoid agonists	Synthetic cannabinoid agonists
• 2-AG (2-arachidonoyl glycerol)	• WIN 55,212–2
• Anandamide (arachidonoyl ethanolamide)	• JWH-133
Cannabidiol (CBD) (isomer of THC)	• HU-210
Cannabinol (CBN) (metabolite of THC)	• CP-55940
Cannabigerol (CBG) (alpha-2-adrenergic receptor agonist)	
Tetrahydrocannabinolic acid (THC biosynthetic precursor)	

Cannabinoid receptors are also found in the liver, gastrointestinal tract, skeletal tissue, and adipose tissue. There are endogenous ligands for cannabinoid receptors (i.e., N-palmitoethanolamide and anandamide) that act like neurotransmitters (26). Part of the complexity of the cannabis issue is the presence of the endogenous endocannabinoid system, and this system is now reviewed.

8.1.2.4 Endocannabinoid system

The endocannabinoid system consists of CNS cannabinoid receptors and their endogenous ligands; ligands (Latin: "binding") are triggering molecules that bind to a target protein site (37). Endocannabinoids (endogenous cannabinoid receptor agonists) include arachidonic acid derivatives: 2-arachidonoyl glycerol (2-AG) and anandamide (arachidonoyl ethanolamide [AEA]) (see table 8.2) (38,39). AEA and 2-AG are the two most researched endocannabinoids. The complex effects of this system on emotional and cognitive behavior may be strongly influenced by various environmental factors (40).

The endocannabinoid system is identified as a cause of psychiatric disorders, but research also suggests that proper manipulation of this system may be pharmacologically useful in management of some psychiatric disorders – such as depression, anxiety, anorexia nervosa, and others (41). For example, CBD may be beneficial in treatment of psychiatric disorders (41).

The endocannabinoid system is involved in processes of brain reward that are related to drug abuse – as noted in animal and human research, this includes cue-induced relapse of drug abuse (42). This CNS system is involved in various functions involving memory, emotions, movement, cell proliferation, and other important cell functions (43). Key neuron classes that express high levels of CB1Rs are GABAergic interneurons in such CNS areas as the cerebral cortex, amygdala, and hippocampus; these areas also contain cholecystokinin, an important neuropeptide (44).

CB1R is mainly found in the central nervous system and CB2R is expressed in immune system cells; both receptors are G-protein–coupled receptors and are involved in adenylate cyclase inhibition (45,46). The CB1R is a G-protein–coupled receptor that is associated with most of the CNS endocannabinoid signaling (47). It is widely found in the cerebellum, basal ganglia, and limbic system; the hippocampus has the highest concentration of cannabinoid receptors. Cannabinoid receptors are found in other tissues including the heart, lungs, endocrine glands, arteries, immune system, sympathetic ganglia, gastrointestinal tract, and reproductive tract (38).

The activation of CB1Rs can inhibit amino acid and monoamine neurotransmitter release. Certain lipid derivatives (i.e., 2-AG and AEA) can function as endogenous ligands for CB1Rs and lead to excitation in such areas as the cerebellum and hippocampus by inhibition suppression (44). Most drugs of abuse alter brain levels of endocannabinoids. Because blockade of this system can change the reward behavior associated with some drugs of abuse, the CNS endocannabinoid system is under active research to develop medications that may be helpful in treatment of drug abuse – including drug relapse (42). Cannabis as potential medication ("medicinal marijuana") is now considered.

8.1.2.5 Use of medical cannabis

Conclusions regarding the "benign" or "malignant" effects of cannabis use influence different countries' policies regarding legalization or criminalization of cannabis use (48). This is also complicated by use of cannabis products in a "medicinal" manner and thus effects to find the most "appropriate" variety or varieties of cannabis that are available (49,50). A plethora of medicinal benefits have been identified with marijuana use over past centuries (51–53) (see table 8.3).

The concern over the addictive and psychomimetic qualities of THC placed active research on potential medical benefits of this plant on the backburner until recently (53). However, increased understanding of the cannabinoid signaling system has led to increased research on potential medicinal uses of cannabis (54); this endocannabinoid system, for example, is being analyzed for use in treatment of various neuropsychiatric diseases (43).

Studies are looking at potential benefits of cannabinoids (phytocannabinoids) in management of neuropathic pain, hypertension, poststroke neuroprotection, multiple sclerosis, epilepsy, cancer, and other disorders (55–62). Cancer research, for example, has identified that cannabinoids can inhibit cancer growth, angiogenesis, and metastasis (62). Cannabinoid-like anti-inflammatory products may be useful as material for wound dressing due to anti-inflammatory effects (63). CBD is under research as a new class of anti-inflammatory bowel disease drug (64).

A number of cannabis products are being manufactured by pharmaceutical companies, including Sativex (THC + CBD), Marinol (dronabinal; THC; Schedule III

Table 8.3: Potential benefits of cannabis based on research studies (see text)

• Remedy for inflammation	• Improvement of anorexia in AIDS patients
• Remedy for pain (including chronic pain and neuropathic pain)	• Treatment for Huntington's disease
• Remedy for diarrhea (as in Crohn's disease)	• Management of inflammatory bowel disease
• Treatment for dystonia	• Beneficial effect on atherosclerosis
• Treatment for multiple sclerosis	• Reduce brain infarct size
• Treatment for rheumatoid arthritis	• Block negative memories in posttraumatic stress disorder
• Treatment for glaucoma	• Reduce cardiac reperfusion injury
• Treatment for emesis due to chemotherapy	• Adjuvant treatment for prostate carcinoma
• Treatment for epilepsy	• Others

drug), and Cesamet (THC, Schedule II) (53). The latter two have been approved for use in the anorexia-cachexia syndrome as well as for nausea and vomiting (53). Dronabinol is a synthesized gelatin capsule that has been used to treat glaucoma by lowering intraocular pressure or relieve chemotherapy-induced emesis (vida infra) (65). Marijuana has been used to treat the wasting syndrome associated with HIV/AIDS (9). A newer tablet formulation of THC is Namisol (>98% THC), which has been studied to ameliorate pain and spasms in adults with multiple sclerosis as well as relieve nausea and emesis in HIV or cancer patients (66).

Though cannabis users noted lowering of anxiety and feelings of anxiety, much research remains to be accomplished to identify which if any cannabinoid products may be therapeutically and safely used in pharmacological management of individuals with anxiety disorders (67). Current research is looking at such anxiety disorders such as social anxiety disorder, posttraumatic stress disorders, panic disorder, and obsessive-compulsive disorder (68,69).

Research suggests that the phytocannabinoid chemical CBD may be useful in blocking negative or fearful memories associated with posttraumatic stress disorder in a process called reconsolidation blockage (70). Some research notes a lower mortality rate among adults with schizophrenia and related psychotic disorders in those who smoked cannabis versus those who did not smoke cannabis (71). Research on smoked, vaporized, and oral cannabis products for potential improvement of health are continuing (72).

8.1.2.6 Synthetic cannabinoids (cannabinoid designer drugs; cannabimimetics)

A number of designer drugs have become available in the 21st century, and cannabis has become involved in this trend as well (see chapter 19). These synthetic cannabinoids (called “legal highs,” “Spice drugs,” “K2” drugs) are similar to THC found in the *C. sativa* plant and produce similar effects to smoking cannabis since they bind to the same cannabinoid brain and peripheral organ receptors as THC (73–79). These herbal blends have been noted since 2008 in various “herbal” smoking products sold via the Internet and in retail outlets (called “head shops”) that focus on drug paraphernalia sold for cannabis and other drug use; brand names include such exotic names as Aroma, Yucatan Fire, Spice Gold, and others (73,80).

Though available in some countries, advertised as “safe” (since they do not resemble the chemical structure of THC), and considered legal in various locations, they are potentially dangerous drugs – having up to 10 times the strength of delta-9-THC (74,81,82). In a moving and dangerous cat-and-mouse game, sellers change the synthetic cannabinoids in attempts to avoid putting up for sale a specific product identified as illegal in a specific country or area. As one synthetic cannabinoid is banned, others are produced to take their place, and as a result, there are more than 140 different Spice drugs that are produced (73). They may be marketed as some type of "incense" or "herbal" product and even "air fresheners," but potential adverse reactions remain (76,77). Toxicology screens looking at THC may miss the presence of these cannabinoid designer drugs (76,78).

They are typically tobacco and cannabis free but produce similar cannabis effects that can include withdrawal symptoms, anxiety, intoxication, psychosis, death, and others (vida infra) (73,83). Some reports suggest that increased hallucinations and paranoia are noted with these "Spice" synthetic cannabinoids (78). Part of the potential danger is that they can contain various added but often unknown chemicals that are part of the manufacturing process. However, some of the products found on the Internet do not have significant amounts of impurities, and adverse effects are due to the synthetic cannabinoids themselves and the potential additives (84).

8.1.3 Cannabis lab testing

Those smoking 3.55% pot develop a peak plasma level near 160 mg/mL 10 minutes after beginning to ingest this product; the THC is removed from the plasma to body tissues leading to its euphoric effects and then to body fat as long-term storage (6). THC is then eliminated over several weeks in the urine and feces. Urine tests can be used to establish the presence of cannabinoid metabolites and can be positive in casual users for up to 10 days versus 14–30 days for chronic pot users (26). Current drug testing (using high-performance liquid chromatography with diode-array detection) can identify low THC content in cannabis seedlings right after germination; however, chemotype determination of THC can occur as the plant ages – at 3 weeks and beyond (85).

Cannabis testing can be used to verify past pot use but not the presence of cannabis intoxication, dependence, or abuse. Testing may also note suppression of testosterone and luteinizing hormone, though it is unclear what such tests actually mean from a clinical viewpoint. Passive inhalation of cannabis does not result in a positive urine test for THC. Urine testing for THC does not identify the presence of synthetic cannabinoids.

THC-COOH (11-nor-9-carboxy-THC) is the main secondary THC metabolite developed after cannabis is taken; it is not psychoactive but has a long-half life and can be detected for days and, in heavy cannabis users, for weeks after consumption. It is an important metabolite used in blood or urine testing for identification of cannabis; urine THC-COOH testing has been used to identify cannabis abstinence, and a positive test can be confirmed with gas chromatography–mass spectrometry THC blood testing that indicates recent cannabis exposure (6). Whole blood and plasma testing can also reveal 11-hydroxy-THC after smoking cannabis. Polymerase chain reaction testing is available to police to identify where specific *C. sativa* samples came from in order to assist with forensic studies and investigations (86). In addition to urine as well as blood testing, saliva and hair testing for cannabis are possible – the latter for evaluation of chronic cannabis exposure (87,88).

8.2 Medical adverse effects

Though some authors question the data on negative effects of cannabis use, most authors conclude that use of cannabis has significant risks for the user in a dose-dependent and/or idiosyncratic fashion (89,90). Identifying adverse effects of cannabis is challenging because studying an illicit drug can be problematic, as can separating out cannabis effects from other drugs that are often taken simultaneously, such as tobacco or alcohol; also, there is variation in the techniques of cannabis consumption (89,91–93).

A case of an infant with altered consciousness after exposure to cannabis smoke (passive inhalation) has been reported (94). Another 10-month-old infant consumed oral cannabis and presented with cannabis poisoning – drowsiness, generalized hypotonia, and restlessness – this infant had high blood as well as urine levels of cannabis products and recovered with symptomatic management that included clinical monitoring for the first 24 hours after the ingestion (95).

A number of side effects are possible for the cannabis consumer including increased mortality rates (see table 8.4). Chronic use can lead to weight gain from overeating and reduced physical activity. Acute pot use can lead to suppression of

Table 8.4: Potential adverse effects of marijuana* (see text)

- Addiction (physiologic)
- Withdrawal syndrome
- Dependence (psychological) and, with heavy use, tolerance
- Variety of negative psychological reactions: anxiety, hallucinations, violent behavior, depression, fear
- Overt precipitation of psychosis or depression
- Insomnia (can be chronic and improved with trazodone)
- Memory spans that are impaired
- Blunted reflexes
- Flu-like reaction (after stopping this drug after 24 to 60 hours, lasting up to 2 weeks)
- Confusion and cognition impairment
- Alteration of time perception
- Amotivational syndrome (lose interest in school or work success)
- Physiologic responses can include cough, bronchospasm, bronchitis
- Amenorrhea
- Immunologic dysfunction

*Used with permission from Greydanus DE, Feucht CL, Hawver EK. Substance abuse disorders. In: DE Greydanus, DR Patel, HA Omar, C Feucht, J Merrick, eds. Adolescent medicine: Pharmacotherapeutics in general, mental, and sexual health. Berlin: De Gruyter, 2012: chap. 10, 180.

rapid eye movement and diffuse slowing of background electroencephalograph activity (26). The smoke of cannabis can be irritating to conjunctival, nasopharyngeal, and bronchial tissue leading to injected conjunctiva, chronic cough, sinusitis, pharyngitis, and (chronic) bronchitis (96). Adolescents or young adults who present with chronic cough should be screened for cannabis use in addition to more classic causes, such as asthma, gastroesophageal reflux, respiratory tract infections, and others (97,98).

Chronic use of cannabis has not been shown to affect thyroid function (99). Acute pancreatitis linked to cannabis use has been reported in a 22-year-old male who presented with epigastric pain, nausea, and emesis (100). Abdominal pain due to colonic perforation and subsequent peritonitis has been reported as a complication of cannabis body packing in attempts to illegally smuggle illicit drugs from one country to another (101).

8.2.1 Cannabis hyperemesis

Cannabinoid hyperemesis is noted in some cannabis users who present with usually sudden, severe, and cyclic (intractable) emesis that resolves with intravenous fluids, antiemetics, and cannabis cessation. There can be cyclic nausea and abdominal pain as well, and after a careful evaluation, the cause is linked to cannabis use (102). It was first described in Australia in 2004 and may be missed in patients presenting with hyperemesis and abnormal patterns of bathing (103). Though cannabinoids have been used to treat chronic nausea and emesis, a paradoxical effect on the gastrointestinal tract in noted in cannabis hyperesis syndrome, and three parts are described: prodromal, hyperemetic, and recovery phases (104).

The hyperemesis phase is usually resolved in 48 hours. Patients may report temporary symptomatic improvement with prolonged hot showers or bath exposure, and thus, compulsive hot water bathing has become part of the cannabis (cannabinoid) hyperemesis complex (102,105–107). Diagnostic confusion with the cyclic vomiting syndrome may occur (104). If cannabis use resumes, the hyperemesis complex may reoccur (104,105,108).

8.2.2 Dental effects of cannabis

Pot users tend to have increased risks for dental caries, oral infections, and periodontal disease (109–111). Dysplastic changes and premalignant lesions can be identified in oral mucosa of cannabis users (109). Use of local anesthetics in patients intoxicated with cannabis intensifies and prolongs pot-induced tachycardia (109).

Exposure to smoking (cannabis or tobacco) leads to contact with many carcinogens (procarcinogens) such as polycyclic aromatic hydrocarbons (112). Cannabis users often smoke tobacco and drink alcohol, which increases carcinogen exposure and risk of oral squamous cell carcinoma, representing 95% of malignant lesions in the mouth (112).

8.2.3 Pulmonary effects

Some research identifies an anti-inflammatory effect from consumption of the *C. sativa* plant. For example, one study of 5,115 adult males that took place over 20 years noted that occasional and low cumulative cannabis use was not associated with adverse effects on pulmonary function (113). Murine studies suggest that CBD has an immunosuppressive and anti-inflammatory effect on acute lung injury because of an increase in extracellular adenosine (114).

However, it is known that marijuana, as well as tobacco, contains a toxic combination of gases and other substances that can be injurious to the pulmonary system (115). Marijuana smokers usually smoke fewer "joints" than tobacco smokers consume cigarettes; however, methods of cannabis smoking may place more cannabis particulate matter into the lungs than noted with typical cigarette smoking (115). Those with cannabis dependence will continue to use it despite chronic cough, excessive sedation, or other marijuana-related problems. Combining marijuana with tobacco leads to known tobacco effects via secondhand smoke.

Pot use can induce some bronchodilation, but regular or heavy cannabis consumption can result in generalized airway inflammation with evidence of respiratory epithelial cell injury and damage to alveolar macrophages, which can lead to pulmonary infection (115). Sharing of cannabis water pipes has led to the development of pulmonary tuberculosis (TB) (116). Smoking cannabis that contains fungal spores can result in pulmonary aspergillosis in those with immune-compromised conditions (116,117).

There is a dose-related large airway dysfunction with hyperinflation and obstruction of airflow; one cannabis joint has been noted to be equivalent to 2.5 to 5 cigarettes in terms of this pulmonary dysfunction (118). Macrophage injury can result in cytokine and nitric oxide impairment. Smokers of cannabis are typically exposed to more carbon monoxide and tar than cigarette smokers; this effect is not related to the THC content (119).

Heavy and/or chronic users of cannabis may have persistent cough, bronchitis, (bullous) emphysema (chronic obstructive lung disease [COLD]), pulmonary dysplasia, pneumothorax, TB, and other respiratory infections (26,115,116,120). Cannabis can lead to increased airway resistance and large airway inflammation, though causal links to COLD or macroscopic emphysema remain controversial and unproven (92,93,118,121). Smoking both tobacco and marijuana increases risks for abnormal tracheobronchial histopathology and COLD (121).

8.2.4 Cannabis and cancer

Marijuana smoke contains toxic chemicals in amounts similar to or higher than that found in tobacco and is linked as a potential respiratory tract carcinogen (26,93,96,120). Chronic inflammatory and precancerous airway changes in a dose-dependent relationship as well as increase in airway cancer are reported in cannabis users (90). Anecdotal reports of upper and lower respiratory airway cancer have been published (116,122). For example, a case of small-cell lung cancer was reported in a 22-year-old male who smoked one marijuana joint three times a week for 3 years (123). However, specific link of cannabis to lung cancer remains unproven (92,93,124). Current literature suggests that cannabis-only smokers are at lower risk of lung cancer than tobacco-only smokers (125). However, some epidemiological data do place an independent role of cannabis smoking in the development of lung cancer (126,127).

8.2.5 Cardiovascular effects

Cannabinoids have complex and varying effects on blood pressure depending on which cannabinoid is being studied (33). Acute effects of cannabis include increase in heart rate along with an increase (usually mild) in blood pressure and then decreased vascular resistance-induced orthostatic hypotension (55,128). Individuals with coronary heart disease may have increased cardiovascular adverse effects from cannabis use (89). Cannabis-induced ST segment elevation mimicking the Brugada syndrome has been reported (129,130). Other drugs, both licit and illicit (i.e., cocaine), have been linked with the Brugada syndrome as well (131).

Reported cardiovascular effects linked to cannabis include anecdotal cases of acute coronary syndrome, congestive heart failure, and arrhythmias (55,96,129, 132–135). Patients with angina may have decreased time with chest pain onset due to the acute effects of cannabis use; also, myocardial infarction may be triggered by the acute effects of cannabis use (55). Patients at high risk for coronary heart disease should be advised to avoid using cannabis (55).

Studies on cannabis also provide evidence of positive or "neutral" effects from cannabis consumption. For example, though inhalation of marijuana may induce acute coronary symptoms, ingestion of cannabinoids may have a positive effect on atherosclerotic heart disease via effects on the endocannabinoid system (134). Also, cannabis use has not been specifically linked to increased hospitalization due to cardiovascular disease or increased mortality from cardiovascular etiology (55). If a patient has a cardiac death and has a positive urine test for cannabinoid, a plasma THC level should also be done before seeking to link the cannabis history with the cardiac death.

8.2.6 Motor vehicle accidents

Adolescents and young adults who drive vehicles under the influence of pot (often combined with alcohol) are at increased risk (two times) of motor vehicle accidents leading to potential death and injury (89,90,96,136,137). Those who consume cannabis without other drugs also place themselves at increased risk for motor vehicle crashes (137). Individuals driving under marijuana influence may experience distortion of oncoming vehicle headlights resulting in motor vehicle crashes. Driving impairment worsens with increasing amounts of cannabis consumed (138–140). The problem of driving while under cannabis influence is increasing, and in some areas of California, for example, the rate of nighttime weekend drivers who tested positive for THC was nearly 20% (139). Unfortunately, tests used in the field to identify if cannabis is involved in motor vehicle accidents may not be sensitive enough to detect the precise presence of this drug. Cannabis consumption is also involved in nontraffic injuries, especially falls in the older adult population (141).

8.2.7 Sports doping

Those involved in sports should understand that cannabis is a drug banned by the World Anti-Doping Agency despite history of pot use in the Olympics, and it has been on the list of prohibited drugs of the International Olympic Committee since 1989 (75,142). Cannabis smoking results in reduced exercise test duration during maximal exercising and increased heart rate at less than maximal exercise levels (55). Cannabis-induced increase in blood pressure and reduced psychomotor activity can also decrease overall athletic performance. Management of urine samples from athletes can be problematic because of the intricacies of interpreting urine samples due to the complexities of prolonged cannabis excretion (143).

8.2.8 Adverse effects: psychiatric

8.2.8.1 Cannabis and neurodevelopment effects

Adverse neuropsychological effects of cannabis use must be separated out from the acute effects of cannabinoids, effects of heavy cannabis consumption, and psychiatric disorders worsened or even caused by cannabinoids (144) (see chapter 16). Specific effects in individual cannabis users are difficult to predict because of the heterogeneity or nonuniformity of different studies that have been done to seek neuroimaging effects in cannabis use; some authors have concluded that it is difficult to prove major effects of cannabis on brain structure (145,146). Some research suggests that identified cannabis-related neurocognitive performance defects disappear after 25 days of cannabis abstinence (147).

However, other recent research studies are noting that cannabis users demonstrate important deficits in prospective memory and executive functioning that exist beyond acute cannabis intoxication (148). The presence of cannabis and nicotine use disorders in parents appears to increase the risk for major depressive disorder in their late adolescent offspring (149). Studies in animals and humans suggest a subtle (vs. gross) effect on cognitive functioning with later development of hyperactivity, reduced attention span, impulsivity, depression, and substance use disorders (150). The most frequently reported adverse effects of cannabis use include mental slowness, reduced reaction times, and increased anxiety (89). Dysfunction occurs to dopamine and opioid neurotransmitter systems (151).

Animal and human research concludes that the developing brain, with its high neuronal plasticity, is vulnerable to exposure to exogenous cannabinoids, particularly in the perinatal/prenatal period and during young adolescence (43,151–154). Animal and human studies suggest that early onset of cannabis use (i.e., early adolescence) can increase risks for cognition dysfunction, CNS changes (i.e., low striatal dopamine release), neuropsychiatric disorders, cannabis dependence, and consumption of additional illicit drugs (152,155). Persistent or problematic marijuana use can lead to major interference with daily life activities whether at work, in school, or in one's home.

Cannabis use often develops in adolescence and early adulthood which, as noted, is a vulnerable time for subsequent adverse brain effects (47). For example, cannabinoid receptors are abundant in the CNS white matter in adolescence as well as young adulthood; long-term cannabis use during this time period can lead to impaired axonal fiber connectivity with negative effects on the white matter of the brain (156). Cannabis use in early adolescence may alter CB1R signaling with potentially increased risk for development of psychiatric disorders (47). Early adolescent cannabis use has been linked with adolescent dropout behavior in some research (157).

Some research links other CNS problems with heavy cannabis use. For example, one study identified regional brain abnormalities (in the hippocampus and amygdale) in long-term, heavy pot users – data found in both human and animal studies (158). Animal studies noted hippocampal-dependent short-term memory deficits that occurred in some but not all rats given chronic cannabinoid administration (159).

8.2.8.2 Cannabis and attention-deficit/hyperactivity disorder (ADHD)

One report of 162 adolescents studied during inpatient management of problems related to drug dependence (i.e., marijuana, heroin, alcohol, or cocaine abuse) revealed ADHD in 34% of them (160). A study from different medical centers that focused on 600 adolescents (ages 13 to 16 years of age) who were undergoing management for marijuana-related problems reported that 38% also had ADHD (161).

Such studies support the theory that ADHD and adolescent substance abuse disorder (including cannabis dependence) can be seen as a developmental disorder with similar underlying physiological mechanisms (19).

8.2.8.3 Cannabis dependence

Psychological dependency and tolerance are classically described in pot smokers. The American Psychiatric Association's (APA) *Diagnostic and Statistical Manual of Mental Disorders*, fourth edition, text revision (*DMS-IV-TR*) describes two cannabis use disorders (cannabis dependence and abuse) and six categories of cannabis-induced disorders (see table 8.5; 26). The 2013 DSM-5 includes the term Cannabis withdrawal while replacing categories of abuse and dependence with substance abuse disorders (mild, moderate, and severe). Some have placed the dependence rate at 7%–10% of regular users (90). A susceptibility gene, NRG1, has been associated with cannabis dependence in African Americans (162).

Those with cannabis dependence can consume cannabis in potent forms for years and spend several hours a day in finding as well as taking it; there can be physiological dependence and also psychological dependence (26). Cannabis intoxication may last longer with oral cannabis versus smoking it. Intoxication may even last up to 24 hours due to the effects of enterohepatic circulation and/or slow release of fat soluble THC and other cannabinoids from fatty tissue. Cannabis use disorders are more common in males versus females and are most prevalent in the 18- to 30-year-old group (26).

Depersonalization and derealization episodes are described in pot users (26). Anecdotal cases of cannabis-induced depersonalization in adolescents have been reported (163). A history of conduct disorder in childhood or adolescence and antisocial personality disorder are risk factors for substance use disorder including cannabis-related disorders (26). Differentiation of cannabis-induced disorders from primary mental health disorders can be difficult. Ataxia and aggression are more likely to be seen with PCP intoxication versus cannabis intoxication; aggression with nystagmus or ataxia is more likely to be from alcohol intoxication (26).

Table 8.5: *DSM-IV-TR* cannabis use and induced disorders (26)

Cannabis use disorders
- Cannabis dependence
- Cannabis abuse

Cannabis-induced disorders
- Cannabis intoxication
- Cannabis intoxication delirium
- Cannabis-induced psychotic disorder, with delusions
- Cannabis-induced psychotic disorder, with hallucinations
- Cannabis-induced anxiety disorder
- Cannabis-related disorder not otherwise specified

Demonstrating a direct link between cannabis use and the development of overt depression has been problematic and not clearly proven (164). Regular cannabis consumption (particularly daily use) in adolescence has been linked with increased risks for anxiety disorders in adolescents and young adults, even after the cannabis was stopped (154). Anxiety is linked to regular or heavy use of cannabis, and further research is needed to unravel this connection in more detail (165). For example, anxiety can arise due to fear of being discovered by law enforcement officials; there can be episodes resembling panic attacks.

8.2.8.4 Cannabis withdrawal syndrome

Chronic pot users can develop psychological addiction and a withdrawal syndrome comparable to heroin addiction (8). A heavy marijuana user, whether an adolescent or adult, who suddenly stops this drug can develop a recognizable withdrawal syndrome as reported by various research studies (166–172). Withdrawal symptoms can develop within 48 hours of cessation and include irritability, restlessness, anxiety, aggression, and sleep difficulties. (89). Withdrawal symptoms tend to subside in 2–12 weeks after cannabis abstention (89). As noted, a cannabis receptor-1 gene (CNR1) has been linked with abstinence-induced withdrawal symptoms (173). Heavy cannabis use has been linked with a smaller amygdala and hippocampus, while those with CNR1 may be predisposed to smaller hippocampal volume following heavy cannabis use (173). Some smoke pot to control problems with anger (169–172).

Withdrawal symptoms are due to the cessation of THC and are relieved with taking delta-9-THC or simply smoking marijuana (166,174). Adolescents undergoing treatment for cannabis dependence experience withdrawal symptoms most acutely during the first week of cannabis absence, and this tends to ease over the next month of abstinence (166,175). Research notes that the majority of heavy pot users report several symptoms after stopping cannabis, and this can complicate effective management, especially since cannabis dependent users may resort to consuming various others drugs to relieve the symptoms of cannabis withdrawal (166,176). Diagnostic criteria for a formal cannabis withdrawal syndrome (CWS) are included in the fifth edition of the APA's *Diagnostic and Statistical Manual of Mental Disorders* (*DSM-5*) (177).

8.2.8.5 Addiction

The identification and isolation of THC in 1964 enhanced specific research into the effects of cannabis on humans and animals (43). Endogenous cannabinoids (particularly CB1R activation) activate neural mechanisms in the CNS similar to how other reward-enhancing drugs induce drug addiction (178–180). This core reward system is part of the addiction mechanism that use of cannabis develops in the unwary pot smoker as well as in users of other illicit drugs of addiction (181,182). This mechanism involves the mesoaccumbens reward circuitry of the CNS as well as neural firing of the neurotransmitter, dopamine. Some research notes that THC can induce striatal effects on dopamine as noted with other drugs of abuse (183). Though some studies suggest that dependence develops faster in cocaine versus cannabis users, recent research concludes there is no such difference (184).

Addiction also involves prefrontal cortex (PFC) dysfunction with frontostriatal dysfunction and the erosion of the ability to stop the addiction; more research is needed to identify potential impact of cannabinoids in the PFC and its potential role in cannabis dependence (185–187). A nucleotide polymorphism has been identified in CNR1 – rs2023239– that is associated with cannabis dependence, cannabis craving, and withdrawal symptoms due to cannabis abstinence (173). Some neuropeptides called orexins (hypocretins) originate in the lateral hypothalamus and are linked to features of drug addiction (i.e., cannabis, nicotine) that include drug craving, relapse, and withdrawal (188).

8.2.8.6 Cannabis and psychosis

Chronic use of cannabis, particularly with the newer synthetic cannabis products, is associated with increased rates of psychosis (189–191). Frequent cannabis use increases the risk by two times for schizophrenia and psychotic symptoms, perhaps by cannabis-induced disruption of the endocannabinoid system in which the normal signaling and functioning of this endogenous system is disturbed (192). Cannabis (marijuana) is commonly used by those with schizophrenia and can cause paranoia in approximately 40% of persons experimenting with this drug (193). Patients with schizophrenia who consume cannabis are hospitalized at rates higher than those who do not use cannabis (194).

Cannabis-induced schizophrenia is currently theorized as being due to dysfunction of late postnatal brain maturation in which glutamatergic transmission dysfunction leads to abnormal prefrontal neurocircuitry (195). Exposure of adolescents to cannabis at certain times in adolescence and at certain doses may lead to prefrontal cortical circuitry abnormalities with the result of inducing schizophrenia in susceptible adolescents (195).

One research group reports a mean time of 7.0 ± 4.3 years between onset of cannabis use and onset of psychosis (190). Those at risk for psychosis may be vulnerable to brain volume loss (i.e., cerebellum, prefrontal cortex, and cingulate) due to use of cannabis (196). Self-mutilation can also occur with cannabis-induced psychosis (197). Those with psychosis who use cannabis may not notice improved psychotic symptoms with cessation of their cannabis (198).

Most cannabis users do not develop psychosis, and this cannabis-psychosis link appears to be via a complex environmental-genetic-molecular interaction possibly involving anandamide dysfunction and other biological factors (191,199,200). Most research suggests a link between cannabis use and risk for suicide in patients with psychosis and also those without psychosis (201). The development of schizophrenia and use of cannabis share a variety of similarities, including neuropsychological deficits, reduced motivation, hallucinations, and initiation in late adolescence (202).

Cannabis is also a very common illicit drug for individuals with psychosis and disruptive disorders to consume (13,203). Those with psychosis have a higher rate of cannabis use than the general population, probably in attempts to utilize the cannabis-induced euphoria to deal with negative aspects of schizophrenia, such as boredom and depression (12). Cannabis can also prompt the onset of psychotic symptoms in otherwise healthy people as well, and this includes paranoia and/or delusional thinking due to effects of THC on striatal and prefrontal function.

Thus, use of marijuana can have opposite effects on different users. Some research fails to find a clear association between use of cannabis and symptoms of psychosis, especially with low or moderate cannabis use (204). A major component of cannabis, CBD, has been shown by some research to have antipsychotic effects (205). The presence of CBD may explain the lack of psychosis development in many cannabis users. Studies with CBD (vs. THC) suggest a modulating effect based on functional magnetic imaging resonance brain imaging (206). Schizophrenic patients using cannabis may be particularly sensitive to brain damage from the cannabis, though CBD may provide a protective effect from brain volume loss (202).

8.2.9 Management

8.2.9.1 Behavioral therapies

The "hedonic" CNS dysregulation seen in drug addiction studies in animals and human subjects underscores the concept of drug addiction as a brain disease and the necessity of prevention before this complex brain dysfunction arises (12,182,207). Indeed, it is difficult to convince an addicted cannabis user to stop smoking this plant, and thus, prevention via intensive and comprehensive education is the best option currently available. Unfortunately, cannabis dependence is difficult to treat successfully, and few who seek to stop their cannabis addiction succeed in long-term cessation (180). One of the ironic reasons for this is that chronic cannabis consumers classically have cognitive impairments that lead to defects in their decision-making skills (208).

However, there are steps that therapists can take in helping this phenomenon of a nation and a world obsessed with smoking pot. Continued education of the dangers of cannabis should take place on a persistent and relentless basis. It should be understood that some literature and some people conclude that the negative impact of smoking cannabis is limited (209). Cannabis consumers may be cognizant of such literature, which may encourage them to continue to use this so-called safe illicit drug. Thus, teaching about the potential problems of cannabis should always be provided by health care providers to help offset this destructive message of "benign" pot consumption.

Treatment specifically for cannabis use is needed as management of other or coexisting drug dependence (e.g., heroin, tobacco, or alcohol) does not necessarily reduce levels of cannabis consumption (210). Comprehensive school-based prevention programs teaching about drug use, including cannabis, can be beneficial in lowering youth drug experimentation and addiction (211,212). Increased education about high-risk adolescent behaviors for adolescents and their parents can be useful in prevention efforts (213). Intense education is needed for groups at high risk for drug abuse, such as males, young adults, and individuals with increased psychological stress (214).

Behavioral principles for management in adolescence can be directed by factors shown to suggest higher risk for cannabis use including genetic factors, family history, minimal parental supervision, drug availability, high-risk peer group, and those with a need for higher thrill-seeking activities (215,216) (see chapter 5). Groups at high risk of mental health problems are those with combined drug use, such as comorbid cannabis and methamphetamine; thus, this group should receive intense management (217). Comprehensive behavioral management can also be of help in reducing cannabis use in those arrested for cannabis possession (218). Screening of these persons for suicide risk is recommended, and lower cannabis use can reduce risks for suicide in those with and without psychosis (201). Patients with psychosis and cannabis smoking should undergo behavioral therapies to improve both problems and not just one (219).

If lifetime abstinence from cannabis is not possible, delaying its use (especially heavy use) as long as possible after adolescence and young adulthood may result in less white matter damage from cannabis consumption than noted during cannabis smoking in the second and third decades of life (156). Management can also focus on reducing cannabis use if abstinence is not possible, since adverse effects tend to be increased with heavy use of cannabis (91). Therapy should seek underlying factors in use of cannabis or other drugs. For example, research notes that socially anxious males are at increased risk for use of cannabis as part of a mechanism to deal with or avoid social situations (220). Thus, therapy can be directed at reasons for this avoidance behavior and the acquisition of successful strategies to improve their social anxiety, which may reduce the need for ongoing cannabis consumption.

Often recommended behavioral management strategies (such as cognitive behavioral therapy [CBT] and contingency management) have their limitations, and combination of these techniques does not increase success in helping those with cannabis dependence (221). However, research notes that youth with cannabis use disorder benefit more from CBT (vs. family therapy) if they are older teenagers (i.e., 17–18 years of age) and do not have preexisting psychiatric disorders; in the same study, multidimensional family therapy was more helpful (vs. CBT) for those who were younger (i.e., under age 17) and/or had a past year history of disruptive disorders (i.e., opposition defiant or conduct disorder) (222).

However, one should continue to provide the cannabis consumer with hope and encouragement that overcoming this drug addiction is possible despite its wide acceptance in society. Research does show that such benefit is more likely with intensive or prolonged behavioral therapy, especially CBT and motivational interviewing (223). Also, it should be understood that even brief (i.e., four) sessions of motivational interviewing with CBT delivered via telephone can be beneficial, at least in the short run, for motivated cannabis users who called in seeking help with treatment (224).

Behavioral therapies can be useful in the motivated cannabis addict, and such counseling seeks to help the cannabis consumer gain control over the addiction at the CNS level by enhancing neuroanatomical progression from ventral striatal (nucleus accumbens) to dorsal striatal control (182). Even brief interventions may have the positive benefit of less cannabis use at 3-month follow-up (3) and in another study at 12-month follow-up (17).

Also, therapy seeks to help the addict deal with cannabis craving and relapse triggers, such as becoming reexposed to various drugs of addiction; it is also important to help this person deal with stress and also with finding and avoiding old cues in his/her milieu, such as key persons, places, or objects (182,207). Genetic factors also have a role in why some develop addiction and are recalcitrant to management strategies (207). Involvement of families, schools, communities, and peer groups are critical in seeking to reduce and prevent cannabis smoking in adolescents. It is unclear what the interactions are between abuse of illicit drugs and use of prescription drugs, but the potential drug interactions should be considered in prevention and treatment plans (225).

8.2.10 Pharmacological therapies

There are no FDA-approved pharmacological agents for management of cannabis dependence. Traditionally, pharmacological agents have not been specifically beneficial in treating marijuana addiction whether dependence or withdrawal symptoms (226). However, a careful assessment of each patient is necessary, and a reduction in cannabis use can be noted in some patients with standard pharmacotherapy (223) (see chapter 6). There is no evidence that one antidepressant, anxiolytic, or antipsychotic is more effective than another. Cannabis use disorders are common in those with schizophrenic spectrum disorders; however, there is no current literature that guides clinicians in the best treatment approaches for this dual diagnosis (227).

Knowledge, however, is slowly emerging to guide pharmacological therapies for cannabis-induced problems in the 21st century.

Individuals with co-occurrence of cannabis and tobacco use tend to have higher abstinence rates if treatment includes measures aimed at dual abstinence (24). Thus, pharmacotherapy for nicotine addiction may help the individual stop marijuana use as well by removing use of, and thus influence of, tobacco. Pot-associated persistent insomnia may be improved with use of trazodone. Research is looking at new methods of treatment that will emerge from the study of the genetics of addiction including gene-milieu interplay and role of genetic variation (228) (see chapter 3).

8.2.11 Cannabis intoxication

Pharmacological management typically centers on use of benzodiazepines or atypical antipsychotics. Propranolol and rimonabant (vida infra) have been reported to be beneficial in the management of acute, physiological effects of cannabis intoxication; use of flumazenil and CBD is under current study in this regard (229).

8.2.12 Cannabis withdrawal

Oral THC (dronabinol) may relieve cannabis *withdrawal* symptoms but not relapse (230,231). Adding dronabinol and lofexidine (alpha-adrenergic receptor agonist) can lower the severity of withdrawal and lower relapse rates in those with cannabis dependence (232). The antidepressant mirtazapine can also help those undergoing cannabis withdrawal.

8.3 Cannabis-associated psychosis

CBD has been shown in animal and human studies to have antipsychotic effects, and it may become a useful pharmacotherapeutic agent for schizophrenia management (205). Research has therapeutically targeted the CB1R since delta-9-THC is a partial CB1R agonist. Treatment of patients with psychotic disorders and cannabis use should include seeking to reduce or stop the cannabis use, perhaps using cannabinoid agonist medication (219). Those with psychosis can be provided with appropriate antipsychotic medications.

8.3.1 Cannabis dependence

Nabilone is a synthetic THC analogue with improved bioavailability over dronabinol and is under current research as a potential medication for marijuana *dependence* because it may lead to a positive mood and limited adverse cognitive effects in marijuana smokers (233) (see chapter 6). Olanzapine can reduce psychomimetic effects of THC in some individuals, and its potential benefit is under study (234). Rimonabant and the anxiolytic buspirone have provided some efficacy in cannabis addicts on maintenance therapy (see chapter 6). Rimonabant is a CB1-selective cannabinoid receptor antagonist/inverse agonist that has been under research for obesity treatment as well as treatment of nicotine and marijuana addiction. It is not available in the United States and was pulled from the European market in October of 2008 due to a high risk-to-benefit ratio; concerns have been identified regarding major psychiatric adverse effects (i.e., depression and suicide) as well as overall efficacy (166).

8.3.1.1 Oxytocin

Animal research notes that various drugs, including cannabis, can induce chronic changes in markers of oxytocin function with resultant social behavior dysfunction. Oxytocin is a neurohypophyseal hormone that has been under research in the regulation of drug abuse (235). This neuropeptide may serve as a neuromodulator on neurotransmission of dopamine in the nucleus accumbens as well as effects on the hippocampus (235). CNS oxytocin pathways may offer a way of improving mood and social deficits found in some individuals with drug addiction (236). Research suggests that use of intranasal oxytocin may be useful in correcting the negative cannabis (and other illicit drug) effect on social behavior and perhaps protect the individual from addictive disorders (237).

8.3.1.2 N-acetylcysteine (NAC)

NAC has been shown to be useful in management of cannabis-dependent adolescents and young adults due to modulation of glutamate in the nucleus accumbens; it is suggested as an adjuvant treatment (1,200 mg per day) along with psychological management (238) (see chapters 6 and 16).

8.3.1.3 Others

Research has failed to validate the use of *naltrexone* for the treatment of cannabis dependence. *Entacapone* is a member of the drug class called nitrocatechols that is used in the management of Parkinson's disease. It is an inhibitor of catechol-O-methyltransferase and is under research as a possible drug for cannabis dependence.

Other drugs under research include lithium, dronabinol, URB597 (fatty acid amide hydrolase inhibitor), methyllycaconitine or MLA (nicotinic alpha-7-receptor antagonist), and endocannabinoid metabolizing enzymes (239).

8.4 Summary

Research must provide more specific information on how cannabis and products derived from cannabis can be useful in medical management of illness or if the cannabis risks simply outweigh any potential benefit (240). Does cannabis have advantages over specific cannabinoids? Can the psychotropic effects of cannabis be reduced while utilizing potential medicinal benefits of CB1R activation? Oral cannabis undergoes changes that produce a narrower therapeutic window and raises questions regarding whether or not medicinal cannabis products can be given orally or must be used as a mist or smoke for positive and optimal benefit. It is difficult to find an oral dose that benefits most without induced unacceptable or unwanted adverse effects in many unwary consumers (240).

Generalized consumption of the unprocessed *C. sativa* plant can lead to considerable public health risks including increased schizophrenia, psychosis, dependence, and other risks as noted in this review (241). A medical role for specific cannabinoid compounds remains under active medical research (242,243). What is well known is that there are many potential medical and psychiatric adverse effects to smoking cannabis and its synthetic derivatives. Links between use of alcohol, cannabis, and other illicit drugs continues to be unveiled by research (244). Research is identifying new techniques of cannabis identification to assist the police and other authorities in forensic investigation (245). Finally, treatment of an individual with cannabis dependence is very difficult and requires more research in the 21st century (246,247). Indeed, *C. sativa*, a controversial plant known for thousands of years, remains disputatious and contentious in the 21st century (248).

References

1. Tashkin DP. Smoked marijuana as a cause of lung injury. Monaldi Arch Chest Dis 2005;63(2): 93–100.
2. Anthony JC. Steppingstone and gateway ideals: A discussion of origins, research challenges, and promising lines of research for the future. Drug Alcohol Depend 2012.
3. Fischer B, Jones W, Shuper P, Rehm J. 12-month follow-up of an exploratory "brief intervention" for high-frequency cannabis use among Canadian university students. Subst Abuse Treat Prev Policy 2012;7(1):15.
4. Shoyama Y, Tamada T, Kurihara K, Takeuchi A, Taura F, Arai S, et al. Structure and function of Δ1-tetrahydrocannabinolic acid (THCA) synthase, the enzyme controlling the psychoactivity of Cannabis sativa. J Mol Biol 2012;423(1):96–105.
5. Greydanus DE, Reed WJ. Substance use and abuse in adolescents. In: Greydanus DE, Patel DR, Pratt HD, Calles JL Jr, eds. Behavioral pediatrics. New York: Nova Science, 2009:426–8.

6. Goullé JP, Saussereau E, Lacroix C. Delta-9-tetrahydrocannabinol pharmacokinetics. Ann Pharm Fr 2008;66(4):232–44.
7. Tsumura Y, Aoki R, Tokieda Y, Akutsu M, Kawase Y, Kataoka T, et al. A survey of the potency of Japanese illicit cannabis in fiscal year 2010. Forensic Sci Int 2012;221(1–3):77–83.
8. Greydanus DE, Patel DR. Substance abuse in the adolescent. In: Greydanus DE, Patel DR, Pratt HD, eds. Essential adolescent medicine. New York: McGraw-Hill, 2006:704–5.
9. Clark PA, Capuzzi K, Fick C. Medical marijuana: Medical necessity versus political agenda. Med Sci Mont 2011;17(12):RA249–61.
10. Steppan M, Kraus L, Piontek D, Siciliano V. Are cannabis prevalence estimates comparable across countries and regions? A cross-cultural validation using search engine query data. Int J Drug Policy 2013;24(1):23–9.
11. Thomas KV, Bijlsma L, Castiglioni S, Covaci A, Emke E, Grabic R, et al. Comparing illicit drug use in 19 European cities through sewage analysis. Sci Total Environ 2012;432:432–9.
12. Kolliakou A, Fusar-Poli P, Atakan Z. Cannabis abuse and vulnerability to psychosis: Targeting preventive services. Curr Pharm Des 2012;18(4):542–9.
13. Teesson M, Slade T, Swift W, Mills K, Memedovic S, Mewton L, et al. Prevalence, correlates and comorbidity of DSM-IV cannabis use and cannabis use disorders in Australia. Aust NZ J Psychiatry 2012;46(12):1182–92.
14. Greydanus DE, Feucht CL, Hawver EK. Substance abuse disorders. In: Greydanus DE, Patel DR, Omar HA, Feucht C, Merrick J, eds. Adolescent medicine: Pharmacotherapeutics in general, mental, and sexual health. Berlin: De Gruyter, 2012:157–99.
15. Greydanus DE, Patel DR. Substance abuse in adolescents: A complex conundrum for the clinician. Pediatr Clin North Am 2003;59(5):1179–223.
16. Greydanus DE, Patel DR. Substance abuse in adolescents: Current concepts. Dis-A-Mon 2005; 51(7):392–431.
17. Fischer B, Dawe M, McGuire F, Shuper PA, Capler R, Bilsker D, et al. Feasibility and impact of brief interventions for frequent cannabis users in Canada. J Subst Abuse Treat 2013;44(1):132–8.
18. Youth Risk Behavior Surveillance (YRBS) – U.S. 2009. MMWR 2010;59(SS-5):1–142.
19. Ivanov I, Pearson A, Kaplan K, Newcorn J. Attention deficit hyperactivity disorder and comorbid substance abuse. In: Greydanus DE, Calles JL Jr, Patel DR, Nazeer A, Merrick J, eds. Clinical aspects of psychopharmacology in childhood and adolescence. New York: Nova Science, 2011:33–49.
20. Bonn-Miller MO, Harris AH, Trafton JA. Prevalence of cannabis use disorders diagnoses among veterans in 2002, 2008, and 2009. Psychol Serv 2012;9(4):404–16.
21. Mehrpour O, Karrari P, Afshari R. Recreational use and overdose of ingested processed cannabis (Majoon Birjandi) in the eastern Iran. Hum Exp Toxicol 2012;31(11):1188–9.
22. Lipperman-Kreda S, Lee JP. Boost your high: Cigarette smoking to enhance alcohol and drug effects among Southeast Asian American youth. J Drug Issues 2011;41(4):509–22.
23. Greydanus DE, Feucht C, Patel DR. Substance abuse disorders in adolescents: Pharmacologic management. In: Greydanus DE, Calles JL Jr, Patel DR, Nazeer A, Merrick J, eds. Clinical aspects of psychopharmacology in childhood and adolescence. New York: Nova Science, 2011:178.
24. Agrawal A, Budney AJ, Lynskey MT. The co-occurring use and misuse of cannabis and tobacco: A review. Addiction 2012;107(7):1221–33.
25. Simmons MS, Tashkin DP. The relationship of tobacco and marijuana smoking characteristics. Life Sci 1995;56(23–24):2185–91.
26. American Psychiatric Association. Diagnostic and statistical manual of mental disorders, 4th ed., text rev. Washington, DC: American Psychiatric Association, 2000.
27. Olthuis JV, Darredeau C, Barrett SP. Substance use initiation: The role of simultaneous polysubstance use. Drug Alcohol Rev 2013;32(1):67–71.
28. Barrett SP, Darredeau C, Pihl RO. Patterns of simultaneous polysubstance use in drug using university students. Hum Psychopharmacol 2006;21(4);255–63.

29. Sartor CE, Agrawal A, Lynskey MT, Duncan AE, Grant JD, Nelson EC, et al. Cannabis or alcohol first? Differences by ethnicity and in risk for rapid progression to cannabis-related problems in women. Psychol Med 2012:1–11.
30. Bowes L, Chollet A, Fombonne E, Galéra C, Melchior M. Lifetime SEP and tobacco and cannabis use. Eur J Public Health 2013;23(2):322–7.
31. Pesce A, West C, Rosenthal M, West R, Crews B, Mikel C, et al. Marijuana correlates with use of other illicit drugs in a pain patient population. Pain Physician 2010;13(3):283–7.
32. O'Brien MS, Comment LA, Liang KY, Anthony JC. Does cannabis onset trigger cocaine onset? A case crossover approach. Int J Methods Psychiatr Res 2012;21(1):66–75.
33. Malinowska B, Baranowska-Kuczko M, Schlicker E. Triphasic blood pressure responses to cannabinoids: Do we understand the mechanism? Br J Pharmacol 2012;165(7):2073–88.
34. Fusar-Poli P, Crippa JA, Bhattacharyva S, Borgwardt SJ, Allen P, Martin-Santos R, et al. Distinct effects of [delta]9-tetrahydrcannabinol ad cannabidiol on neural activation during emotional processing. Arch Gen Psychiatry 2009;66(1):95–105.
35. Borgwardt SJ, Allen P, Bhattacharyya S, Fusar-Poli P, Cirppa JA, Seal ML, et al. Neural basis of Delta-9-tetrahydrocannabinol and cannabidiol: Effects during response inhibition. Biol Psychiatry 2008;64(11):966–73.
36. Bergamaschi MM, Queiroz RH, Zuardi AW, Crippa JA. Safety and side effects of cannabidiol: A Cannabis sativa constituent. Curr Drug Saf 2011;6(4):237–49.
37. Solinas M, Yasar S, Goldberg SR. Endocannabinoid system involvement in brain reward processes related to drug abuse. Pharmacol Res 2007;56(5):393–405.
38. Grotenhermen F. Cannabinoids. Curr Drug Targets CNS Neurol Disord 2005;4(5):507–30.
39. Mechoulam R, Parker LA. The endocannabinoid system and the brain. Annu Rev Psychol 2013; 64:21–47.
40. Zanettini C, Panlilio LV, Alicki M, Goldberg SR, Haller J, Yasar S. Effects of endocannabinoid system modulation on cognitive and emotional behavior. Front Behav Neurosci 2011;5:57–62.
41. Marco EM, Garcia-Gutiérrez MS, Bermúdez-Silva FJ, Moreira FA, Guimarães F, Manzanares J, et al. Endocannabinoid system and psychiatry: In search of a neurobiological basis for detrimental and potential therapeutic effects. Front Behav Neurosci 2011;55:63–70.
42. Fattore L, Spano MS, Deiana S, Melis V, Cossu G, Fadda P, et al. An endocannabinoid mechanism in relapse to drug seeking: A review of animal studies and clinical perspectives. Brain Res Rev 2007;53(1):1–16.
43. Trezza V, Cuomo V, Vanderschuren LJ. Cannabis and the developing brain: Insights from behavior. Eur J Pharmacol 2008;585(2–3):441–52.
44. Iversen L. Cannabis and the brain. Brain 2003;26(Pt 6):1252–70.
45. Marriott KS, Huffman JW. Recent advances in the development of selective ligands for the cannabinoid CB (2) receptor. Curr Top Med Chem 2008;8(3):187–204.
46. Guindon J, Hohmann AG. The endocannabinoid system and cancer: Therapeutic implication. Br J Pharmacol 2011;163(7):1447–63.
47. Caballero A, Tseng KY. Association of cannabis use during adolescence, prefrontal CB1 receptor signaling, and schizophrenia. Front Pharmacol 2012;3:101–4.
48. Hall W. The adverse health effects of cannabis use: What are they, and what are their implications for policy? Int J Drug Policy 2009;20(6):458–66.
49. Hazelkamp A, Fischedick JT. Cannabis-from cultivar to chemovar. Drug Test Anal 2012;4(7–8): 660–7.
50. Cannabis-based medicines – GW pharmaceuticals: High CBD, high THC, medicinal cannabis – GW pharmaceuticals, THC:CBD. Drugs R D 2003;4(5):306–9.
51. Naftali T, Lev LB, Yablecovitch D, Half E, Konikoff FM. Treatment of Crohn's disease with cannabis: An observational study. Isr Med Assoc J 2011;13(8):455–8.
52. Collen M. Prescribing cannabis for harm reduction. Harm Reduct J 2012;9(1):1.

53. Fernandez-Ruiz J. Cannabinoid drugs for neurological diseases: What is behind? Rev Neurol 2012;54(10):613–28.
54. Kraft B. Is there any clinically relevant cannabinoid-induced analgesia? Pharmacology 2012;89 (5–6):237–46.
55. Sidney S. Cardiovascular consequences of marijuana use. J Clin Pharmacol 2002;42(11 Suppl): 64S–70S.
56. Zajicek JP, Hobart JC, Slade A, Barnes D, Mattison PG, Multiple sclerosis and extract of cannabis of the MUSIC Group. J Neurol Neurosurg Psychiatry 2012;83(11):1125–32.
57. Hofmann ME, Frazier CJ. Marijuana, endocannabinoids, and epilepsy: Potential and challenges for improved therapeutic intervention. Exp Neurol 2011;233:112–25.
58. Calvaruso G, Pellerito O, Notaro A, Giuliano M. Cannabinoid-associated cell death mechanisms in tumor models (review). Int J Oncol 2012;41(2):407–13.
59. Corey-Bloom J, Wolfson T, Gamst A, Jin S, Marcotte TD, Bentley H, et al. Smoked cannabis for spasticity in multiple sclerosis: A randomized, placebo-controlled study. CMAJ 2012;184(10): 1143–50.
60. Wade D. Evaluation of the safety and tolerability profile of Sativex: Is it reassuring enough? Expert Rev Neurother 2012;12(4 Suppl):9–14.
61. Jones NA, Glyn SE, Akiyama S, Hill TD, Hill AJ, Weston SE, et al. Cannabidiol exerts anti-convulsant effects in animal models of temporal lobe and partial seizures. Seizure 2012;21(5):344–52.
62. Caffarel MM, Andradas C, Pérez-Gómez E, Guzmán M, Sánchez C. Cannabinoids: A new hope for breast cancer therapy? Cancer Treat Rev 2012;38(7):911–8.
63. Styrczewska M, Kulma A, Ratajczak K, Amarowicz R, Szope J. Cannabinoid-like anti-inflammatory compounds from flax fiber. Cell Mol Biol Lett 2012;17(3):479–99.
64. Esposito G, Filippis DD, Cirillo C, Luvone T, Capoccia E, Scuderi C, et al. Cannabidiol in inflammatory bowel diseases: An overview. Phytother Res 2012;27(5):633–6.
65. De Vries K, Green AJ. Therapeutic use of cannabis. Nurs Times 2012;108(9):12–5.
66. Klumpers LE, Beumer TL, van Hasselt JG, Lipplaa A, Karger LB, Kleinloog HD, et al. Novel delta-9-tetrahydrocannabinol formulation Namisol has beneficial pharmacokinetics and promising phamacodynamics effects. Br J Clin Pharmacol 2011;72(12):810–6.
67. Tambaro S, Bortolato M. Cannabinoid-related agents in the treatment of anxiety disorders: Current knowledge and future perspectives. Recent Pat CNS Drug Discov 2012;7(1):25–40.
68. Schier AR, Ribeiro NP, Silva AC, Hallak JE, Crippa JA, Nardi AE, et al. Cannabidiol, a Cannabis sativa constituent, as an anxiolytic drug. Rev Bras Psiquiatr 2012;34(Suppl 1):104–10.
69. Passie T, Emrich HM, Karst M, Brandt SD, Halpern JH. Mitigation of post-traumatic stress symptoms by Cannabis resin: A review of the clinical and neurobiological evidence. Drug Test Anal 2012;4(7–8):649–59.
70. Stern CA, Gazarini L, Takahashi RN, Guimarães FS, Bertolglio LJ. On disruption of fear memory by reconsolidation blockage: Evidence from cannabidiol treatment. Neuropsychopharmacology 2012;37(9):2132–42.
71. Kolliakou A, Ismail K, Atakan Z. Why do psychotic patients use cannabis? Case series. Curr Pharm Des 2012;18(32):4950–9.
72. Grant I, Atkinson JH, Gouaux B, Wilsey B. Medical marijuana: Clearing away the smoke. Open Neurol J 2012;6:18–25.
73. Fattore L, Fratta W. Beyond THC: The new generation of cannabinoid designer drugs. Front Behav Neurosci 2011;5:60–4.
74. Berkovitz R, Arieli M, Marom E. Synthetic cannabinoids – the new "legal high" drugs. Harefuah 2011;150(12):884–7.
75. Hilderbrand RL. High-performance sport, marijuana, and cannabimimetics. J Anal Toxicol 2011;35(9):624–37.

76. Castellanos D, Thornton G. Synthetic cannabinoid use: Recognition and management. J Psychiatr Pract 2012;18(2):86–93.
77. Seely KA, Lapoint J, Moran JH, Fattore L. Spice drugs are more than harmless herbal blends: A review of the pharmacology and toxicology of synthetic cannabinoids. Prog Neuropsychopharmacol Biol Psychiatry 2012;39(2):234–43.
78. Bebarta VS, Ramirez S, Varney SM. Spice: A new "legal" herbal mixture abused by young active duty military personnel. Subst Abus 2012;33(2):191–4.
79. Karila Petit A, Cottencin O, Coscas S, Reynaud M. Synthetic drugs: The new low-cost landscape of drugs. Rev Prat 2012;62(5):664–6.
80. Rosenbaum CD, Carreiro SP, Babu KM. Here today, gone tomorrow . . . back again? A review of herbal marijuana alternatives (K2, Spice), synthetic cathinones (bath salts), Kratom, Salvia divinorum, methoxetamie, and piperazines. J Med Toxicol 2012;8(1):15–32.
81. Funada M. Pharmacological properties and dependence liabilities of synthetic cannabinoids. Nihon Arukoru Yakubutsu Igakkai Zasshi 2010;45(3):167–74.
82. Johnson LA, Johnson RL, Alfonzo C. Spice: A legal marijuana equivalent. Mil Med 2011;176(6):718–20.
83. Schneir AB, Cullen J, Ly BT. "Spice" girls: Synthetic cannabinoid intoxication. J Emerg Med 2011;40(3):296–9.
84. Ginsburg BC, McMahon LR, Sanchez JJ, Javors MA. Purity of synthetic cannabinoids sold online for recreational use. J Anal Toxicol 2012;36(1):66–8.
85. De Backer B, Maebe Verstraete AG, Charlier C. Evolution of the content of THC and other major cannabinoids in drug-type cannabis cuttings and seedlings during growth of plants. J Forensic Sci 2012;57(4):918–22.
86. Köhnemann S, Nedele J, Schwotzer D, Morzfeld J, Pfeiffer H. The validation of a 15 STR multiplex PCR for Cannabis species. Int J Legal Med 2012;126(4):601–6.
87. Mura P, Saussereau E, Brunet B, Goulié JP. Workplace testing of drugs of abuse and psychotropic drugs. Ann Pharm Fr 2012;70(3):120–32.
88. Salomone A, Gerace E, E'Urso F, Di Corcia D, Vincenti M. Simultaneous analysis of several synthetic cannabinoids, THC, CBD, and CBN, in hair by ultra-high performance liquid chromatography tandem mass spectrometry: Method validation and application to real samples. J Mass Spectrom 2012;47(5):604–12.
89. Adverse effects of cannabis. Prescrire Int 2011;20(112):18–23.
90. Kalant H. Adverse effects of cannabis on health: An update of the literature since 1996. Prog Neuropsychopharmacol Biol Psychiatry 2004;28(5):849–63.
91. Monshouwer K, Van Dorsselaer S, Verdurmen J, Bogt TT, De Graaf R, Vollegergh W. Cannabis use and mental health in secondary children: Findings from a Dutch survey. Br J Psychiatry 2006;188:148–53.
92. Lee MH, Hancox RJ. Effects of smoking cannabis on lung function. Expert Rev Respir Med 2011;5(4):537–46.
93. Howden ML, Naughton MT. Pulmonary effects of marijuana inhalation. Expert Rev Respir Med 2011;5(1):87–92.
94. Zarfin Y, Yefet E, Abozaid S, Nasser WM, Finkelstein Y. Infant with altered consciousness after cannabis passive inhalation. Child Abuse Negl 2012;36(2):81–3.
95. Molly C, Mory O, Basset T, Patural H. Acute cannabis poisoning in a 10-month-old infant. Arch Pediatr 2012;19(7):729–32.
96. Mallaret M, Dal'Bo-Rohrer D, Demattéis M. Adverse effects of marijuana. Rev Prat 2005;55(1):41–9.
97. Davis GP, Gunderson EW. Evaluation of chronic cough should consider cannabis use. Am Fam Physician 2012;85(7):680–2.

98. Benich JJ III, Carek PJ. Evaluation of the patient with chronic cough. Am Fam Physician 2011; 84(8):887–92.
99. Bonnet U. Chronic cannabis abuse, delta-9-tetrahydrocannabinol and thyroid function and thyroid function. Pharmacopsychiatry 2013;46(1):35–6.
100. Fatma H, Mouna B, Leila M, Radhouane D, Taoufik N. Cannabis: A rare case of acute pancreatitis. Clin Res Hepatol Gastroenterol 2013;37(1):e24–5.
101. Spadari M, Canioni D, Gregoire E, Drouet G, Bourdon JA, Arditti J, et al. Cannabis body packing: Two case reports. Clin Toxicol (Phila) 2011;49(9):862–4.
102. Simonetto DA, Oxentenko AS, Herman ML, Szostek JH. Cannabinoid hyperemesis: A case series of 98 patients. Mayo Clin Proc 2012;87(2):114–9.
103. Fleig S, Brunkhorst R. Hyperemesis and a high water bill. Z Gastroenterol 2011;49(11):1479–81.
104. Galli JA, Sawaya RA, Friedenberg FK. Cannabinoid hyperemesis syndrome. Curr Drug Abuse Rev 2011;4(4):241–9.
105. Wallace EA, Andrews SE, Garmany CL, Jelley MJ. Cannabinoid hyperemesis syndrome: Literature review and proposed diagnosis and treatment algorithm. South Med J 2011;104(9):659–64.
106. Nicolson SE, Denysenko L, Mulcare JL, Vito JP, Chabon B. Cannabinoid hyperemesis syndrome: A case series and review of previous reports. Psychosomatics 2012;53(3):212–9.
107. Luther V, Yap L. A hot bath to calm what ails you: The cannabis hyperemesis syndrome. Acute Med 2012;11(1):23–4.
108. Wild K, Wilson H. Cannabinoid hyperemesis. Emerg Med J 2012;29(1):67–9.
109. Cho CM, Hirsch R, Johnstone S. General and oral health implications of cannabis use. Aust Dent J 2005;50(2):70–4.
110. Maloney WJ. Significance of cannabis use to dental practice. J Mich Dent Assoc 2011;93(11): 44–8.
111. Maloney WJ. Significance of cannabis use to dental practice. Today's FDA 2012;24(1):43–5.
112. Lopes CF, de Angelis BB, Prudente HM, de Souza BV, Cardoso SV, de Azambuja Ribeiro RI. Concomitant consumption of marijuana, alcohol, and tobacco in oral squamous cell carcinoma development and progression: Recent advances and challenges. Arch Oral Biol 2012;57(8):1026–33.
113. Pletcher MJ, Vittinghoff E, Kalhan R, Richman J, Safford M, Sidney S, et al. Association between marijuana exposure and pulmonary function over 20 years. JAMA 2012;307(2):173–81.
114. Ribeiro A, Ferraz-de-Paula V, Pinheiro ML, Vitoretti LB, Mariano-Souza DP, Quinteiro-Filho WM, et al. Cannabidiol, a non-psychotropic plant-derived cannabinoid, decreases inflammation in a murine model of acute lung injury: Role for the adenosine A (2A) receptor. Eur J Pharmacol 2012;678(1–3):78–85.
115. Tashkin DP. Airway effects of marijuana, cocaine, and other inhaled illicit agents. Curr Opin Pulm Med 2001;7(2):43–61.
116. Pfeifer AK, Lange P. Pulmonary consequences of marijuana smoking. Ugeskr Laeger 2006; 168(1):1743–6.
117. Szyper-Kravitz M, Lang R, Manor Y, Lahav M. Early invasive pulmonary aspergillosis in a leukemia patient linked to aspergillus contaminated marijuana smoking. Leuk Lymphoma 2001; 42(6):1433–7.
118. Aldington S, Williams S, Nowitz M, Weatherall M, Pritchard A, McNaughton A, et al. Effects of cannabis on pulmonary structure, function, and symptoms. Thorax 2007;62(12):1058–63.
119. Wu TC, Tashkin DP, Djahed B, Rose JE. Pulmonary hazards of smoking marijuana as compared with tobacco. N Engl J Med 1988;318(6):347–51.
120. Reid PT, Macleod J, Robertson JR. Cannabis and the lung. JR Coll Physicians Edinb 2010; 40(4):328–33.
121. Tan WC, Lo C, Jong A, Xing L, Fizgerald MJ, Vollmer WM, et al. Marijuana and chronic obstructive lung disease: a population-based study. CMAJ 2009;180(8):814–20.

122. Van Hoozen BE, Cross CE. Marijuana: Respiratory tract effects. Clin Rev Allergy Immunol 1997;15(3):243–69.
123. Kothadia JP, Chhabra S, Marcus A, May M, Saraiya B, Jabbour SK. Anterior mediastinal mass in a young marijuana smoker: A rare case of small-cell lung cancer. Case Report Med 2012 Apr 1; 2012:754231.
124. Quoix E. Novel epidemiology in lung cancer-nonsmokers, women and cannabis. Rev Mal Respir 2007;24(8 Pt 2):6S20–5.
125. Chen AL, Chen TJ, Braverman ER, Acuri V, Kemer M, Varshavskiy M, et al. Hypothesizing that marijuana smokers are at significantly lower risk of carcinogenicity relative to tobacco-non-marijuana smokers: Evidence based on statistical reevaluation of current literature. J Psychoactive Drugs 2008;40(3):263–72.
126. Quoix E. What is new in the epidemiology of lung cancer: Non-smokers, women, and the role of cannabis. Rev Pratt 2009;59(7):920–4.
127. Quoix E, Lemarié E. Epidemiological novelties in lung cancer. Rev Mal Respir 2011;28(8):1048–58.
128. Montecucco F, Di Marzo V. At the heart of the matter: The endocannabinoid system in cardiovascular function and dysfunction. Trends Pharmacol Sci 2012;33(6):331–40.
129. Pratap B, Komiyenko A. Toxic effects of marijuana on the cardiovascular system. Cardiovasc Toxicol. 2011;11:4–10.
130. Romero-Puche AJ, Trigueros-Ruiz N, Cerdán-Sánchez MC, Pérez-Lorente F, Roldán D, Vicente-Vera T. Brugada electrocardiogram pattern induced by cannabis. Rev Esp Cardiol 2012;65(9): 856–8.
131. Irani F, Kasmani R, Kanjwai Y. Hyperkalemia and cocaine induced Brugada-type electrocardiogram. Eur J Emerg Med 2010;17(2):113–5.
132. Bailly C, Merceron O, Hammoudi N, Dorent R, Michel PL. Cannabis induced acute coronary syndrome in a young female. Int J Cardiol 2010;143(1):e4–6.
133. Cappelli F, Lazzeri C, Gensini GF, Valente S. Cannabis: A trigger for acute myocardial infarction? A case report. J Cardiovasc Med 2008;9(7):725–8.
134. Singla S, Sachdeva R, Mehta JL. Cannabinoids and atherosclerotic coronary heart disease. Clin Cardiol 2012;35(6):329–35.
135. Yurtdas M, Aydin MK. Acute myocardial infarction in a young man; Fatal blow of the marijuana: A case report. Korean Circ J 2012;42(9):641–5.
136. Asbridge M, Hayden JA, Cartwright JL. Acute cannabis consumption and motor vehicle collision risk: Systemic review of observational studies and meta-analysis. BMJ 2012;9;344:e536.
137. Li MC, Brady JE, DiMaggio CJ, Lusardi AR, Tzong KY, Li G. Marijuana use and motor vehicle crashes. Epidemiol Rev 2012;34(1):65–72.
138. Drabek M, Andysz A. Effects of marijuana and amphetamine (and its derivatives) on driving performance based on the driving simulator studies. Med Pr 2011;62(5):551–63.
139. Johnson MB, Kelley-Baker G, Voas RB, Lacey JH. The prevalence of cannabis-involved driving in California. Drug Alcohol Depend 2012;123(1–3):105–9.
140. Drummer OH, Kourtis I, Beyer J, Tayler P, Boorman M, Gerostamoulos D. The prevalence of drugs in injured drivers. Forensic Sci Int 2012;215(1–3):14–7.
141. Barrio G, Jimenez-Mejias E, Pulido J, Lardelli-Claret P, Bravo MJ, de la Fuenta L. Association between cannabis use and non-traffic injuries. Accid Anal Prev 2012;47:172–6.
142. Campos DR, Yonamine M, de Moraes Moreau RL. Marijuana as doping in sports. Sports Med 2003;33(6):395–9.
143. Saugy M, Avois L, Saudan C, Robinson N, Giroud C, Mangin P, et al. Cannabis and sports. Br J Sports Med 2006;40(Suppl 1):13–5.
144. Pope HG Jr, Gruber AJ, Yurgelun-Todd D. The residual neuropsychological effects of cannabis: the current status of research. Drug Alcohol Depend 1995;38(1):25–34.

145. Martin-Santos F, Fagundo AB, Crippa JA, Atakan Z, Bhattacharyya S, Allen P, et al. Neuroimaging in cannabis use: A systemic review of the literature. Psychol Med 2010;40(3):383–98.
146. Crippa JA, Lacerda AL, Amaro E, Busatto Filho G, Zuardi AW, Bressan RA. Brain effects of cannabis – neuroimaging findings. Rev Bras Psiquiatr 2005;27(1):70–8.
147. Schreiner AA, Dunn ME. Residual effects of cannabis use on neurocognitive performance after prolonged abstinence: A meta-analysis. Exp Clin Psychopharmacol 2012;20(5):420–9.
148. Montgomery C, Seddon AL, Fisk JE, Murphy PN, Jansari A. Cannabis-related deficits in real-world memory. Hum Psychopharmacol 2012;27(2):217–25.
149. Marmorstein NR, Iacono WG, McGue M. Associations between substance use disorders and major depression in parents and late adolescent-emerging adult offspring: An adoption study. Addiction 2012;107(11):1965–73.
150. Harvey MA, Sellman JD, Porter RJ, Frampton CM. The relationship between non-acute adolescent cannabis use and cognition. Drug Alcohol Res 2007;26(3):309–19.
151. Sundram S. Cannabis and neurodevelopment: Implications for psychiatric disorders. Hum Psychopharmacol 2006;21(4):245–54.
152. Schneider M. Puberty as a highly vulnerable developmental period for the consequences of cannabis exposure. Addict Biol 2008;13(2):253–63.
153. Dinieri JA, Hurd YL. Rat models of prenatal and adolescent cannabis exposure. Methods Mol Biol 2012;829:231–42.
154. Degenhardt L, Coffey C, Romaniuk H, Swift W, Carlin JB, Hall WD, et al. The persistence of the association between adolescent cannabis use and common mental disorders into young adulthood. Addiction 2013;108(1):124–33.
155. Urban NB, Slifstein M, Thompson JL, Xu X, Grigis RR, Raheja S, et al. Dopamine release in chronic cannabis uers: A [(11) C] raclopride positron emission tomography study. Biol Psychiatry 2012;71(8):677–83.
156. Zalesky A, Solowij N, Yücel M, Lubman DI, Takagi M, Harding IH, et al. Effect of long-term cannabis use on axonal fibre connectivity. Brain 2012;135(Pt 7):2245–55.
157. Leach LS, Butterworth P. The effect of early onset common mental disorders on educational attainment in Australia. Psychiatry Res 2012;199(1):51–7.
158. Yücel M, Solowij N, Respondek C, Whittle S, Fornito A, Pantelis C, et al. Regional brain abnormalities associated with long-term heavy cannabis use. Arch Gen Psychiatry 2008;65(6):694–701.
159. Abushi H, Akirav I. Short-and long-term cognitive effects of chronic cannabinoids administration in late-adolescence rats. PLoS One 2012;7(2):e31731.
160. Gordon SM, Tulak F, Troncale J. Prevalence and characteristics of adolescent patients with co-occurring ADHD and substance dependence. J Addict Dis 2004;23:31–40.
161. Dennis M, Godley SH, Diamond G, Tims FM, Babor T, Donaldson J, et al. The Cannais Youth Treatment (CYT) Study: Main findings from two randomized trials. J Subst Abuse Treat 2004;27(3):197–213.
162. Han S, Yang BZ, Kranzler HR, Oslin D, Anton R, Farrer LA, et al. Linkage analysis followed by association shown NRG1 associated with cannabis dependence in African Americans. Biol Psychiatry 2012;15;72(8):637–44.
163. Hürlimann F, Kupferschmid S, Simon AE. Cannabis-induced depersonalization disorder in adolescence: Cannabis-induced depersonalization disorder in adolescents. Neuropsychobiology 2012;65(3):141–6.
164. Horwood LJ, Fergusson DM, Coffey C, Patton GC, Tait R, Smart D, et al. Cannabis and depression: An integrative data analysis of four Australasian cohorts. Drug Alcohol Depend 2012;126(3):369–78.
165. Van Dam NT, Bedi G, Earleywine M. Characteristics of clinically anxious versus non-anxious regular, heavy marijuana users. Addict Behav 2012;37(11):1217–23.

166. Budney AJ. Should cannabis withdrawal disorder be included in DSM-5? Psychiatric Times 2011;28(2):48–50.
167. Budney AJ, Hughes JR, Moore BA, Vandrey R. Review of the validity and significance of cannabis withdrawal syndrome. Am J Psychiatry 2004;161:1967–77.
168. Budney AJ, Hughes JR. The cannabis withdrawal syndrome. Curr Opin Psychiatry 2006;19: 233–8.
169. Crowley TJ, MacDonald MJ, Whitmore EA. Cannabis dependence, withdrawal, and reinforcing effects among adolescents with conduct symptoms and substance use disorders. Drug Alcohol Depend 1998;50:27–37.
170. Vandrey RG, Budney AJ, Hughes JR, Liguoria A. A within-subject comparison of withdrawal symptoms during abstinence from cannabis, tobacco, and both substances. Drug Alcohol Depend 2008;92(1–3):48–54.
171. Arendt M, Rosenberg R, Fjordback L, Brandholdt J, Foldager L, Sher L, et al. Testing the self-medication hypothesis of depression and aggression in cannabis-dependent subjects. Psychol Med 2007;37(7):935–45.
172. Calles JL Jr, Nazeer A. Aggressive and violent behavior. In: Greydanus DE, Calles JL Jr, Patel DR, Nazeer A, Merrick J, eds. Clinical aspects of psychopharmacology in childhood and adolescence. New York: Nova Science Publishers, 2011:106.
173. Schacht JP, Hutchinson KE, Filbey FM. Associations between cannabinoid-receptor-1 (CNR1) variation and hippocampus and amygdale volumes in heavy cannabis users. Neuropsychopharmacology 2012;37(11):2368–76.
174. Haney M, Hart CL, Vosburg KD. Marijuana withdrawal in humans: Effects of oral THC or divalproex. Neuropsychopharmacology 2004;29:158–70.
175. Milin R, Manion I, Dare G, Walker S. Prospective assessment of cannabis withdrawal in adolescents with cannabis dependence: A pilot study. J Am Acad Child Adolesc Psychiatry 2008;47:174–8.
176. Cornelius JR, Chung T, Martin C, et al. Cannabis withdrawal is common among treatment seeking adolescents with cannabis dependence and major depression, and is associated with rapid relapse to dependence. Addict Behav 2008;103:787–99.
177. Gorelick DA, Levin KH, Copersino ML, Heishman SJ, Liu F, Boggs DL, et al. Diagnostic criteria for cannabis withdrawal syndrome. Drug Alcohol Depend 2012;123(1–3):141–7.
178. Gardner EL. Addictive potential of cannabinoids: The underlying neurobiology. Chem Phys Lipids 2005;31;121(1–2):267–90.
179. Cooper ZD, Haney M. Cannabis reinforcement and dependence: Role of cannabinoid CB1 receptor. Addict Biol 2008;13(2):188–95.
180. Cooper ZD, Haney M. Actions of delta-9-tetrahydrocannabinol in cannabis: Relation to use, abuse, dependence. Int Rev Psychiatry 2009;2192:104–12.
181. Gardner EL. Endocannabinoid signaling system and brain reward: Emphasis on dopamine. Pharmacol Biochem Behav 2005;81(2):263–84.
182. Gardner EL. Addiction and brain reward and antireward pathways. Adv Psychosom Med 2011;30:22–60.
183. Bossong MG, van Berckel BN, Boellaard R, Zuurman L, Schuit RC, Windhorst AD, et al. Delta 9-tetrahydrocannabinol induces dopamine release in the human striatum. Neuropsychopharmacology 2009;34(3):759–66.
184. Horey JT, Mariani JJ, Cheng WY, Bisaqa A, Sullivan M, Nunes E, et al. Comparison of substance use milestones in cannabis-and cocaine-dependent patients. J Addict Dis 2012;31(1):60–6.
185. Goldstein RZ, Volkow ND. Dysfunction of the prefrontal cortex in addiction: Neuroimaging findings and clinical implications. Nat Rev Neurosci 2011;12(11):652–69.
186. Goldstein RZ, Volkow ND. Drug addiction and its underlying neurobiological basis: Neuroimaging evidence for the involvement of the frontal cortex. Am J Psychiatry 2002;159(10):1642–52.

187. Feil J, Sheppard D, Fitzgerald PB, Yücel M, Lubman DI, Bradshaw JL. Addiction, compulsive drug seeking, and the role of frontostriatal mechanisms in regulating inhibitory control. Neurosci Biobehav Rev 2010;35(2):248–75.
188. Rotter A, Bayerlein K, Hansbauer M, Weiland J, Sperling W, Kornhuber, et al. Orexin A expression and promoter methylation in patients with cannabis dependence in comparison to nicotine-dependent cigarette smokers and nonsmokers. Neuropsychobiology 2012;66(2):126–33.
189. Schafer G, Feilding A, Morgan CG, Agathangelou M, Freeman TP, Valerie Curran H. Investigating the interaction between schizotypy, divergent thinking, and cannabis use. Conscious Cogn 2002.
190. Galvez-Buccollini JA, Proal AC, Tomaselli V, Trachtenberg M, Coconcea C, Chun J, et al. Association between age at onset of psychosis and age at onset of cannabis use in non-affective psychosis. Schizophr Res 2012;139(1–3):157–60.
191. Giovanni M, Giuseppe DI, Gianna S, Domenico DB, Luisa DR, Massimo DG. Cannabis use and psychosis: Theme introduction. Curr Pharm Des 2012;18(32):4991–8.
192. Leweke FM, Koethe D. Cannabis and psychiatric disorders: It is not only addiction. Addict Biol 2008;13(2):264–75.
193. Nazeer A, Calles JL Jr. Schizophrenia in children and adolescents. In: Greydanus DE, Calles JL Jr, Patel DR, Nazeer A, Merrick J, eds. Clinical aspects of psychopharmacology in childhood and adolescence. New York: Nova Science, 2011:152.
194. Van Dijk D, Koeter MW, Hijman R, Kahn RS, van den Bring W. Effect of cannabis use on the course of schizophrenia in male patients: A prospective cohort study. Scizophr Res 2012; 137(1–3):50–7.
195. Bossong MG, Niesink RJ. Adolescent brain maturation, the endogenous cannabinoid system, and the neurobiology of cannabis-induced schizophrenia. Prog Neurobiol 2010;92(3):370–85.
196. Rapp C, Bugra H, Riecher-Rössler A, Borgwardt S. Effects of cannabis use on human brain structure in psychosis: A systematic review combining in vivo structural neuroimaging and post-mortem studies. Curr Pharm Des 2012;18(32):5070–80.
197. Khan MK, Usmani MA, Hanif SA. A case of self amputation of penis by cannabis induced psychosis. J Forensic Leg Med 2012;19(6):355–7.
198. Barrowclough C, Emsley R, Eisner E, Beardmore R, Wykes T. Does change in cannabis use in established psychosis affect clinical outcome? Schizophr Bull 2013;39(2):339–48.
199. Leweke FM. Anandamide dysfunction in prodromal and established psychosis. Curr Pharm Des 2012;18(32):5188–93.
200. Decoster J, van Os J, Myin-Germeys I, De Hert M, van Winkel R. Genetic variation underlying psychosis-inducing effects of cannabis: critical review and future directions. Curr Pharm Des 2012; 18(32):5015–23.
201. Serafini G, Pompili M, Innamorati M, Rihmer Z, Sher L, Girardi P. Can cannabis increase the suicide risk in psychosis? A critical review. Curr Pharm Des 2012;18(32):5165–87.
202. Hermann D, Schneider M. Potential protective effects of cannabidol on neuroanatomical alterations in cannabis users and psychosis: A critical review. Curr Pharm Des 2012;18(32):4897–905.
203. Lev-Ran S, Aviram A, Braw Y, Nitzan U, Ratzoni G, Fennig S. Clinical correlates of cannabis use among adolescent psychiatric inpatients. Eur Psychiatr 2012;27(6):470–5.
204. Auther AM, McLaughlin D, Carrión RE, Naqachandran P, Correll CU, Cornblatt BA. Prospective study of cannabis use in adolescents at clinical high risk for psychosis: Impact of conversion to psychosis and functional outcome. Psychol Med 2012;30:1–13.
205. Zuardi AW, Crippa JA, Bhattacharyya S, Atakan Z, Martin-Santos R, et al. A critical review of the antipsychotic effects of Cannabidiol: 30 years of translational investigation. Curr Phar Des 2012;18(32):5131–40.
206. Bhattacharyya S, Crippa JA, Allen P, Martin-Santos R, Borgwardt S, Fusar-Poli P, et al. Induction of psychosis by δ9-tetrahydrocannabinol reflects modulation of prefrontal and striatal function during attentional salience processing. Arch Gen Psychiatry 2012;69(1):27–36.

207. Blum K, Gardner E, Oscar-Berman M, Gold M. "Liking" and "wanting" linked to reward deficiency syndrome (RDS): Hypothesizing differential responsivity in brain reward circuitry. Curr Pharm Des 2012;18(1):113–8.
208. Bailén AJR, Quesada PS, Valladares MA. Decision making in cannabis users. Adicciones 2012; 24(2):161–72.
209. Van Ours JC, Williams J. The effects of cannabis use on physical and mental health. J Health Econ 2012;31(4):564–77.
210. Schifano F, Martinotti G, Cunniff A, Reissner V, Scherbaum N, Ghodse H. Impact of an 18-month, NHS-based, treatment exposure for heroin dependence: Results from the London Area Treat 2000 Study. Am J Addict 2012;21(3):268–73.
211. Porath-Waller AJ, Beasley E, Beirness DJ. A meta-analytic review of school-based prevention for cannabis use. Health Educ Behav 2010;37(5):709–23.
212. Teesson M, Newton NC, Barrett EL. Australian school-based prevention programs for alcohol and other drugs: A systemic review. Drug Alcohol Rev 2012;31(6):731–6.
213. De Looze M, Harakeh Z, van Dorsselaer SA, Raaijmakers QA, Vollebergh WH, Bogt TF. Explaining educational differences in adolescent substance use and early sexual debut: The role of parents and peers. J Adolesc 2012;35(4):1035–44.
214. Yap MB, Reavley NJ, Jorm AF. Young people's beliefs about the harmfulness of alcohol, cannabis, and tobacco for mental disorders: Findings from two Australian national youth surveys. Addiction 2012;107(4):838–47.
215. Gillespie NA, Lubke GH, Gardner CO, Neale MC, Keanler KS. Two-part random effects growth modeling to identify risks associated with alcohol and cannabis initiation, initial average use, and changes in drug consumption in s sample of adult, male twins. Drug Alcohol Depend 2012;123(1–3):220–8.
216. Abdoul H, Le Faou AL, Bouchez J, Touzeau D, Lagrue G. Cannabis cessation interventions offered to young French users: Predictors of follow-up. Encaphale 2012;38(2):141–8.
217. Scott LA, Roxburgh A, Bruno R, Matthews A. Burns L. The impact of comorbid cannabis and methamphetamine use on mental health among regular ecstasy users. Addict Behav 2012; 37(9):1058–62.
218. Friedmann PD, Green TC, Taxman FS, Harrington M, Rhodes AG, Katz E, et al. Collaborative behavioral management among parolees: Drug use, crime & re-arrest in the Step'n Out randomized trial. Addiction 2012;107(6):1099–108.
219. Baker AL, Thornton LK, Hides L, Dunlop A. Treatment of cannabis use among people with psychotic disorders: A critical review of randomised control trials. Curr Pharm Des 2012;18(32):4923–37.
220. Buckner JD, Zvolensky MJ, Schmidt NB. Cannabis-related impairment and social anxiety: the roles of gender and cannabis use motives. Addict Behav 2012;37(11):1294–7.
221. Carroll KM, Nich C, Lapaglia DM, Peters EN, Easton CJ, Petry NM. Combining cognitive behavioral therapy and contingency management to enhance their effects in treating cannabis dependence: Less can be more, more or less. Addiction 2012;107(9):1650–9.
222. Hendriks V, van der Schee E, Blanken P. Matching adolescents with a cannabis use disorder to multidimensional family therapy or cognitive behavioral therapy: Treatment effect moderators in a randomized controlled trial. Drug Alcohol Depend 2012;125(1–2):119–26.
223. Baker AL, Hides L, Lubman DI. Treatment of cannabis use among people with psychotic or depressive disorders: A systemic review. J Clin Psychiatry 2010;71(3):247–54.
224. Gates PJ, Norberg MM, Copeland J, Digiusto E. Randomised controlled trial of a noval cannabis use intervention delivered by telephone. Addiction 2012;107(12):2149–58.
225. Lindsey WT, Stewart D, Childress D. Drug interactions between common illicit drugs and prescription therapies. Am J Drug Alcohol Abuse 2012;38(4):334–43.
226. Vandrey R, Haney M. Pharmacotherapy for cannabis dependence: How close are we? CNS Drugs 2009;23:543–53.

227. Hjorthøj C, Fohlmann A, Nordentoft M. Treatment of cannabis use disorders in people with schizophrenia spectrum disorders-a systemic review. Addict Behav 2009;34(6–7):520–5.
228. Agrawal A, Verweil KJ, Gillespie NA, Health AC, Lessov-Schlaggar CN, Martin CN, et al. The genetics of addiction – a translational perspective. Transl Psychiatry 2012;2:e140.
229. Crippa JA, Derenusson GN, Chagas MH, Atakan Z, Matin-Santos R, Zuardi AW, et al. Pharmacologic interventions in the treatment of the acute effects of cannabis: A systemic review of literature. Harm Reduct J 2012;9(1):7.
230. Crippa JA, Hallak JE, Machado-de-Sousa JP, Queiroz RH, Bergamaschi M, Chagus MH, et al. Cannabidol for the treatment of cannabis withdrawal syndrome: A case report. J Clin Pharm Ther 2013;38(2):162–4.
231. Vandrey R, Stitzer ML, Mintzer MZ, Huestis MA, Murray JA, Lee D. The dose effects of short-term dronabinol (oral THC) maintenance in daily cannabis users. Drug Alcohol Depend 2013; 128(1–2):64–70.
232. Haney M, Hart CL, Vosburg KD. Effects of THC and lofexidine in a human laboratory model of marijuana withdrawal and relapse. Psychopharmacology (Berl) 2008;197:157–68.
233. Bedi G, Cooper ZD, Haney M. Subjective, cognitive and cardiovascular dose-effect profile of nabilone and dronabinol in marijuana smokers. Addict Biol 2012;17:33–39.
234. Kleinloog D, Liem-Moolenaar M, Jacobs G, Klaassen E, de Kam M, Hijman R, et al. Does olanzapine inhibit the psychomimetic effects of [Delta] 9-tetrahydrocannabinol? J Psychopharmacol 2012.
235. Sarnyai Z. Oxytocin and neuroadaptation to cocaine. Prog Brain Res 1998;119:449–66.
236. Baskerville TA, Douglas AJ. Dopamine and oxytocin interactions underlying behaviors: Potential contributions to behavioral disorders. CNS Neurosci Ther 2010;16(3):e92–123.
237. McGregor IS, Bowen MT. Breaking the loop: Oxytocin as a potential treatment for drug addiction. Horm Behav 2012;61(3):331–9.
238. Gray KM, Carpenter MJ, Baker NL, Desantis SM, Kryway E, Hartwell KJ, et al. A double-blind randomized controlled trail of N-acetylcysteine in cannabis-dependent adolescents. Am J Psychiatry 2012;169(8):805–12.
239. Weinstein AM, Gorelicki DA. Pharmacologic treatment of cannabis dependence. Curr Pharm Des 2011;17(14):1351–8.
240. Pertwee RG. Cannabis and cannabinoids: Pharmacology and rationale for clinical use. Foresch Komplementarmed 1999;Suppl 3:12–15.
241. Svrakic DM, Lustman PJ, Mallya A, Lynn TA, Finney R, Svrakic NM. Legalization, decriminalization & medicinal use of cannabis: A scientific and public health perspective. Mo Med 2012; 109(2):90–8.
242. Beaulieu P, Rice AS. The pharmacology of cannabinoids derivatives: Are there applications to treatment of pain? Ann Fr Anesth Rhanim 2002;21(6):493–508.
243. Lee MC, Ploner M, Wiech K, Bingel U, Wanigasekera V, Brooks J et al. Amygdala activity contributes to the dissociative effect of cannabis on pain perception. Pain 2013;154(1):124–34.
244. Richardson GA, Larkby C, Goldschmidt L, Day NL. Adolescent initiation of drug use effects of prenatal cocaine exposure. J Am Acad Child Adolesc Psychiatry 2013;52(1):37–46.
245. Mercolini L, Mandrioli R, Sorella V, Somaini L, Giocondi D, Serpelloni G, et al. Dried blood spots: Liquid chromatography-mass spectrometry analysis of delta-9-tetrahydrocannabinol and its main metabolites. J Chromatogr A 2013;1271(1):33–40.
246. Danovitch I, Gorelick DA. State of the art treatments for cannabis dependence. Psychiatr Clin No Amer 2012;35(2);309–26.
247. Forray A, Sofuoglu M. Future pharmacologic treatments for substance use disorders. Br J Clin Pharmacol 2012. doi: 10.1111/j.1365–2125.2012.04474.x.
248. Greydanus DE, Feucht C, Hawver EK. Substance abuse and adolescence. Int J Child Health Hum Dev 2012;5(2):149–79.

9 Primary care management of alcohol use disorders of adolescents and young adults

Angela Nash and Oscar G Bukstein

Prevalence of drinking by adolescents increases dramatically from the stages of late elementary through young adulthood, and most engage in dangerous patterns of binge drinking. Problems and disorders associated with alcohol use are responsible for a significant portion of the morbidity and mortality of individuals ages 12–24. Primary care providers (PCPs) are in unique positions to identify and influence the alcohol use of their patients. This chapter provides information on the spectrum of alcohol use and abuse by adolescent and college-age youth and gives practical empirically sound advice on screening, brief interventions (BIs), and referral to higher levels of treatment for youth of this age. It also touches on the identification and treatment of sedative and hypnotics abuse by adolescents.

9.1 Introduction

Alcohol use by high school and college-age students is prevalent and is associated with substantial harm and an increased risk for the development of alcohol abuse and dependence. According to national surveys in 2011, 15% of 8th graders and 51% of 12th graders report having been drunk or ridden in a car driven by someone who had been drinking at least once in their life (1–2). Of seniors in high school, 31% admit to binge drinking, and more than 13% report having driven a vehicle while under the influence of alcohol at least once in the past month (1–2). Alcohol contributes to all four of the major causes of death for people ages 10–24 (motor vehicle crashes [26%], other unintentional injuries [17%], homicide [16%], and suicide [13%]) (1–4). Even in the absence of concern for alcohol use disorders (AUDs), alcohol use should be a priority topic for pediatric PCPs to address with their adolescent patients (see chapter 13). During the transition from child to adult, adolescents are exercising autonomy over many of the decisions that influence their health. PCPs have the privilege of influencing many of the health care choices their young patients make.

The purpose of this chapter is to provide the PCP with empirically sound and clinically useful information on the spectrum of alcohol use and associated problems among adolescent and college-age youth. Information on rapid screening and risk assessment will be provided. An introduction to screening, brief intervention, and referral to treatment (SBIRT), an effective office-based intervention for youth at low or moderate risk, will be presented. The chapter will conclude with a brief overview of treatment issues for benzodiazepine abuse.

9.2 Epidemiology: Drinking patterns and beverage preferences

9.2.1 Drinking patterns

According to the Monitoring the Future (MTF) annual survey, alcohol use by youth is widespread despite its being illegal for all secondary school students and most college-age "young adults" (5,6). Alcohol has been tried by 33% of current 8th graders, 69% of 10th graders, 79% of 12th graders, 81% of college students, and 87% of young adults (19–28 years old). Nationally, 20.5% of youth report having first consumed alcohol prior to the age of 13 (1,2,5,6). Current use is also widespread. More important is the prevalence of occasions of binge drinking, or drinking to intoxication (drinking enough in a 2-hour period to reach a blood alcohol concentration [BAC] of at least 80 mg/dL [the adult legal limit]) (7) (see chapter 16). The number of standard drinks required to reach this BAC varies by age and gender but has been defined as five drinks for older male youth and adults, four drinks for females older than age 17, three or more drinks for female youth up to age 17, and male youth up to age 15.

Children ages 9–13 who consume five or more drinks on one occasion would achieve a BAC estimated to be twice the legal adult limit (7). Binge drinking at least once in the past 2 weeks was reported by 6% of 8th graders, 15% of 10th graders, 22% of 12th graders, 36% of college students, and 37% of young adults who were surveyed in 2011 (5–6). Heavy drinking peaks in the early 20s and recedes with age after that, reflected by the 30% rate found among 29- to 30-year-olds. College students have generally had daily drinking rates that were slightly lower than their same age noncollege peers (4.6% vs. 4.9% in 2011), suggesting that they were more likely to confine their drinking to weekends (5–6).

9.2.2 Drinking preferences

An analysis of data from a subset of the adolescents who completed the Youth Risk Behavior Survey and reported drinking at least one alcoholic beverage in the last 30 days (N = 7,723) revealed that adolescents prefer hard liquor twice as much as other beverages (median = 43.8%). Beer was the second most commonly preferred beverage (median = 19.4%), followed by malt beverages (17.4%). Wine and wine coolers were reported as the beverage of choice by < 5% (8). Preferences for liquor and beer were associated with riskier drinking patterns (binge and heavier use) and the associated risky behaviors (driving under the influence or use of other substances) (8).

Almost a quarter of self-reported drinking college students (N = 2,886) surveyed reported consumption of alcohol mixed with an energy drink (AmED) (9). Reasons given for mixing energy drinks with alcohol were to hide the flavor of the alcohol, to be able to drink more without feeling the effects of drunkenness, to drink more and not appear intoxicated, and to avoid a hangover (9). Students who consumed AmEDs reported twice as many binge-drinking days (6.4 vs. 3.4 days) and twice as many episodes of weekly drunkenness (1.4 days vs. 0.73 days per week), and they reported drinking 36% more drinks per occasion than those who drank alcohol only (8.3 vs. 6.1 drinks) (9).

People who drink AmEDs compared with those who drink the same dose of alcohol without an energy drink perform with equal deficits of motor skills and reaction times; however, those who consume the energy drink report less subjective symptoms of drunkenness (9). Even after adjusting for alcohol consumption, those who consumed AmEDs were twice as likely to be the victim of unwanted sexual activity (Adjusted Odds Ratio (AOR) = 2.18), ride in a car with someone who had been drinking (AOR = 2.25), or need medical attention (AOR = 2.17) than their drinking peers who did not mix alcohol with energy drinks (9).

9.3 Confidentiality in primary care

Prior to consideration of screening, it is important to emphasize the significance of confidentiality for the establishment of an influential patient provider relationship with adolescent patients (see chapter 13). Parents are considered key informants for child and adolescent psychopathology, particularly for symptoms of externalizing disorders or negative consequences related to substance misuse (10); however, they are usually unaware of the extent of substance use in which their child has been involved (10). Screening adolescents for mental and behavioral health problems during routine health visits with the use of psychometrically strong instruments is effective in identifying those in need of services (11) (see chapter 14). Studies suggest youth have concerns about behavioral risks and that they are willing to discuss them if confidentiality is assured (12). A national study of adolescent health concerns revealed that adolescents who engage in risky behaviors have admitted to foregoing needed care due to confidentiality concerns (13).

Most states have laws allowing minors to consent for assessment and treatment for conditions involving substance use or substance dependence and, with some exceptions, requiring that providers maintain confidentiality (14). Arranging the pediatric practice culture to facilitate confidential consultation for a portion of the history and visit with youth ages 12–20 (scope increasing with age) encourages a trusting provider patient relationship and magnifies the odds that the concerns and advice of the provider will be well received (12).

Adolescents are more likely to reveal information on paper or computer-assisted devices. In a study of more than 1,000 youth attending five primary care offices, adolescents were given handheld PDAs to complete behavioral risk surveys prior to the visit (15). The survey included questions and scales relating to the subjects' interest in discussing a wide range of risk behaviors (from unhealthy eating to suicidal ideation). Cues from positive answers led to further questioning regarding depth of involvement in the behavior as well as motivation to quit. The number of behavioral risk factors discussed during adolescent visits increased, and providers reported improved satisfaction with adolescent well visits because they spent less time inquiring about sensitive topics and were able to prioritize their advice based on the issues marked.

Patients reported a greater sense of being heard, being treated with confidentiality, and overall satisfaction with the visit (15). When providers discussed sensitive topics during primary care visits, youth reported positive impressions of the PCP, and felt more empathy in their care (12).

9.4 Screening in primary care

SBIRT is a comprehensive, integrated, public health approach to the delivery of early interventions for individuals with risky alcohol and drug use, as well as the timely referral to more intensive substance abuse treatment for those who have substance use disorders (SUDs) (16). SBIRT consists of three basic elements: screening to identify the degree of risky alcohol involvement and the level of intervention called for; a brief nonconfrontational, patient-centered counseling intervention (usually based on motivational interviewing [MI]); and referral to specialty treatment for those adolescents or young adults identified as needing more extensive treatment (4,16–18).

9.4.1 Screening

In order to reduce the public health problem of substance abuse disorders, the U.S. Preventive Services Task Force (19), the Substance Abuse Mental Health Services Administration (SAMHSA), and the American Academy of Pediatrics (AAP) Committee on Substance Abuse recommend universal screening of all older children, adolescents, and adults for alcohol and substance use (16–20) (see chapters 4 and 13). SBIRT is ideal as an intervention for adolescent behavior change because of its focus on personalization, brevity, and respect for patient autonomy (4). Despite the availability of the SBIRT concept and resources (17), PCPs identify a number of barriers to screening for alcohol problems (4,16,18,21). These barriers include lack of sufficient time and knowledge of how to manage a positive screen; lack of resources for referral; the implicit acceptance of adolescent drinking in rural and other communities, combined with fears of loss of confidentiality in a small community; and the related stigma attached to the labeling of youth with an "alcohol problem" (16,18,21).

9.4.2 Screening tools

The AAP Task Force on Mental Health recommends screening all adolescents for substance use at each health maintenance visit and when injuries or history suggest the possibility of substance abuse, as studies show adolescents are more likely to report risky behaviors at these visits (16,22,23). Empirically established instruments should be used because research that compared providers' clinical impressions of adolescents' level of substance use with the diagnostic classification obtained by use of a structured diagnostic interview found that providers' clinical impressions grossly underestimated the prevalence of substance use pathology (24). Screening is not meant to diagnose, but to guide decision making. Two basic screening goals related to alcohol include (1) evaluation of alcohol use in the past year and (2) determination of the level of risk for alcohol problems or substance abuse disorders (16).

In 2011, a work group of experts convened by the National Institute on Alcohol Abuse and Alcoholism (NIAAA) developed a practitioner's guide to use of SBIRT with youth ages 12–20 (4,25,26). In recognition of the challenges faced by PCPs because of time pressures in clinical practice, one goal was to develop an empirically based, simple, and reliable prescreening tool (consisting of one or two questions) to use with youth for predicting drinking and AUDs (4,16). The two questions found to have the most predictive value for identifying alcohol misuse or problems for children and youth ages 12–20 were the following:

- "Do you have **any friends** who drank beer, wine, or any drink containing alcohol in the past year?"
- "In the past year, **on how many days have you had** more than a few sips of beer, wine, or any drink containing alcohol?" (Exclude drinking for religious reasons.) (4,25,26)

Developmental stage determines the order and wording of the questions. Children ages 11–13 should have the question about friends posed first. Any drinking by friends is a red flag, so a positive response should be followed by the second question. Youth ages 14 and older (or in high school) should have the personal question posed first ("How many days in the past year have you had . . ."). If the response is positive, rephrase the friends question as follows:

- "If your friends drink, **how many drinks** do they usually drink at one occasion?"

If friends are binge drinking, it may be fruitful to ask the youth to elaborate on how he or she manages to abstain when friends are drinking (4). Positive answers on the prescreening questions should be followed by formal screening or a full psychosocial interview based on the level of risk identified (16). Two empirically supported, brief screening instruments are the alcohol use disorders identification test (AUDIT) and the CRAFFT (4,16). Both instruments fit well into the broader psychosocial interview scheme – home, education, activities, drugs and alcohol, sexuality, and safety (HEADSS) (16) – and both can be completed privately by the adolescent in computer or paper/pencil formats (4). The AUDIT, a 10-item screen that focuses on alcohol-related behaviors, includes 3 consumption items and 7 problem items with up to five response options for each item (27). Adolescent studies of the AUDIT have yielded sensitivity rates ranging from 54% to 87%, specificity rates from 65% to 97%, and optimal scores ranging from 2 to 10 (27).

When directly compared, other methods have typically not been found to improve on the AUDIT for identification of AUDs (28). Even the use of one question on the frequency of drinking episodes and using a threshold of three or more episodes per month was found to identify adolescents with AUD at 90% sensitivity and 84% specificity (29). Similarly, the endorsement of at least one of two AUD items (i.e., hazardous use and drinking more or longer than intended) from the *Diagnostic and Statistical Manual of Mental Disorders*, fourth edition (*DSM-IV*), identified adolescents with AUD at 88% sensitivity and 90% specificity (29). The CRAFFT is a six-item questionnaire designed to screen for alcohol and other drug use disorders. The CRAFFT consists of six questions that can be administered verbally or in written form.

C: Have you ever ridden in a **CAR** driven by someone (including yourself) who was "high" or had been using alcohol or drugs?
R: Do you ever use alcohol or drugs to **RELAX**, feel better about yourself, or fit in?
A: Do you ever use alcohol or drugs while you are by yourself, **ALONE**?
F: Do you ever **FORGET** things you did while using alcohol or drugs?
F: Do your family or **FRIENDS** ever tell you that you should cut down on your drinking or drug use?
T: Have you ever gotten into **TROUBLE** while you were using alcohol or drugs? (4,16,30)

The score on the CRAFFT was compared to concurrently administered substance use problem scales and a structured diagnostic interview for patients seen for routine care in an adolescent clinic (30). A score of 2 or higher was able to identify any problem (sensitivity, 0.76; specificity, 0.94), any disorder (sensitivity, 0.80; specificity, 0.86), and dependence (sensitivity, 0.92; specificity, 0.80). The instrument has been implemented into the AAP SBIRT policy statement (4,16). The CRAFFT demonstrated acceptable psychometric properties in some studies (30,31) but poor specificity in some settings (28).

9.5 Assessment of risk

Providers faced with a positive substance use screen along with a significant list of other problems must use the standard for problem triage by addressing the most pressing issues first and then either reschedule the patient for a follow up visit to more fully address the remaining issues or to refer them to a behavioral health provider or program for more detailed assessment and intensive intervention. Those youth at highest risk include those with past-year drinking of 1 or more days (under age 12), 6 days (ages 12–15); 12 days (age 16); 24 days (age 17), and weekly for age 18 (4). National data show that any drinking by youth ages 12–15 is considered to be at least moderate risk, and half of 12- to 15-year-old drinkers fit the high-risk category (4). Approximately one-third of drinkers between the ages of 16 and 18 fit in the moderate-risk category, and almost half drink enough to be considered highest risk (4). The AAP SBIRT algorithm recommends that all those who answer yes to having ridden in a car with someone under the influence receive education on the associated dangers, and that they should be willing to commit to a safety contingency plan that prevents them from ever riding in a car with someone who has been drinking (16).

Red flags that require a break in confidentiality and immediate referral include signs of alcohol dependence (CRAFFT score of > 2 in youth less than 15 years old or > 5 for youth 15 or older; near daily use of any substance; or blackouts) or dangerous alcohol- or drug-related behavior (use of intravenous drugs or the combination of alcohol with substances that are potentially life threatening, fights, assaults, or driving under the influence). It is important to maintain lists of specialty substance-related treatment or mental health providers proficient with treatment of adolescent AUDs. Suggested provider response based on identified level of risk is given in table 9.1.

Table 9.1: Suggested provider response based on identified level of risk (4,16)

Risk level	Provider response based on risk
None	Praise the patient's good choices and explore his or her plans to stay alcohol free, particularly in settings where friends may be drinking. Affirm and educate regarding the risks of riding in cars driven by others under the influence of alcohol.
Lower	• Explore the drinking behavior of friends. • Ask about use of other substances. • If response is negative: o Educate on the risks of alcohol use during the time of rapid brain development. Give clear medical advice promoting abstinence. o List the possibility of harmful consequences that may occur when in the presence of binge-drinking friends (fights, unwanted sexual encounters, accidents, etc.)
Moderate	• Explore the use of other substances and/or substance-related problems. • If none, reinforce strengths and praise any positives. o Give clear brief advice encouraging abstinence as for lower-risk patients. o Express empathetic concern regarding the frequency of drinking and encourage cessation.

(*Continued*)

Table 9.1: Suggested provider response based on identified level of risk (4,16) (*Continued*)

Risk level	Provider response based on risk
	• If problems, reinforce strengths and praise any positives. o Give brief motivational interview (discussed later). o Ask if parents know. o Elicit commitment for at least one goal for behavior change; praise and emphasize your belief in the youth's ability to keep the commitment. o Schedule a follow-up for a full psychosocial interview within 2–4 weeks.
Highest	• Reinforce strengths and praise any positives. o Give brief motivational interview (described later). o Based on your estimate of severity and risk for acute danger, consider immediate referral for further evaluation and treatment. o Ask if parents know. o Based on your estimate of severity, ask for permission or inform of the need to break confidentiality to share recommendations for referral with parents.

9.5.1 Screening the college student

The NIAAA Task Force of the National Advisory Council on Alcohol Abuse and Alcoholism (32) recommends incorporating alcohol screening into standard practice at college student health centers (see chapter 16). The student health center provides an ideal opportunity to intervene with students who are identified as high-risk drinkers and who are experiencing alcohol-related harms. Without a systematic approach to routine alcohol screening, student health centers must rely on episodic alcohol-history information, often obtained after a significant harm has occurred, thereby missing the majority of students in need of identification and intervention. Despite recommendations for routine screenings of high-risk drinking, only 32% of student health centers conduct them, and only 12% use standardized screening instruments (33).

There is limited information on alcohol-screening instruments specifically used in college populations (32). Alcohol-screening instruments such as the 10-question AUDIT have been promoted for routine use in primary health care settings, although their psychometric properties are based on general adult samples (34). Further information on screening and risk assessment can be found in the Appendix.

9.6 BIs for the primary care office

In primary care, the term *brief intervention* (BI) includes a range of responses to the results of screening (16). For those adolescents who report no alcohol use, the "intervention" is to provide brief positive feedback and reinforcement of their current healthy choices, along with advice to not ride in cars with others who have been drinking. When the screening process reveals alcohol use, the BI expands from providing brief advice to the use of a brief negotiated interview based on motivational techniques to encourage the behavior change or acceptance of a referral for treatment (4,16,20).

BIs are defined in various ways but generally refer to the use of motivational enhancement counseling (such as motivational interviewing) in a limited number of concise sessions (can range from one to four) that incorporate common features that can be remembered with the acronym *FRAMES*: (a) give assessment and personalized norm-referenced FEEDBACK; (b) emphasize personal RESPONSIBILITY for change; and (c) offer brief ADVICE given as (d) a MENU of options with (e) an attitude of EMPATHY and (f) promoting SELF-EFFICACY (20). The attitude of the provider should be that of positive regard and collaboration, with a genuine interest in understanding the clients' perceived needs, wishes, and desires (35). MI is believed to be particularly useful for promotion of motivation to change problem behaviors for youth since developmentally they are seeking autonomy and resist pressure from authority figures (35,36).

9.7 MI

MI was developed as a way to help people work through their ambivalence over changing their drinking behavior (36,37) (see chapter 5). Ambivalence over change of reinforcing behaviors is natural for all people. For youth who have not yet experienced many alcohol-related problems, resistance to change is to be expected. Because MI techniques respect the autonomy and potential self-efficacy of adolescents, it is consistent with the developmental tasks faced by youth (36).

- **Promote autonomy: Ask permission before giving advice.** The first lesson a provider must learn in order to be proficient in MI is that no one can make these young patients *want* to change anything. The goal of MI is to elicit and enhance the patient's own motivation for change. Research has repeatedly shown that it is the respectful combination of concern, empathy, collaboration, and respect for autonomy (*the "spirit" of MI*) that is considered the most influential aspect of MI's success (35,37).
- **Do more listening than talking.** Seek information regarding patients' interests, goals, and dreams. Ask what they find appealing about drinking; how they began, and what keeps them doing it. Use active-listening skills to encourage young patients to continue (35). Follow this by asking them to discuss some of the "not so good things" about drinking. Adolescents love to feel that a concerned adult really cares about what they think.
- **Develop a discrepancy.** Listen carefully, and respectfully highlight ways that continuing to drink may interfere with one of your patient's valued interests,

goals, or dreams. One way to approach this might be to say, "*I hear you telling me that you love the closeness you feel with all your buddies when you guys party after football games. You all laugh and have a good time and seem to like each other more when you're drunk. But I also heard you say you worry that some of your friends get kind of mean and you've had to 'get in the middle' of some fights, and that once a couple of the guys pulled out knives. Studies say that many assaults and even deaths that occur happen as a result of drunken people doing things they wouldn't ordinarily do if they were sober. Have you ever thought about what it would be like if you were in the middle of a brawl like that, trying to stop a fight and someone pulled a knife or a gun?*" The patient's response may be one of reflection or resistance. Either way, the seed will have been planted for the patient to consider.

- **Resistance** is immediate feedback from your patient that can teach you that you've crossed the boundaries between the "spirit of MI" and the less successful strategy of acting as the "expert who knows everything he [or she] needs" (36). Pushing back against resistance tends to amplify it. The more you argue for change, the more the patient will think of reasons *not* to change. It's best to "*roll with resistance*," refuse to argue or push, acknowledge the patient's autonomy, and focus on something else. Your goal is to elicit and reinforce the patient's own reasons for changing, not to force yours on the patient (35,36).
- **Listen for "change talk" and reinforce it.** MI was derived from the theory that people tend to become committed to that which they defend themselves (36,37). Often the process of giving feedback from the assessment can provoke conversation that elicits statements from patients that include expressions of their own desires, goals, or needs to change. Listen carefully for those statements, and reflect them back.
- **Listen for and affirm the patient.** Listen for any character strengths, challenges the patient faces, or good choices you hear the patient speak to (36).
- **Support self-efficacy.** Summarize what you heard, emphasizing any "change talk" and including a statement of concern for the patient and confidence in the patient's ability to change (36,37).

9.8 A clinical vignette

This 17-year-old teen boy has been in your practice since he was 10 years of age. He is bright, and you and he have developed a great relationship through the years since he is an avid athlete and has unfortunately suffered quite a few minor injuries. He is captain of the football team and is now in his senior year. He lives with his mom and younger brother, but both his parents have regular contact with him, and there are no major relationship issues in the family. A maternal uncle is in recovery from alcoholism, but there are no other family mental health issues. He revealed that his grades are mostly As and Bs, but he is struggling with his precalculus class. He hopes to get a football scholarship to a state university since his parents would have a hard time supporting him if he left his hometown. He recently started working. He drives but does not own his own car. Other than sports injuries, he is healthy.

He revealed to you that he began drinking the previous summer, when he went to a university-sponsored football camp. He drinks "only now and then; at parties, or after football games with the team." He does not use other drugs. He drinks three to four beers and has never blacked out or driven under the influence. He says they use "DDs" (designated drivers). Since football season started, he has been drinking every Friday, "since that's when we have games." He does not see consider himself a heavy drinker: "It's too expensive to drink all the time!" He does not think his parents know about his drinking. They only drink occasionally when they go out.

PCP: *So you love partying on Fridays after football games. But you have a job now and it has become really hard for you to get to work on time on Saturday mornings, and when you do get there, you have a headache and feel terrible. How badly do you need this job?*

Teen: My parents won't let me get a car until I've saved at least $2000.00 and 6 months' worth of insurance.

PCP: *That's a lot of money. How much do you have so far?*

Teen: Well, it took me 5 months to get the job. I have about $450. But last week my boss told me I better not be late anymore. Something about "plenty more where you came from." I really need a car. I can't go into my senior year riding the bus to school!

PCP: *Hmm . . . Sounds like you really need this job. What do you think it will take for you to keep it?*

Teen: I guess I could stop partying so much. Maybe.

PCP: *Well, you've always been one to set good goals for yourself. What is a reasonable goal for you to set with me today so you can assure you get to work on time for the next 4 weeks?*

Teen: I don't know. I guess I can go home after games and tell my friends I have to work. Maybe I can party with them on holidays or days I don't have to work.

PCP: *So I hear you say that you plan to tell your friends you have to go home after the game because you have to work early in the morning. Right? Is there anything you can do to help keep yourself motivated? Like, what kind of car are you going to get?*

Teen: My dad says I can get an old Jeep or a 4-Runner, as long as it's in good condition. I kind of know a little about cars and I know I can pimp it; uh you know . . . make it custom. I can't wait!

PCP: *Well, sounds as if you have a big goal! And you are a very talented young man. I want you to let me see your new ride when you finish, OK? I'm going to schedule you to follow up for your acne in 3 weeks so we can talk about how you're doing. I feel certain you have what it takes to do this. We won't talk to your parents about this as long as you give me your word that you will* NOT EVER *drive or ride with anyone under the influence. OK?*

MI sounds simple, but it's not easy (36). It requires a major paradigm shift for most pediatric providers, who develop relationships with these kids and care so much for their well-being. The risks and the potential outcomes of adolescents' risky choices are alarming. Pediatric PCPs have been trained, even socialized to believe that their education and paternal anticipatory guidance will prevent accidents, harm, and suffering. Giving advice is almost like a reflex! And in cases of acute illness, it is sought and valued. The problem is, behavior change does not respond well to that metric! Motivation is amenable to influence, but collaboration and gentle leading, rather than paternal advice and pressure, seem to be most effective for motivating adults and youth with AUDs to seek treatment for and to change their alcohol misuse behaviors (4,36,37). Information on training in the use of MI can be found in the Appendix.

9.9 Specific BIs for college students

Brief motivational interventions (BMIs) that combine cognitive-behavioral skills with personalized feedback, norms clarification, risk-reduction strategies, and motivational enhancement have been effective for reducing both alcohol amount, frequency, and problems related to use (38,39). The NIAAA Task Force on College Drinking (40) lists BMI as a "Tier One" preventive strategy with demonstrated effectiveness among college students. Previous trials conducted in nonmedical settings have shown that interventions combining cognitive-behavioral skills and MI lead to reduced alcohol consumption by college students (39,41,42). The existing literature suggests the use of a personalized approach addressing expectancies and normative use (e.g., information about the percentage of students who binge drink) employing a motivational interview style (43).

Those interventions having the best evidence to help identify and assist problem student drinkers include the Alcohol Skills Training Program (44) and the Brief Alcohol Screening and Intervention for College Students program (41,42). Each of these programs involved enhancing motivation to change drinking; changing the college drinker's expectancies about alcohol's effects; clarifying norms through feedback on the drinker's alcohol use in comparison with other students; providing cognitive-behavioral skills training, including how to monitor daily alcohol consumption and stress management; and developing a personalized plan for reducing alcohol use (41,42).

Clinicians should be prepared to refer any college-age students found to have more severe levels of alcohol use, indicated by the presence of physical sequelae of alcohol use and/or withdrawal symptoms, to professionals or specific treatment programs for adults with AUDs.

9.10 Sedative/hypnotics

9.10.1 Epidemiology

Currently, this group of drugs includes primarily the benzodiazepines, which are listed under Schedule IV by the Drug Enforcement Administration as an indication of their potential for abuse and dependence (45). A substantial decrease in the use of these drugs from the mid-1970s through the early 1990s was noted, followed by a steady increase in use from the early 1990s. Illicit use of sedatives and hypnotics continued to rise, even after the increase in use of most other illegal drugs began to reverse in the late 1990s. Annual prevalence of tranquilizer use among 12th graders saw a long and substantial decline from 11% in 1977 to 2.8% in 1992 but eventually increased to a peak of 7.7% in 2002 and settled slightly to 5.6% in 2011 (6,46). Reported tranquilizer use among 8th graders in 2011 was 2.0%. Lifetime prevalence rates were 3.4%, 6.8%, and 8.7% for grades 8, 10, and 12, respectively. Similarly, after a period of stability, college student use showed an increase between 1994 and 2003 (to 6.9%), before a decline to 4.2% by 2011 (5,46). For the young adult sample, after a long period of decline, annual prevalence more than doubled between 1997 and 2002, with minimal change since then (5.9% in 2011) (5). Most of the reported tranquilizer use in recent years in the MTF sample has involved diazepam and alprazolam. Perceived risk for use tends to be relatively low for these prescription drugs, which we believe is a major reason why their use is relatively high (6).

Misuse of prescription sedatives or anxiolytics is highly correlated with other illicit substance use among adolescents (46). Among a group of antisocial youth in residential treatment, those with comparatively high levels of anxiety and depression reported significantly more intensive sedative/anxiolytic misuse than their counterparts and may be at high risk for sedative/anxiolytic abuse and dependence (47).

9.10.2 Associated problems

Although regular sedative/hypnotic use is relatively infrequent among youth, misuse can contribute to impaired judgment, impulsive or disinhibited behavior, substance dependence, and adverse medical outcomes such as respiratory depression and arrest (particularly in combination with alcohol) (45). Long-term sedative/hypnotic use may result in cognitive deficits that persist even when the drugs are discontinued (48). The primary acute danger for sedative/hypnotic use is the frequent concurrent use of these agents with other drugs and particularly alcohol.

Because of the infrequency of use of sedative/hypnotics by adolescents, even by those with other substance use problems, the challenge for primary care clinicians is to include this group of drugs in any screen of illicit substances. Reports of regular use of these agents with or without alcohol should prompt evaluation for possible withdrawal symptoms and planning for the treatment of abstinence syndrome. While there are no studies for treatments specifically for youth with sedative/hypnotic disorders, clinicians are advised to use intervention approaches (described previously) and treatment programs for SUDs in general.

9.11 Conclusions

For primary care clinicians, the SBIRT model provides a useful outline for tasks related to screening for and intervening with high school and college-age youth with alcohol use and problems related to use. Screening involves the systematic use of questions or brief instruments that measure frequency and/or problems related to use. Once problem users are identified, BIs, usually based on motivational enhancement techniques and ranging from advice to structured sessions, can be employed. Primary care clinicians should be prepared to refer those youth with more severe problems to SUD treatment professionals or programs for more detailed and intensive assessment and interventions.

References

1. Centers for Disease Control and Prevention. Youth risk behavior surveillance: United States, 2011. MMWR 2012;61:SS-4. Accessed July 25, 2012. URL: http://www.cdc.gov/mmwr/pdf/ss/ss6104.pdf
2. Johnston L, O'Malley P, Bachman J, Schulenberg J. Monitoring the future national results on adolescent drug use: Overview of key findings, 2011. Ann Arbor, MI: Institute Social Research, University Michigan, 2012.
3. U.S. Department of Health and Human Services, Office of the Surgeon General. The surgeon general's call to action to prevent and reduce underage drinking: A guide to action for educators. 2007. Accessed July 25, 2012. URL: http://www.surgeongeneral.gov/library/calls/underagedrinking/communityguide.pdf
4. U.S. National Institute on Alcohol Abuse and Alcoholism (NIAAA). Alcohol screening and brief intervention for youth: A practitioner's guide, 2011. Accessed July 25, 2012. URL: http://pubs.niaaa.nih.gov/publications/Practitioner/YouthGuide/YouthGuide.pdf
5. Johnston LD, O'Malley PM, Bachman JG, Schulenberg, JE. Monitoring the future national survey results on drug use, 1975–2011. Vol. 2, College students and adults ages 19–50 years. Ann Arbor: Institute Social Research, University Michigan, 2012.

6. Johnston LD, O'Malley PM, Bachman JG, Schulenberg, JE. Monitoring the future national survey results on drug use, 1975–2011. Vol. 1, Secondary school students. Ann Arbor: Institute Social Research, University Michigan, 2012.
7. Donovan JE. Estimated blood alcohol concentrations for child and adolescent drinking and their implications for screening instruments. Pediatrics 2009;123(6):975–81.
8. Siegel MB, Naimi TS, Cremeens JL, Nelson DE. Alcoholic beverage preferences and associated drinking patterns and risk behaviors among high school youth. Am J Prev Med 2011;40(4): 419–26.
9. O'Brien MC, McCoy TP, Rhodes SD, Wagoner A, Wolfson M. Caffeinated cocktails: Energy drink consumption, high-risk drinking, and alcohol-related consequences among college students. Acad Emerg Med 2008;15(5):453–60.
10. Latimer WW, Winters KC, D'Zurilla T, Nichols M. Integrated family and cognitive-behavioral therapy for adolescent substance abusers: A stage I efficacy study. Drug Alcohol Depend 2003; 71(3):303–17.
11. Ko S. Screening in primary care settings for illicit drug use: Assessment of screening instruments – A supplemental evidence update for the U.S. Preventive Services Task Force. Evidence Synthesis No. 58, Part 2. AHRQ Publication No. 08–05108-EF-2. Rockville, MD: Agency Healthcare Research Quality, 2008.
12. Brown JD, Wissow LS. Discussion of sensitive health topics with youth during primary care visits: Relationship to youth perceptions of care. J Adolesc Health 2009;44(1):48–54.
13. Lehrer JA, Pantell R, Tebb K, Shafer, MA. Forgone health care among U.S. adolescents: Associations between risk characteristics and confidentiality concern. J Adolesc Health 2007;40(3): 218–26.
14. Texas Department of State Health Services. Adolescent health: A guide for providers. 2011. Accessed July 25, 2012. URL: http://www.dshs.state.tx.us/thsteps/Adolescent-Guide.doc
15. Olson AL, Gaffney CA, Hedberg VA, Gladstone GR. Use of inexpensive technology to enhance adolescent health screening and counseling. Arch Pediatr Adolesc Med 2009;163 (2):172–7.
16. American Academy of Pediatrics. Substance use screening, brief intervention, and referral to treatment for pediatricians. Pediatrics 2011;128:e1330–40.
17. Substance Abuse and Mental Health Services Administration. Screening, brief intervention and referral to treatment (SBIRT) in behavioral healthcare, 2011. Accessed July 25, 2012. URL: http://www.samhsa.gov/prevention/sbirt/SBIRTwhitepaper.pdf
18. Gordon AJ, Ettaro L, Rodriguez KL, Mocik J, Clark DB. Provider, patient, and family perspectives of adolescent alcohol use and treatment in rural settings. J Rural Health 2011;27(1):81–90.
19. U.S. Preventive Services Task Force. Guide to clinical preventive services, recommendations of the U.S. Preventive Services Task Force. AHRQ Publication No. 06–05882006. Rockville, MD: Agency Healthcare Research Quality, 2006.
20. Levy S, Vaughan BL, Knight JR. Office-based intervention for adolescent substance abuse. Pediatr Clin North Am 2002;49(2):329–43.
21. Van Hook S, Harris SK, Brooks T, Carey P, Kossack R, Kulig J, et al. The "six T's": Barriers to screening teens for substance abuse in primary care. J Adolesc Health 2007;40(5):456–61.
22. American Academy of Pediatrics. The case for mental health screening. In: Addressing mental health concerns in primary care: A clinician's toolkit, 1st ed. Elk Grove Village, IL: American Academy Pediatrics, 2010. Accessed July 25, 2012. URL: http://www.teenscreen.org/images/stories/CaseforRoutineMentalHealthScreening.pdf
23. Windle M, Zucker RA. Reducing underage and young adult drinking: How to address critical drinking problems during this developmental period. Accessed July 25, 2012. URL: http://pubs.niaaa.nih.gov/publications/arh40/29-44.htm

24. Wilson CR, Sherritt L, Gates E, Knight JR. Are clinical impressions of adolescent substance use accurate? Pediatrics 2004;114(5):e536–40.
25. Smith GT, Chung T, Martin CS, Donovan JE, Windle M. Youth alcohol screening workgroup I: Measuring consumption of alcohol as a screener in children and adolescents. Alcohol Clin Exp Res 2010;34:276A.
26. Brown SA, Donovan JE, McGue MK, Shulenberg JE, Zucker RA, Goldman, MA. Youth alcohol screening workgroup II: Determining optimal secondary screening questions. Alcohol Clin Exp Res 2010;34:267A.
27. Reinert DF, Allen JP. The alcohol use disorder identification test: An update of research findings. Alcohol Clin Exp Res 2007;31:185–99.
28. Cook RL, Chung T, Kelly TM, Clark DB. Alcohol screening in young persons attending a sexually transmitted disease clinic: Comparisons of AUDIT, CRAFFT, and CAGE instruments. J Gen Intern Med 2005;20:1–6.
29. Kelly TM, Donovan JE, Chung T, Bukstein OG, Cornelius JR. Brief screens for detecting alcohol use disorder among 18–20 year old young adults in emergency departments: Comparing AUDIT-C, CRAFFT, RAPS4-QF, FAST, RUFT-Cut, and DSM-IV 2-item scale. Addict Behav 2009; 34:668–74.
30. Knight JR, Sherritt L, Shrier LA, Harris SK, Chang G. Validity of the CRAFFT substance abuse screening test among adolescent clinic patients. Arch Pediatr Adolesc Med 2002;156(6):607–14.
31. Knight JR, Harris SK, Sherritt L, Van Hook S, Lawrence N, et al. Prevalence of positive substance abuse screen results among adolescent primary care patients. Arch Pediatrics Adolesc Med 2007;161:1035–41.
32. Task Force of the National Advisory Council on Alcohol Abuse and Alcoholism. A call to action: Changing the culture of drinking at U.S. colleges. Bethesda, MD: National Institute Alcohol Abuse Alcoholism, 2002.
33. Foote J, Wilkens C, Vavagiakis P. A national survey of alcohol screening and referral in college health centers. J Am Coll Hlth 2004;52:149–57.
34. Saunders JB, Aasland OG, Babor TF, de la Fuente JR, Grant M. Development of the alcohol use disorders identification test (AUDIT): WHO collaborative project on early detection of persons with harmful alcohol consumption-II. Addiction 1993;88(6):791–804.
35. Moyers TB, Miller WR, Hendrickson SML. How does motivational interviewing work? Therapist interpersonal skill predicts client involvement within motivational interviewing sessions. J Consult Clin Psychol 2005;73(4):590–8.
36. Miller WR, Rose GS. Toward a theory of motivational interviewing. Am Psychol 2009;64(6): 527–37.
37. Hettema J, Steele J, Miller WR. Motivational Interviewing. Annu Rev Clin Psychol 2005;1:91–111.
38. Larimer ME, Cronce JM. Identification, prevention and treatment: A review of individual-focused strategies to reduce problematic alcohol consumption by college students. J Stud Alcohol 2002;14:148–63.
39. Larimer ME, Cronce JM. Identification, prevention, and treatment revisited: Individual-focused college drinking prevention strategies 1999–2006. Addict Behav 2007;32:2439–68.
40. Dejong W, Larimer ME, Wood MD, Hartman R. NIAAA's rapid response to college drinking problems initiative: Reinforcing the use of evidence-based approaches in college alcohol prevention. J Stud Alcohol Drugs 2009;16:5–11.
41. Baer JS, Kivlahan DR, Blume AW, McKnight P, Marlatt GA. Brief intervention for heavy-drinking college students: 4-year follow-up and natural history. Am J Publ Hlth 2001;91:1310–16.
42. Marlatt GA, Baer JS, Kivlahan DR, Dimeff LA, Larimer ME, Quigley LA, et al. Screening and brief intervention for high-risk college student drinkers: Results from a 2-year follow-up assessment. J Cons Clin Psychol 1998;66:604–15.

43. Fager JH, Melnyk BM. The effectiveness of intervention studies to decrease alcohol use in college undergraduate students: An integrative analysis. World News Evid Based Nurs 2004;1:102–19.
44. Baer JS, Marlatt GA, Kivlahan DR, Fromme K, Larimer ME, Williams E. An experimental test of three methods of alcohol risk reduction with young adults. J Cons Clin Psychol 1992;60:974–9.
45. National Institute on Drug Abuse. Selected prescription drugs with potential for abuse 2005. Accessed July 25, 2012. URL: http://www.nida.nih.gov.ezproxyhost.library.tmc.edu/PDF/Prescription Drugs.pdf
46. McCabe SE, Boyd CJ, Young A. Medical and nonmedical use of prescription drugs among secondary school students. J Adolesc Hlth 2007;40:76–83.
47. Hall MT, Howard MO, McCabe SE. Subtypes of adolescent sedative/anxiolytic misusers: A latent profile analysis. Addict Behav 2010;35:882–9.
48. Stewart, SA. The effects of benzodiazepines on cognition. J Clin Psychol 2005;66:9–13.

Appendix

Bright Futures in Practice: Mental Health (Includes Substance Abuse)

Excellent free resource for PCPs. Includes information on mental health issues in a developmental context. This two-volume resource includes practice guidelines and tools for screening and early recognition, care management, and patient teaching materials: http://www.brightfutures.org/mentalhealth/

Confidential Care for Adolescents

Center for Adolescent Health and the Law website: http://www.cahl.org/

The NIAAA's *Alcohol Screening and Brief Intervention for Youth: Practitioner's Guide* and pocket guide contain more detailed information and prompts and are available free of charge from: http://www.niaaa.nih.gov/YouthGuide

The American Academy of Pediatrics policy on SBIRT for pediatricians contains an empirically based algorithm and many practical aids for implementing SBIRT in practice.

It is available online at: http://pediatrics.aappublications.org/content/128/5/e1330.full.pdf

Motivational Interviewing

Supported by SAMHSA, this site is full of resources including training opportunities, manuals, a bibliography, case studies, and contacts for personal clinical coaching. http://www.motivationalinterview.org/

10 Opioids and prescription drugs

Joseph L. Calles, Jr.

Over time, synthetic opioids have migrated from legitimate medical settings to the street, where they are increasingly being used by young people for recreational purposes. This chapter provides an overview of the misuse of opioids and other prescription drugs, over-the-counter (OTC) drugs, and heroin by adolescents and young adults. The scope of the problem is discussed, as are available pharmacotherapeutic interventions.

10.1 Introduction

As discussed throughout this book, the abuse of drugs by adolescents is an increasing public health concern. As law enforcement efforts to eradicate drug use have focused on illicit substances, one aspect of the drug problem that has been underappreciated until fairly recently is the inappropriate use of prescription and OTC drugs by adolescents. In order to accurately gauge the extent of an adolescent's drug-use problem, it is important to classify the use as belonging to one of three categories: misuse, abuse, or dependence (1). Misuse implies that a drug was not prescribed to the person using it or is being used for the purpose of altering the person's feelings or perceptions (i.e., "getting high"). Abuse is similar in its objective to experientially alter the user, but it is also associated with significant impairments in functioning and/or negative consequences (e.g., legal). Dependence is the ultimate stage of inappropriate drug use because it includes increasing tolerance to the desired effects of the drug and/or withdrawal effects (when drug use is decreased or terminated), as well as more time being spent procuring and using the drug, to the exclusion of life goals and obligations. Therapeutic intervention at the misuse stage provides the best opportunity to help adolescents to stop using drugs. What follows is an overview of the misuse of prescription drugs, OTC drugs, and illicit opioids by young people, as well as options for therapeutic intervention.

10.2 Prescription drugs

Data from the 2010 National Survey on Drug Use and Health (NSDUH) help to put the nonmedical use of prescription drugs (NMUPD) by adolescents into perspective (2). In that survey year, the misuse of psychotherapeutics (i.e., analgesics, tranquilizers, stimulants, or sedatives) began for 2.4 million persons aged ≥ 12 years, an average of 6,600 new users per day. A more recent survey of 8th, 10th, and 12th graders identified prescription drugs as the second-most abused category of drugs after marijuana (3). A question that is often asked is, Where are these young people getting their prescription drugs from? The answer is that, at least in North America, the most common source is diversion from family or friends (4). In order to put this problem into social and clinical perspectives, what follows are overviews of the NMUPD by specific medication groups and descriptions of selected pharmacotherapeutic agents to use in their treatment.

10.3 Analgesics

In the 2010 NSDUH, the most commonly misused prescription medications were pain relievers (i.e., narcotics), represented by 17.3% of those who used illicit drugs for the first time (2). In 55.0% of all nonmedical users of pain relievers, the drug they most recently used was obtained from a friend or relative for free. The easy availability of prescription opioids is hardly surprising, given that it has been estimated that 1/25 of those medications end up being diverted for nonmedical use (5). In younger people, the nonmedical use of prescription opioids seems to peak in the 12th grade (6). This is a critical time of life, associated with graduation from high school and the beginning of college or full-time employment. Complicating that transition is the association of the NMUPD, specifically opioids, and the use of alcohol, tobacco, marijuana, and other illicit drugs (6). In a similar manner, the heavier the nonmedical use of prescription opioids, the heavier the use of all other substances. The detection of opioid misuse may be missed during the early phase of the disorder or attributed to other psychiatric disorders. For example, opioid intoxication, with its associated psychomotor and cognitive slowing, could be mistaken for depression. Conversely, the psychomotor agitation of opioid withdrawal could be misdiagnosed as an anxiety disorder. If opioid misuse is suspected, drug testing can help to identify it or to rule it out. As opioids, and their metabolites, tend to clear from blood and saliva fairly quickly, detection is best accomplished by examining a patient's urine (the drug is present up to 1–3 days after use) or hair (up to 7–90 days after use) (7).

Once adolescent opioid analgesic misuse, abuse, or dependence is discovered, the next step should be treatment. However, there may be barriers to treatment. Using data from the 2005–2008 NSDUH, Wu et al. examined various treatment factors in 1,788 adolescents (ages 12–17 years) who met at least one of the past-year criteria for prescription opioid abuse or dependence (8). In those with a perceived need for treatment, only 13% reported any use of substance abuse treatment or services in the past year. The most common reasons for not seeking treatment were not being ready to stop using (34%), not wanting others to find out (22%), thinking that treatment might cause neighbors to have negative opinions of them (22%), and believing that they could handle the problem without treatment (21%). (Note: Subjects could endorse more than one factor contributing to nontreatment.) Fewer African American youth (1.8%) had a perceived need for treatment than did Hispanic (5.5%) or Caucasian (5.2%) youth. Smaller numbers of adolescents went untreated due to insurance not covering treatment or having concerns about cost (10%) and not knowing where to get treatment (8%).

Assuming that barriers to treatment are eliminated, therapeutic interventions for prescription opioid use disorders can include psychopharmacological agents. In the United States, there are currently three approved medications for the treatment of opioid dependence: methadone (a long-acting opioid), combined buprenorphine-naloxone (an opioid partial agonist with an opioid antagonist), and injectable naltrexone (an opioid antagonist). In the combination medication, naloxone is not absorbed orally and is added to block the effects of the buprenorphine should it be used intravenously in an attempt to "get high." All three medication options are used for maintenance therapy (i.e., to try and prevent craving for, withdrawal from, and/or use of illicit opioids and, by extension, overuse of prescription opioids). Neither naltrexone nor methadone is approved for use in individuals younger than age 18 years; buprenorphine is approved for use in those ages ≥ 16 years. There have been only a few studies of pharmacological agents for opioid dependence in adolescents, likely due, in part, to the ethical limitations inherent in working with minors.

One study from Australia compared rates of treatment retention (time in treatment) and relapse (return to treatment) in 61 adolescents (ages 14–17 years at the onset of treatment) with heroin dependence (9). Of the three treatment groups – buprenorphine, methadone, and nonopioid medications (control group) – those in the buprenorphine and methadone groups stayed in treatment longer and, if they dropped out of treatment, took longer to return to treatment when compared to the control group. When comparing subjects in the buprenorphine versus methadone groups, those in the latter group had a significantly longer retention in the initial treatment episode and a longer time to treatment reentry. Despite the seeming superiority of methadone, the authors initiate the treatment of heroin dependence with buprenorphine and consider a subsequent switch to methadone if patients drop out of that phase of treatment. This seems like a reasonable approach to take with adolescents who are dependent on prescription opioids, especially given that buprenorphine can be prescribed in a routine clinical setting. In the United States, methadone for the treatment of opioid dependence must be prescribed in a government-licensed facility and only to patients who are adults (10). In the noted Australian study (9), daily doses of buprenorphine ranged from 4 to 16 mg (mean 9.3 mg); daily doses of methadone ranged from 20 to 90 mg (mean 52.3 mg).

Another medication used in the United States for the prevention of relapse to opioid dependence in adults is the extended-release, injectable form of naltrexone. There are very limited data on its use in addicted youth. One study examined a convenience sample of the first 16 consecutive patients (ages 16–20 years; mean 18.5 years) with opioid dependence treated with extended-release naltrexone (11). Results were encouraging: of the 14 patients who attended at least two outpatient visits, 12 received at least two doses of the medication, 10 stayed in treatment for 4 months, and 9 (56%) had a "good" outcome, defined as no or less frequent opioid use, no new drug-related problems, and improvement in psychosocial functioning. The medication was well tolerated. A major barrier to treatment was cost of the medication ($800–$900 monthly), which was not necessarily covered by insurance plans.

In summary, the pharmacological treatment of opioid dependence should start with the buprenorphine-naloxone combination, which is relatively safe and easy to manage and is very effective, especially when combined with psychological and psychosocial treatments. Dosing should follow the guidelines established for adults. The use of methadone is not an option unless the patient is of legal age, and then it must be dispensed at an authorized treatment facility. Injectable naltrexone does not have legal restrictions, but its use may be limited by high costs, which may not be covered by health insurance or may not be reimbursable.

10.4 Tranquilizers

The 2010 NSDUH found that the second-most commonly misused prescription medications were the tranquilizers (predominantly benzodiazepines [BZPs]), represented by 4.6% of those who used illicit drugs for the first time (2) (see chapters 6 and 9). In a study of 7th- to 12th-grade students in southeast Michigan (12), the use of sedative-anxiety medications was small compared to the use of pain medications; however, sedative or anxiety medications had one of the highest illicit-to-medical use ratios. Similar to the diversion of opioids, the diversion of tranquilizer medications is related to their increased availability. In the years 1994–2001, the numbers of anxiolytics prescribed to youth (14- to 18-year-olds) greatly increased, as reported in the National Ambulatory Medical Care Survey (13). In that survey, the numbers of prescriptions for antidepressants, stimulants, and other drugs were compared. The "other" category, which included at least 23 antipsychotics and 17 antianxiety medications, recorded the highest percentage growth (385.4%) over the years surveyed.

The treatment of BZP dependence has been both confusing and disappointing, especially when compared to the progress that has been made in the treatment of dependence on alcohol, which has several effects in common with the BZPs. A 2006 comprehensive review of pharmacological interventions for BZP monodependence mostly compared strategies using short-acting versus long-acting BZPs for tapering and maintenance treatment and briefly discussed the use of adjunctive medications, such as antidepressants, serotonergic anxiolytics (e.g., hydroxyzine), anticonvulsants, beta-blockers, and benzodiazepine antagonists (14). It was noted that carbamazepine demonstrated modest benefit in reducing BZP withdrawal severity (in conjunction with a BZP taper). After BZP discontinuation, the maintenance of a BZP-free state when treated with carbamazepine versus placebo was statistically significant at 5-week follow-up (95% vs. 62% of respective participants), but not at

12-week follow-up (74% vs. 52%, respectively). These results suggest that carbamazepine may have clinical significance for abstinence from BZPs in some individuals.

Another anticonvulsant that is used to treat BZP withdrawal is pregabalin (PGB) (15). There have been several studies of PGB in adults with generalized anxiety disorder (GAD) that have demonstrated significant reductions in somatic and psychic anxiety symptoms (16,17,18) and at least one study in adults with social anxiety disorder that had similar results (19). To date, there are no published studies on the use of PGB to prevent relapse in individuals who have BZP abuse or dependence and no studies of its use as an anxiolytic in adolescents, in whom PGB is not approved for any indication. However, in adolescents in whom their BZP overuse began as self-medication for GAD or social anxiety disorder, a trial of PGB may be reasonable, especially if other interventions (e.g., selective serotonin reuptake inhibitors [SSRIs] or serotonin-norepinephrine reuptake inhibitors [SNRIs]) are ineffective and if the continued use of the BZPs is having significant negative consequences.

In summary, the pharmacological treatment of BZP dependence will largely depend on the presence of premorbid or comorbid anxiety disorders that are not responding to treatment with SSRIs or SNRIs, such as venlafaxine. Of interest is that in one of the previously cited adult studies (17), PGB worked faster, was better tolerated, and was more effective at reducing the symptoms of GAD than was extended-release venlafaxine. Since the safe use of medications is always a consideration, especially in younger patients, use of PGB for BZP abuse or dependence in adolescents should begin at a low dose (i.e., 75 mg daily, divided into two or three doses) and then be titrated slowly for tolerance and clinical response.

10.5 Stimulants

Ranked third on the 2010 NSDUH list of the most commonly misused prescription medications were the stimulants, represented by 2.5% of those who used illicit drugs for the first time (2) (see chapters 11 and 16). The 2011 Monitoring the Future (MTF) survey (3) reported that there has been a downward trend in the nonmedical use of amphetamines, which includes the brand-name attention-deficit/hyperactivity disorder (ADHD) medications Ritalin and Adderall. Unfortunately, for a small number of adolescents, the inappropriate use of prescription stimulants continues to be a problem, one deserving of identification and treatment.

The search for effective pharmacological treatments for stimulant abuse/dependence has itself been problematic. One approach is to treat with a "safer" alternative stimulant (20,21), a strategy not recommended for adolescent stimulant misusers, even those with comorbid ADHD.

Another approach is to use a nonstimulant medication, of which several have been tried (20), but of which only three – modafinil, bupropion, and naltrexone – have shown some efficacy in adults with methamphetamine abuse/dependence

(22). Although similar studies in adolescents have not been conducted, clinicians could reasonably decide to try modafinil, bupropion, or naltrexone for prescription amphetamine, or methylphenidate, abuse/dependence. This approach would also be appropriate if comorbid ADHD were present, especially regarding the use of modafinil (23) and possibly the use of bupropion (24).

In summary, the absence of clinical trials of psychopharmacological agents to treat stimulant abuse/dependence in adolescents should not deter their cautious use in patients who are not responding to other interventions. Modafinil dosing should begin low (100 mg) and in the morning, with gradual titration (in 50–100 mg increments) up to a maximum of 400 mg a day. The use of bupropion should also begin in the morning and at a low dose (150 mg) of the extended-release formulation, with increases (in 150 mg increments) up to a maximum daily dose of 450 mg. Dosing of oral naltrexone was only 50 mg daily in one study of adults with amphetamine dependence (25). Given the high cost of modafinil, bupropion is the more cost-effective medication of first choice, with naltrexone a comparably priced second choice.

10.6 Others

The final category of prescription drugs reported on in the 2010 NSDUH were the sedatives (including barbiturates and hypnotics), represented by only 1.9% of those who used illicit drugs for the first time (2). The MTF survey found that in 12th graders the lifetime prevalence of nonmedical use of barbiturates was 6.8%–8.3% (3).

There is a paucity of medical literature on the treatment of sedative-hypnotic abuse and dependence. This may be related to the steady decline in numbers of prescriptions for those agents since the introduction of the BZPs into clinical practice. Nonetheless, a review of the use of valproic acid (VPA) for sedative-hypnotic withdrawal and relapse prevention concluded that VPA may be useful for both of those purposes (26). The authors caution that the data presented were extrapolated from studies in adult patients with dependence on alcohol or BZPs. Further studies are needed to identify safe and effective pharmacological treatments for sedative-hypnotic abuse and dependence.

10.7 OTC drugs

Although OTC drugs can include many different types of compounds, including steroids and herbal products, in this chapter OTC drugs refer to medications – either brand name or generic – that are produced by pharmaceutical companies to treat such nonspecific symptoms as cough and rhinitis (27). Of the many OTC preparations available for retail, nonprescription purchase, the two most commonly misused are dextromethorphan (DXM) and the antihistamines.

10.8 DXM

DXM is a semisynthetic morphine derivative (the dextrorotatory stereoisomer of the left-handed codeine analogue levorphanol) that is used clinically as an antitussive and is widely contained in many OTC cough and cold preparations (28,29). Despite its easy availability, DXM is a potentially dangerous dissociative agent, similar in its effects to ketamine and phencyclidine, and it is that particular property that contributes to its abuse potential. A recent study, from the state of Texas, looked at intentional ingestions of DXM (for nonmedical purposes) reported to poison centers during the years 2000–2009 (30). Not counting a decline during the years 2003–2005, the misuse of DXM-containing preparations remained steady. More than half of the reports involved the use of Coricidin products, with the majority of users being males, ages 13–19 years. A similar report from poison centers in Illinois found that the predominant abusers of Coricidin products were adolescents (mean age 15.7 years; 55.4% male), the peak use was during the fall months, and the total hospital charges to treat DXM-related adverse events were about $353,313.65/year (31).Clearly, the misuse of DXM has profound effects on individuals, as well as on society.

There are no specific therapeutic interventions for DXM abuse, and it appears to not proceed to physical dependency, although psychological withdrawal can occur (32). Most DXM abusers can be treated in a community setting, using traditional psychosocial interventions. In those individuals who do not respond to routine care, more intensive treatment in a detoxification and rehabilitation program may be necessary.

10.9 Antihistamines

Many OTC cold and allergy preparations contain antihistamines, often in combination with other OTC medications, such as analgesics and antitussives. Some antihistamines are also used as antiemetics. There are reports in the medical literature that cyclizine, diphenhydramine (DPH), and dimenhydrinate (this is an equimolar combination of DPH and 8-chlorotheophylline) have been abused to "get high," mostly related to their associated anticholinergic effects (33–35).

As with DXM, there are no specific treatments for antihistamine/anticholinergic abuse. Community-based psychosocial therapies should be tried first before considering a more intensive – and restrictive – treatment program.

10.10 Illicit opioids

As discussed earlier in this chapter, the most common opioids abused by youth are controlled, prescription drugs that are diverted from legitimate use. There is one opioid, however, that is a nonprescription medication and that has high addiction potential: heroin. In the previously cited MTF study, for the year 2011, heroin use was low, with only 1.2% of 8th–12th graders having tried it at some point during their lifetimes, 0.7% having tried it that year, and 0.4% having tried it within 30 days of responding to the survey (3). Of concern is that the availability of heroin was perceived by 20.8% of 12th graders to be "fairly easy" or "very easy" to get. On a positive note, 94.3% of that same class disapproved of adults (and also, presumably, their peers) trying heroin as little as only once or twice.

A government report (for year 2007) described the characteristics of adolescent heroin users who were admitted for substance abuse treatment (36). Not surprisingly, the highest number of referrals (33%) was made by the criminal justice system. A low number of referrals (7%) came from other (i.e., clinicians not involved in alcohol or drug care) care providers, which includes primary care physicians. This speaks to the need for pediatricians to be aware of heroin-using patients in their practices and for timely referral to formal detoxification and treatment services. Recent data highlight the need for ongoing treatment of heroin-dependent adolescents with either buprenorphine or methadone (37). In order to maintain abstinence, treatment will be necessary beyond 1 year for almost one-half of patients.

10.11 Conclusion

This chapter highlights the ready availability and abuse of prescription, OTC, and illicit opioid drugs, with an emphasis on adolescents and young adults. Several treatment options are discussed in terms of theoretical rationale and clinical applicability. Further research is needed to identify more effective pharmacological agents for use in relapse prevention.

References

1. Ford JA, Lacerenza C. The relationship between source of diversion and prescription drug misuse, abuse, and dependence. Subst Use Misuse 2011;46(6):819–27.
2. Substance Abuse and Mental Health Services Administration. Results from the 2010 National Survey on Drug Use and Health: Summary of national findings. NSDUH Series H-41, HHS Publication No. (SMA) 11-4658. Rockville, MD: Substance Abuse and Mental Health Services Administration, 2011. Accessed December 20, 2012. URL: http://www.samhsa.gov/data/NSDUH/2k10NSDUH/2k10Results.pdf
3. Johnston LD, O'Malley PM, Bachman JG, Schulenberg JE. Monitoring the future national results on adolescent drug use: Overview of key findings, 2011. Ann Arbor: Institute for Social Research, The University of Michigan, 2012. Accessed February 26, 2012. URL: www.monitoringthefuture.org/pubs/monographs/mtf-overview2011.pdf
4. Fischer B, Bibby M, Bouchard M. The global diversion of pharmaceutical drugs non-medical use and diversion of psychotropic prescription drugs in North America: A review of sourcing routes and control measures. Addiction 2010;105(12):2062–70.

5. Katz NP, Birnbaum HG, Castor A. Volume of prescription opioids used nonmedically in the United States. J Pain Palliat Care Pharmacother 2010;24(2):141–4.
6. Catalano RF, White HR, Fleming CB, Haggerty KP. Is nonmedical prescription opiate use a unique form of illicit drug use? Addict Behav 2011;36(1–2):79–86.
7. Fareed A, Stout S, Casarella J, Vayalapalli S, Cox J, Drexler K. Illicit opioid intoxication: Diagnosis and treatment. Subst Abuse Res Treat 2011;5:17–25.
8. Wu LT, Blazer DG, Li TK, Woody GE. Treatment use and barriers among adolescents with prescription opioid use disorders. Addict Behav 2011;36(12):1233–9.
9. Bell J, Mutch C. Treatment retention in adolescent patients treated with methadone or buprenorphine for opioid dependence: A file review. Drug Alcohol Rev 2006;25(2):167–71.
10. Parrino M. State methadone treatment guidelines. TIPS Series 1. DHHS Publication No. (SMA) 93–1991. Rockville, MD: Department of Health and Human Services, 1993.
11. Fishman MJ, Winstanley EL, Curran E, Garrett S, Subramaniam G. Treatment of opioid dependence in adolescents and young adults with extended release naltrexone: Preliminary case-series and feasibility. Addiction 2010;105(9):1669–76.
12. Boyd CJ, McCabe SE, Cranford JA, Young A. Prescription drug abuse and diversion among adolescents in a southeast Michigan school district. Arch Pediatr Adolesc Med 2007;161(3):276–81.
13. Thomas CP, Conrad T, Casler R, Goodman E. Trends in the use of psychotropic medications among adolescents, 1994 to 2001. Psychiatr Serv 2006;57(1):63–9.
14. Denis C, Fatseas M, Lavie E, Auriacombe M. Pharmacological interventions for benzodiazepine mono-dependence management in outpatient settings. Cochrane Database Syst Rev 2006;(3): CD005194.
15. Oulis P, Konstantakopoulos G, Kouzoupis AV, Masdrakis VG, Karakatsanis NA, Karapoulios E, et al. Pregabalin in the discontinuation of long-term benzodiazepines' use. Hum Psychopharmacol 2008;23(4):337–40.
16. Bandelow B, Wedekind D, Leon T. Pregabalin for the treatment of generalized anxiety disorder: A novel pharmacologic intervention. Expert Rev Neurother 2007;7(7):769–81.
17. Kasper S, Herman B, Nivoli G, Van Ameringen M, Petralia A, Mandel FS, et al. Efficacy of pregabalin and venlafaxine-XR in generalized anxiety disorder: Results of a double-blind, placebo-controlled 8-week trial. Int Clin Psychopharmacol 2009;24(2):87–96.
18. Montgomery SA, Herman BK, Schweizer E, Mandel FS. The efficacy of pregabalin and benzodiazepines in generalized anxiety disorder presenting with high levels of insomnia. Int Clin Psychopharmacol 2009;24(4):214–22.
19. Feltner DE, Liu-Dumaw M, Schweizer E, Bielski R. Efficacy of pregabalin in generalized social anxiety disorder: Results of a double-blind, placebo-controlled, fixed-dose study. Int Clin Psychopharmacol 2011;26(4):213–20.
20. Grabowski J, Shearer J, Merrill J, Negus SS. Agonist-like, replacement pharmacotherapy for stimulant abuse and dependence. Addict Behav 2004;29(7):1439–64.
21. Herin DV, Rush CR, Grabowski J. Agonist-like pharmacotherapy for stimulant dependence: Preclinical, human laboratory, and clinical studies. Ann NY Acad Sci 2010;1187:76–100.
22. Karila L, Weinstein A, Aubin HJ, Benyamina A, Reynaud M, Batki SL. Pharmacological approaches to methamphetamine dependence: A focused review. Br J Clin Pharmacol 2010;69(6):578–92.
23. Mann N, Bitsios P. Modafinil treatment of amphetamine abuse in adult ADHD. J Psychopharmacol 2009;23(4):468–71.
24. Elkashef AM, Rawson RA, Anderson AL, Li SH, Holmes T, Smith EV, et al. Bupropion for the treatment of methamphetamine dependence. Neuropsychopharmacology 2008;33(5):1162–70.
25. Jayaram-Lindström N, Hammarberg A, Beck O, Franck J. Naltrexone for the treatment of amphetamine dependence: A randomized, placebo-controlled trial. Am J Psychiatry 2008; 165(11):1442–8.

26. Harris JT, Roache JD, Thornton JE. A role for valproate in the treatment of sedative-hypnotic withdrawal and for relapse prevention. Alcohol Alcohol 2000;35(4):319–23.
27. Lessenger JE, Feinberg SD. Abuse of prescription and over the counter medications. J Am Board Fam Med 2008;21(1):45–54.
28. Boyer EW. Dextromethorphan abuse. Pediatr Emerg Care 2004;20(12):858–63.
29. Akerman SC, Hammel JL, Brunette MF. Dextromethorphan abuse and dependence in adolescents. J Dual Diagnosis 2010;6:266–78.
30. Forrester MB. Dextromethorphan abuse in Texas, 2000–2009. J Addict Dis 2011;30(3):243–7.
31. Yin S, Wahl M. Intentional Coricidin product exposures among Illinois adolescents. Am J Drug Alcohol Abuse 2011;37(6):509–14.
32. Romanelli F, Smith KM. Dextromethorphan abuse: Clinical effects and management. Pharmacy Today 2009;15(3):48–55.
33. Bassett KE, Schunk JE, Crouch BI. Cyclizine abuse by teenagers in Utah. Am J Emerg Med 1996;14(5):472–4.
34. Thomas A, Nallur DG, Jones N, Deslandes PN. Diphenhydramine abuse and detoxification: A brief review and case report. J Psychopharmacol 2009;23(1):101–5.
35. Rowe C, Verjee Z, Koren G. Adolescent dimenhydrinate abuse: Resurgence of an old problem. J Adolesc Health 1997;21(1):47–9.
36. Substance Abuse and Mental Health Services Administration. The TEDS Report: Characteristics of adolescent heroin admissions. Rockville, MD: Substance Abuse Mental Health Services Administration, 2009.
37. Smyth BP, Fagan J, Kernan K. Outcome of heroin-dependent adolescents presenting for opiate substitution treatment. J Subst Abuse Treat 2012;42(1):35–44.

11 Illicit stimulant abuse in adolescents and young adults

Marc Lener, Sarah Ann Anderson, and Iliyan Ivanov

There has been a decline in cocaine and methamphetamine abuse in all ages in the United States, but a substantial number of adolescents and young adults continue to use and abuse illicit stimulants. Identification of early warning signs can allow for timely medical, psychological, and programmatic interventions. Understanding how to communicate with the patient as well as the patient's family is an extremely powerful preventative strategy, and understanding risk factors and comorbidities in patients who are abusing stimulants allows for appropriate risk management during clinical visits. Once stimulant abuse has been identified, clinicians need to also identify available treatment resources and make referrals to ensure proper management. Stimulant abuse, as well as drug abuse overall, is a multisystem-wide problem and a shared responsibility between various health care providers, the patient, the family of the patient, and any individuals who interact with the patient out of the home, at work, school, or other places where the individual interacts with others. This chapter will review the current literature and summarize recommendations for diagnosis and management of illicit stimulant use, abuse, and dependence in adolescents and young adults that are applicable for physicians in primary care.

11.1 Introduction

Illicit stimulant abuse is increasingly prevalent among the U.S. adolescent and young adult population. As such, up-to-date perspectives on the epidemiology, neurobiology, and clinical aspects of illicit stimulant abuse in the adolescent population may enhance efficacious treatment. In contrast to prescription stimulants, whereby rigorous pharmacological and clinical testing is regulated by the FDA, methamphetamine and cocaine production is free from the same rigor. As a consequence, the chemical composition is largely unknown and can lead to unpredictable physiological outcomes making it a challenge to identify and treat in the clinical setting.

The burden of identification and engagement in treatment often falls in the hands of primary care physicians with limited clinical experience on the matter. Accordingly, this chapter discusses methamphetamine and cocaine abuse in the adolescent and young adult populations with emphasis on identification, diagnosis, and clinical management in primary care settings. Identification of acute intoxication and/or chronic abuse relies heavily on the treating physician, whereas long-term management requires the coordination of multiple system-wide resources and providers. In consideration of the negative health, psychological, and social aspects of cocaine and methamphetamine use, abuse, and dependence, we provide recommendations to primary care clinicians who treat and manage this patient population. Data were selected from articles and published texts as recent as 2012 using the search terms *stimulants, methamphetamines, cocaine, neurobiology, gateway theory, adolescents,* and *adolescence.* The cited publications include both reviews of the literature as well as original research articles published in English.

11.2 History of cocaine and methamphetamine

The earliest recorded origins for the medicinal use of cocaine predate the 16th century (see the introduction to this book). During this era, Andean natives would chew the leaves of the *Erythroxlon coca* plant to physiologically increase respiratory rate in an effort to meet the greater oxygen demands at higher altitudes (1). Sixteenth-century colonization of South America led to the biosynthesis and distribution of cocaine for its utility in ophthalmic surgery, local anesthesia, and treatment for sexual impotence and depression (2). Cocaine's euphorigenicity was a widely known characteristic of the plant extract and was therefore marketed and sold in tonics and nonalcoholic soft drinks, most notably in Coca Cola (3).

The emergence of the first cocaine epidemic in the United States (as evidenced by a 790% increase in cocaine use from 1890 to 1902) was a result of its widespread use, high abuse liability, lack of stringent legal restrictions on manufacturing and sales, and lack of adequate biological research into the effects of cocaine abuse (4). This epidemic brought awareness to the unintended physiological and psychiatric side effects of cocaine use and abuse leading to the Harrison Narcotics Act in 1914, banning the nonmedical use of cocaine. In 1922, cocaine was assigned as a narcotic substance and subsequently labeled a Schedule II drug under the Controlled Substances Act in 1970. Although the onset of cocaine prohibition led to a transient decrease of cocaine use, a reemergence of illegal consumption in the 1960s in addition to the synthesis and widespread abuse of crack cocaine in the 1980s spurred a renewed interest in research of the long-term effects of cocaine abuse (4).

Unlike the plant-derived production of cocaine, methamphetamine was developed as a synthetic alternative to the bioactive compound of the *Ephedra sinica* plant, named ephedra (ephedrine). Ephedrine was discovered nearly five centuries ago in Chinese medicine and is currently used in the Western world as a decongestant for asthma, hay fever, and the common cold. At the turn of the 20th century, ephedrine was isolated in the laboratory, whereupon it was found that the chemical structure was most similar to epinephrine. At that time, an orally administered pill formulation was manufactured that had a longer duration of action and larger therapeutic index and produced a more robust and dependable stimulant effect in the central nervous system (5). It is for the latter reason that ephedrine, and its chemically related compounds such as amphetamine and methamphetamine, became sought-after agents to be distributed and sold as illicit drugs of abuse.

During the 1960s, a large rise in the illegal sales of amphetamine and methamphetamine led to the Drug Abuse Control Amendments of 1965. These amendments were the first critical steps in controlling the manufacturing, distribution, prescription, and sales of amphetamines and amphetamine-like substances. The instatement of these amendments led to the Comprehensive Drug Abuse Prevention and Control Act of 1970, which limited the accepted medical uses for prescribed amphetamines and classified them as Schedule II medications (5). The United States experienced a short-lived decline in methamphetamine sales and distribution, until the most recent rise over the past 20 years reflecting an eastward growing market, in part due to the advent of small, home laboratories. A rising adolescent subpopulation of methamphetamine users presents a challenge to pediatricians and internists who must diagnose and manage the majority of adolescents who abuse stimulants.

Both cocaine and methamphetamine are currently experiencing a resurgence among young adults as popular "club drugs" due to their ability to induce euphoria, bringing about feelings of interpersonal and spiritual connectedness (6). Although cocaine has a strong history with club culture, the significant increase in manufacturing of methamphetamines through an underground culture of "clandestine methamphetamine laboratories" has brought them to the forefront of club drug use. Approximately 80% of methamphetamines distributed are synthesized in these "meth labs" and develop out of homes and other secluded closed spaces (7).

Most recently brought to popular culture through the AMC show *Breaking Bad*, these hidden laboratories perpetuate an underground culture in which instructions for chemical synthesis are shared via the Internet or other means of communication. Manufacturers (aka "cooks") commonly derive methamphetamine by using the chemical precursor, phenyl-2-propanone (P2P). In 1980, the Drug Enforcement Administration made P2P a Schedule II controlled substance leading to the illicit manufacturing of P2P from precursors – namely, ephedrine and pseudoephedrine – both of which can be found over the counter. Given this use of ephedrine, the Combat Methamphetamine Epidemic Act of 2005 enforced additional restrictions on the purchasing of ephedrine over the counter.

11.3 Epidemiology

Cocaine is distributed and marketed illegally under the following names: "coke." "C," "snow," "blow," "white girl," "flake," "rock," "yayo," and "toot" (8). Smoked cocaine is often called "crack cocaine," which derives its name from the crackling sound emitted when the cocaine crystals are heated (9). Cocaine remains one of the most highly abused illicit drugs in all age groups and is the number one cause for illicit drug-related visits to the emergency department (ED) (9). This statistic reflects both the harmful physiological effects of cocaine use/abuse and its enduring popularity. The age group 18–24, representative of late adolescence and young adulthood, reportedly has the highest rate of current cocaine use compared with any other group (9–10), which is also reflected by inconsistent increases of cocaine-related ED visits in this age group. Of note, there is an eightfold increase of cocaine-related ED visits in individuals 21 and older as compared to those 20 and younger, suggesting a strong age association of serious cocaine use and early adulthood (10).

The increased prevalence of cocaine use in later adolescence is also represented in national middle and high school studies that show that approximately 2.0% of high school seniors had used cocaine in the past month with percentages half of that found in 8th and 10th graders, a trend that has been apparent since 1980 (11). These data trends indicate a larger reflection of decreased perceived drug harmfulness evident in all grade levels (12). Although cocaine usage in adolescence and early adulthood is substantial, there has been an overall decline in usage, which some studies support is due to decreased availability of the drug (12).

Methamphetamine is also known as “meth,” “speed,” “crank,” “chalk,” “ice,” “glass,” “crystal,” “batu,” “poor man’s cocaine,” “glass uppers,” “tina biker’s,” “go-fast black beauties,” “stove top,” “methlies quick,” “yaba,” and “yellow barn” (13). According to a report from the Community Epidemiology Work Group, the methamphetamine epidemic continues to grow on the West Coast of the United States, with persisting high levels in Honolulu, San Diego, Seattle, San Francisco, and Los Angeles (14–16). However, there has been a fast-growing eastward trend of methamphetamine abuse in rural and urban sections of the South and Midwest, especially in metropolitan Atlanta (7,14–16).

In 2010, approximately 13 million people 12 years and older had abused methamphetamine in their lifetimes, and, in 2010, approximately 353,000 were current users (9). A 2011 national survey of roughly 46,700 students in 400 public and private schools showed prevalence rates of 0.8%, 1.4%, and 1.4% for 8th, 10th, and 12th graders, respectively. All of these levels are down considerably from similar estimates taken in 1999, when they were 3.2%, 4.6%, and 4.7% (12). The perceived risk of crystal methamphetamine use has risen considerably since 2003, which may have contributed to the decline in use since then. Perceived availability has been falling in all three grades since 2006, perhaps in part because there are fewer users. These figures are similar to those from the National Survey on Drug Use and Health, taken from 2002 to 2008, showing that past-month use of methamphetamine declined significantly among youths aged 12 to 17, from 0.3% to 0.1%, and young adults aged 18 to 25 also reported significant declines in past-month use, from 0.6% in 2002 to 0.4% in 2008 (17). Although the existing evidence suggests that the use of illicit stimulants in adolescents and young adults may be declining, the rates of young people transitioning from experimentation to problem use is still unacceptably high given the serious complications associated with these drugs.

11.4 Risk factors and comorbidity

Medical and psychiatric comorbidities reflect either predisposing factors or sequelae of longstanding drug abuse and should be distinguished from intoxication or toxicological emergency, which will be discussed in more detail later. In the literature, risk factors have been associated with cocaine more so than with methamphetamine abuse. This is unsurprising given that at present the body of literature on cocaine addiction far supersedes that of methamphetamine addiction, owing largely to the longer history of use, the larger variance in users, and research funding interests.

The risk factors for both methamphetamine and cocaine abuse are largely similar. These may include the following: male sex, exposure to drug abuse at an earlier age, psychiatric history, criminal history, family history of drug abuse, and personality traits such as impulsivity and risk-taking behavior (18–20). Both males and females have equal rates of lifetime exposure to cocaine; however, females were exposed at an early age as opposed to males who were exposed at a later age (21). The gender specificity of early exposure to crack/cocaine in females may be due to the strong association between female adolescent sexual abuse and lifetime crack/cocaine abuse and dependence (22). Early life trauma (sexual and nonsexual) also plays a significant role in cocaine dependence especially if trauma sequelae persist in adulthood (23,24). Rates of methamphetamine and cocaine use are high among homosexual males and appear to be linked to high rates of HIV transmission in this subpopulation (25), which is at particular health risk given the continually high incidence and prevalence of HIV infection rates.

Comorbid substance use disorders (SUDs) have been of particular research interest in the cocaine addiction literature. The “gateway drug theory” suggests that precedent drug using behavior may potentiate more risky and dangerous drug use (26). This theory has been applied to adolescent nicotine and cannabis use as a predictor for later abuse of cocaine. Recent epidemiological studies of drug using behavior in high school seniors support that 84.9% of student cocaine users initiate cocaine use after the onset of nicotine smoking (27), a trend that also predicts increased risk of cocaine dependency (28). Animal studies have shown that adolescent nicotine exposure may confer long-lasting epigenetic changes in the brain, giving rise to an enhancement of emotional and behavioral responses to cocaine (29).

These epigenetic changes may provide an explanation for the increased liability of later cocaine abuse in adulthood. Adolescent marijuana use, particularly before the age of 15, is also strongly correlated with lifetime cocaine abuse (27). While nicotine and cannabis use in and of itself does not necessarily cause cocaine abuse, the reasons for such an association may in part be due to selection of peer group and neurobiological mechanisms involved in craving and reward-seeking behaviors. Therefore, it may be clinically relevant to have frank discussions with adolescents about peer-group selection during middle school/high school transitions.

Psychiatric comorbidity in cocaine and methamphetamine abuse, and drug abuse overall, is generally accepted as the rule rather than the exception (30–31). A causal association between drug abuse and psychiatric illness is often difficult to delineate given that an intrinsic psychiatric disorder can contribute toward drug-abusing behavior and drug-abuse behavior can induce a psychiatric condition (30); this applies to both Axis I major psychiatric conditions and Axis II personality disorders. Studies have shown that cocaine users are at a threefold higher lifetime risk for anxiety and depression at any age, although adolescent cocaine users have a higher comorbidity with anxiety (30).

Severity of depressive and anxiety symptoms have been associated with more severe drug abuse patterns before treatment and with poorer alcohol and drug use outcomes, increased health service utilization, and higher levels of psychiatric symptomatology, including suicidality in follow-up studies after successful treatment (32,33). In a study comparing methamphetamine and cocaine users, cocaine users were more likely to have a psychiatric diagnosis and were also more likely to be HIV-positive and engage in high-risk behaviors for HIV transmission such as using and sharing needles (34).

11.5 Pharmacology and pathophysiology

Cocaine can be administered intranasally, intravenously, or via inhalation. Common adulterants of cocaine are procaine, amphetamine, methylephedrine, diltiazem, hyrdoxyzine, baking soda, talcum, and cornstarch (35). Intranasal administration results in a slow increase in concentration of cocaine in plasma resulting in a euphoric "high" that may last between 15 and 30 minutes and is associated with perforation of the nasal septum, epistaxis, anosmia, or rhinorrhea (8).

Intravenous delivery of cocaine is achieved by dissolution of cocaine salts in a water vehicle and injection producing a rapid increase in concentration in plasma and resulting in a high that lasts 5–10 minutes. "Crack" cocaine is the inhaled form of cocaine.

Methamphetamine can also be administered intranasally, intravenously, and via inhalation. Although methamphetamine's slightly higher lipophilicity allows it to cross the blood-brain barrier faster than that of cocaine, methamphetamine is absorbed to a large degree in the lung, and in turn, peak plasma levels are not reached until 2.5–6.3 hours after inhalation of vapor. Crystalline S-methamphetamine hydrochloride is mainly metabolized by the liver, does not have any psychoactive metabolites, and is excreted by the kidneys (36).

This is largely similar to that of cocaine; however, plasma cholinesterases have an additional role in cocaine metabolism (37). Methamphetamine remains in the brain for a much longer time than cocaine with subjective highs lasting between 4 and 14 hours. As in all euphorigenic substances, the route of administration is related to abuse liability (intravenous followed by smoke inhalation and then intranasal) as well as risk for comorbid conditions such as HIV and hepatitis C with intravenous use (8), although stimulant-induced euphoria may also be responsible for this association (38).

Cocaine and methamphetamine are central- and peripheral-acting psychostimulants that affect monamine neurotransmitter systems (which include dopamine, norepinephrine, and serotonin) (see chapter 2). Although both agents act on the presynaptic terminals by altering monoamine transport, they have two different modes of action. Cocaine acts as a reuptake inhibitor that blocks the presynaptic reuptake of monoamine neurotransmitters leading to an influx of all three monoamines in the synapse (39).

In contrast, amphetamines bind reuptake transporters and are directly transported into the presynaptic cytoplasm to induce monoamine neurotransmitter release in the synapse. Amphetamines have a higher affinity for dopamine and serotonin transporters than norepinephrine, whereas cocaine shows equal affinity to all three transporters (39). As a result of these effects, postsynaptic monoaminergic receptors are continuously activated based on the duration of action of the drug. Given the central role of monoamines such as dopamine in the reward circuitry of the brain, the transient increase of dopamine from psychostimulants significantly contributes to the abuse liability of these drugs.

Furthermore, human imaging studies have indicated that increased dopamine in the dorsal striatum correlates with individual assessment of reward and euphoria (40). This is particularly relevant in the adolescence brain, which has been shown to undergo an increase of dopaminergic receptors before later pruning in adulthood, suggesting that they are a particularly vulnerable population to the effects of psychostimulants (41).

11.6 Clinical manifestations of intoxication, overdose, and withdrawal

One of the main concerns for clinicians in any field is related to the acute effects of stimulant intoxication, which may be unpredictably fatal. The effects of stimulants on the cardiovascular system are of primary importance, and acute cardiovascular episodes in young individuals with no family or prior personal history should always raise suspicions about potential stimulant overdose. While acute subjective effects may diminish over 4 hours, the cardiovascular effects tend to remain elevated. In turn, as the marked acute tachyphylaxis to subjective effects may drive repeated use within intervals of 4 hours, cardiovascular risk will increase. When used concomitantly, alcohol and cocaine may produce the metabolite cocaethylene, which intensifies cocaine euphoria and is also associated with greater rates of sudden death (42). Additional symptoms may include dilated pupils, overall hyperactivity and euphoric mood, irritability, and anxiety.

During intoxication, a person may experience bursts of energy and a lack of hunger and may go long periods of time without eating or sleeping, leading to weight loss and mucosal dryness. Whereas acute intoxication is associated with episodes of excessive talking and physical activity, a stimulant withdrawal syndrome may present as depression, excessive and irregular sleep, and decreased activity. A summary of these symptoms is presented in table 11.1 and reflects the *Diagnostic and Statistical Manual of Mental Disorders*, fourth edition, text revision (*DSM-IV-TR*) (43), criteria for acute intoxication and withdrawal (see table 11.2 and figures 11.1 and 11.2).

Table 11.1: Signs of acute intoxication, withdrawal, and chronic abuse of illicit stimulants*

	Signs of acute intoxication	Signs of withdrawal	Signs of chronic drug abuse (dependence)
General	• Dehydration • Diaphoresis • Hunger suppression • Hyperactivity • Hyperthermia	• Fatigue • Generalized malaise • Increased appetite • Psychomotor retardation or agitation	• Eroded dentition (methamphetamines) • Negligent of personal hygiene • Failure to fulfill major role obligations at work, school, or home • Weight changes • Halitosis
Cardiac	• Dysrhythmia • Increased blood pressure • Increased heart rate • Sudden death • Myocardial infarction	• Arrhythmias	• Heart disease • Myocardial infarction • Pulmonary hypertension (methamphetamines) • Sudden death (cocaine)
Neurological	• Dilated pupils • Dystonia • Dyskinesias • Seizures	• Lack of coordination • Vivid unpleasant dreams • Insomnia or hypersomnia	• Ischemic or hemorrhagic stroke • Seizures • Slurred speech • Tremor
Psychiatric	• Agitated delirium (hostility, paranoia, hyperactivity, and aggression) • Changes in personality • Confusion • Depression	• Depression • Dysphoria • Increased anxiety • Irregular sleeping patterns	• Abrupt changes in relationships • Depression • Impulsive • Increased anxiety • Paranoid psychosis

(*Continued*)

Table 11.1: Signs of acute intoxication, withdrawal, and chronic abuse of illicit stimulants* (*Continued*)

	Signs of acute intoxication	Signs of withdrawal	Signs of chronic drug abuse (dependence)
	• Excessive talking • Increased anxiety • Mood lability • Psychosis		
Musculoskeletal	• Muscular edema • Muscular weakness • Postural changes	• No musculoskeletal symptoms noted in literature	• Cocaine-associated rhabdomyolisis
Gastrointestinal	• Nausea • Vomiting	• Nausea • Vomiting	• Cocaine-associated rhabdomyolisis

*Amphetamines and cocaine manifest themselves similarly physiologically, and where they differ is specified explicitly within the table.

Table 11.2: Differential diagnosis of cocaine and methamphetamine intoxication

Toxicological	• Amphetamine or other stimulant abuse • Lysergic acid diethylamide (LSD) intoxication • Phencyclidine (PCP) intoxication • Neuroleptic malignant syndrome • Anticholinergic drug exposure • Theophylline • Tricyclic antidepressants • Serotonin syndrome • Caffeine • Salicylates
Neurological	• Trauma • Stroke • Intracranial hemorrhage • Brain lesion • Epilepsy (frontal or temporal lobe)
Psychiatric	• Schizophrenia • Bipolar depression • Depression
Endocrine	• Adrenal hyperplasia or adenoma • Hyperthyroidism
Infectious	• Meningitis (infectious or from monoamine oxidase inhibitors) • Encephalitis
Other syndromes	• Delirium • Malignant hypertension • Malignant hyperthermia • Sepsis

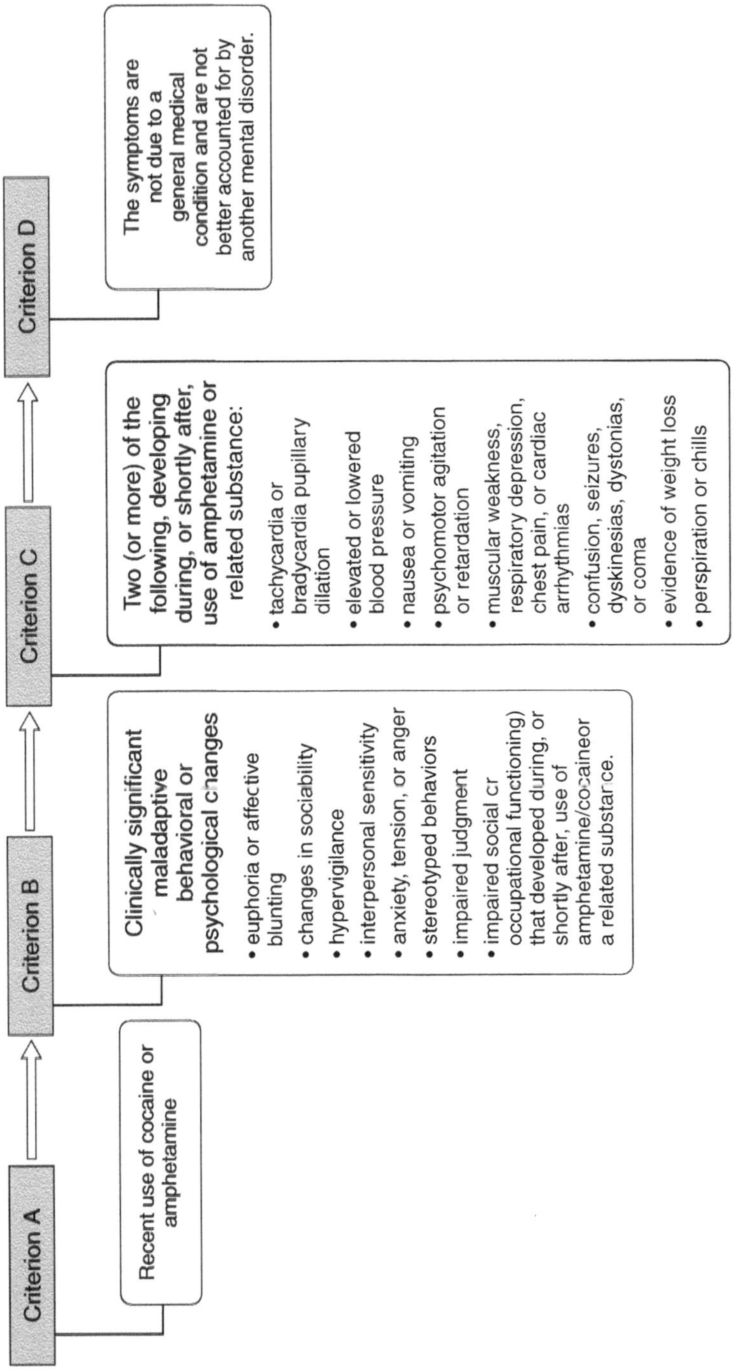

Figure 11.1: Diagnostic criteria for acute cocaine or amphetamine intoxication (adapted from American Psychiatric Association. Diagnostic and statistical manual of mental disorders, 4th ed., text rev. Washington, DC: APA, 2000)

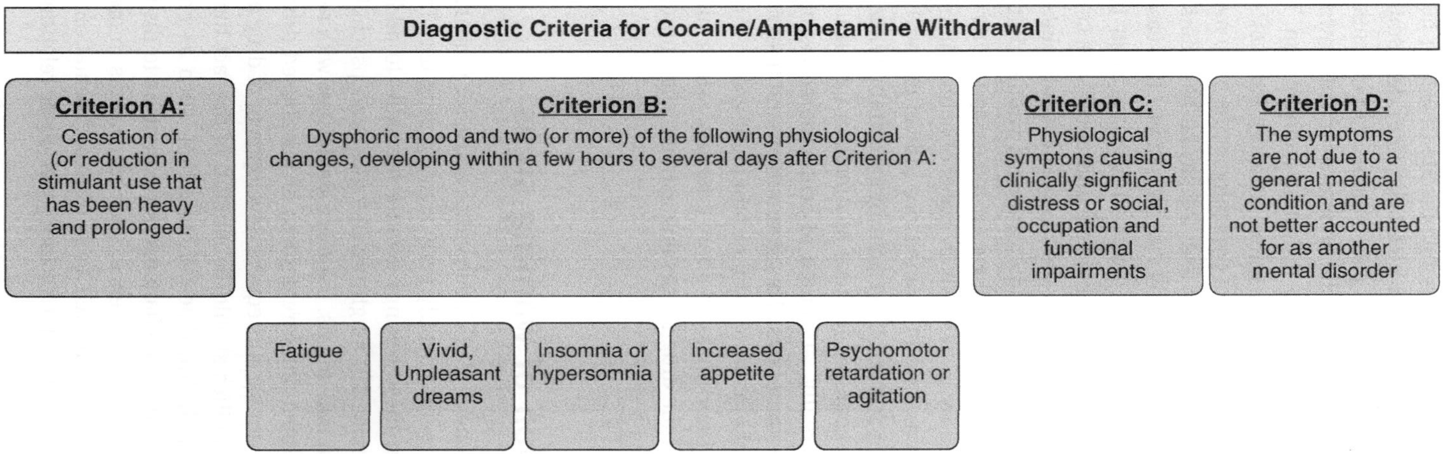

Figure 11.2: Diagnostic criteria for stimulant withdrawal (adapted from American Psychiatric Association. Diagnostic and statistical manual of mental disorders, 4th ed., text rev. Washington, DC: APA, 2000)

Mild acute intoxication signs and symptoms are transient; however, due to increased activity levels and accelerated metabolic rate, dehydration is a common complicating factor, and severe cases may require hospitalization and treatment with intravenous (IV) fluids. Similarly, the symptoms of withdrawal are mostly managed with supportive measures such as hydration and nutrition. The psychological effects of stimulant withdrawal may manifest as acute onset of severe depression and are thought to be due to depletion of dopamine in the brain mesolimbic circuits. Although uncommon, these states may lead to suicidal behaviors and may require acute psychiatric hospitalization. Lastly, in rare cases, the vasoconstrictive and chronotropic effect of stimulants may result in heart or brain infarcts, requiring acute treatment in hospital setting; in some circumstances, this can lead to immediate death. These complications may be used as educational points when discussing the deleterious effects of drugs with adolescents and young adults.

It should be also emphasized that there are increased reports of episodes of extreme violence committed by individuals in states of acute stimulant intoxication, a phenomenon that becomes troublesome since individuals with no prior history of violent behaviors often commit these acts. Since irritability, hostility, and paranoid thinking are well-recognized features of stimulant intoxication, these violent acts may be, at least partially, attributed to acute alterations of the individual's mental state after use of stimulants. This intermittent and unexpected onset of violence goes along with the pattern of binge stimulant use as individuals may intake multiple doses of the drug(s) in short intervals, which may result in very high cumulative doses of the drug(s), causing extreme and unpredictable changes in mental state.

11.7 Identification of warning signs

The most relevant component of illicit substance abuse for primary care physicians is the ability to recognize and identify early signs of drug use. Therefore, it is essential that clinicians in these settings acquire the skills to address such issues with the patient and family. Although physiological and psychological effects of drug abuse vary between individuals, there are similarities with respect to changes in behavior and social functioning regardless of the abused drug. Given the fact that early use is a risk factor for subsequent development of drug abuse and dependence, physicians and families should be mindful of the fact that risk for experimentation is more likely during times of transition, such as change in school, relocation, or family conflict. The challenge for parents is to distinguish between the normal characteristics of adolescence, such as changes in mood and the propensity for impulsive actions, and red flags of experimentation with substances and potential drug abuse. The latter include new onset relationship difficulties, abrupt changes in peer group, impulsive break ups of romantic relationships, neglect of previously established responsibilities, and abrupt personality and behavioral changes.

Social interactions are of great importance in adolescence, and therefore changes of peers groups and affiliations are normative. However, an abrupt discard of an established group of friends for new associates should raise parents' and clinicians' concern, especially when it is done secretively and the individual becomes evasive about new interests and activities. Similarly, establishment and turnover of romantic partners in adolescents can vary widely; however, frequent, impulsive, and explosive breakups may be suggestive of more than just a "difficult personality" and should signal to parents and clinicians to initiate discussion about friends and romantic partners and the possibility of concomitant drug use.

When concerns about potential drug use are raised, parents and clinicians may need to obtain additional information about their child's academic work as well as their social behavior at school and during other out-of-home activities. Often there may be declining grades, new onset delinquency, behavioral problems with authorities at school, and increased frequency of risky behaviors such as reckless driving, promiscuity, and engaging in unprotected sex. It is not unusual that affected teens will start neglecting extracurricular activities or may lie about attending practices and competitions when in reality they will be missing such activities. It is even more challenging to assess behavioral changes in situations where there is a lack of regular contacts with close family members. This is typically experienced when young adults move away from home to live on campus during college matriculation or to live on their own when they have established financial independence. Since physicians may not be able to contact collaterals without patients' consent, involvement of the family is crucial in these situations as they may have access to friends or employers.

A different set of warning signs of drug abuse include abrupt changes in physical appearance such as acute changes in weight, deterioration in personal hygiene, and unusual smells on breath, body, or clothing (44). A person abusing drugs may begin exhibiting tremors, demonstrate abnormal movements, or be seen with an altered level of alertness or even slurring of speech. Psychological changes such as unexplained change in personality or attitude, mood liability, irritability, or angry outbursts should be noted and examined. Wide fluctuations of emotions and activity level such as periods of unusual hyperactivity, agitation, or giddiness followed by lack of motivation and/or unprovoked episodes of intense anxiety, fearfulness, and paranoia may indicate more serious drug involvement. This, in turn, may be accompanied by more serious legal problems such as arrests for disorderly conduct, driving under the influence, or stealing to support a drug habit. Most disconcerting is the increasing number of reports of violence leading to fatal injuries all in the context of illicit stimulants use (45).

11.8 Problem use (abuse and dependence)

It should be acknowledged that the line between initial experimentation and more consistent chronic use is blurry, and, in reality, drug abuse in adolescents and young adults may remain unidentified for a considerable amount of time. Theoretically, the progression from innocuous to more overtly problematic behaviors could be interrupted with timely interventions; however, in practice this can prove to be more challenging. Not surprisingly, justifications for inaction could be linked to misconceptions about the nature of drug use–related problems and the ability to influence the outcomes. Such "myths" about substance abuse are linked to beliefs such as one can overcome addiction as a matter of willpower, and therefore "one can stop using drugs if they really want to."

A growing accumulation of evidence shows that prolonged exposure to drugs alters the brain in ways that result in powerful cravings and a compulsion to use, and therefore cessation of drug use is extremely difficult to accomplish even by choice (46). Alternatively, some believe that if addiction is a disease, then "there's nothing that a person can do about it." While most experts agree that addiction is a brain disease, they also recognize that brain changes associated with addiction can be treated and may be reversed through therapy, medication, exercise, and other treatments. In relation to treatment, it is commonly accepted by the public that affected individuals have to "hit rock bottom before they can get better." In reality, recovery can begin at any point in the addiction process, and the longer that drug abuse continues, the harder it becomes to treat. This highlights the importance of engagement, particularly with otherwise physically healthy adolescents and young adults.

The initial steps of their engagement are often difficult and can be further compromised by adopting the attitude that "you can't force someone into treatment; they have to want help." No evidence exists in the literature supporting the notion that treatments have to be voluntary in order to be successful. People who are pressured into treatment by their family, employer, or the legal system are just as likely to benefit as those who choose to enter treatment on their own. More often than not, as the physiological effects of drugs wear off, much of the resistance becomes easier to overcome, and individuals seek change. However, successful outcomes cannot be guaranteed, and it is not unusual for clinicians to be faced with the argument that "treatment didn't work before, so there's no point trying again." One sensible response is that relapse doesn't mean that treatment has failed, but rather, it's a signal to get back on track, either by reengaging in treatment or adjusting the current treatment approach.

In cases when the warning signs were missed or when proactive measures failed, some individuals may develop problematic drug use that can then be designated by *DSM-IV-TR* criteria for abuse or dependence (43). The criteria for illicit stimulant abuse and dependence are the same as the criteria for abuse and dependence for any other substance. Overall, these two conditions differ mainly on the severity of the drug use and its impact on the individual's social functioning. The clinical picture could be complicated by drug-induced mood and anxiety or psychotic disorders or by psychological trauma related to drug use experiences. These conditions may require long-term treatments that will address in parallel symptoms related to drug use (compulsive drug seeking and taking, intense craving, and relapse) as well as symptoms of depression, anxiety, and psychosis. There is also evidence that low striatal dopamine function in methamphetamine addicts is associated with increased risk for relapse during treatment (47).

11.9 Treatment of illicit stimulant abuse and dependence

Behavioral therapy and pharmacotherapy have both been investigated for the treatment of stimulant abuse/dependence (see chapters 5 and 6). While effectiveness of some behavioral interventions has been demonstrated, most medication trials have failed to demonstrate compelling evidence for efficacy. However, an expanding literature supports the use of agonist-like medications to treat stimulant abuse/dependence, a strategy that has been effective for nicotine and opiate dependence. The conceptualization for treating stimulant dependence with agonist-like agents posits that medications with properties similar to that of the abused drug, but possessing lesser abuse liability, may be able to normalize neurochemistry and stabilize behavior and, in turn, may reduce drug use. This concept is supported by findings showing that stimulant-dependent individuals treated with dexamphetamine and heroin-dependent patients treated with methadone exhibited an equivalent reduction in illicit IV drug use.

11.10 Biological treatments

Review of the available literature shows that a range of medications, from l-dopa/carbidopa to antidepressants and amphetamine preparations, have been used to treat adults with stimulant abuse and dependence (48). It should be noted, however, that no data are available for the treatment of individuals younger than 18 with any of these compounds. Although prescription amphetamines have been used as a first-line treatment for attention-deficit/hyperactivity disorder (ADHD), as augmentation for depression, and as cognitive enhancement, there is growing evidence that supports the use of these agents to safely wean dependent patients off of stimulants.

Although some of the protocol samples are rather small, these studies are informative as proof of concept for the utility of these types of treatments. For instance, one study treated seven cocaine-dependent patients with dexamphetamine maintenance and reported blunted effects of cocaine when the drug was administered in the lab (49). In another trial that followed 30 cocaine IV users, 16 of whom were treated with dexamphetamine and 14 with a placebo, cocaine-positive urine tests in the dexamphetamine group fell from 94% to 56%, while the placebo group showed no change after 14 weeks of treatment (50). In a randomized, double-blind, placebo-controlled study, 82 cocaine-dependent individuals were evaluated when treated with placebo and immediate- and sustained-release methamphetamine. Those in the sustained-release condition exhibited consistently lower rates of cocaine-positive urine samples and reported the greatest reduction in craving for cocaine (51).

Modafinil, a nonamphetamine stimulant that is approved by the U.S. Food and Drug Administration (FDA) for the treatment of narcolepsy and other sleep disorders, has also been studied for the treatment of illicit stimulant dependence (52). Modafinil does not carry the same risk for misuse as prescriptions stimulants, making it a promising alternative as a maintenance drug. Data largely support the utility of modafinil in reducing cocaine use in dependent adults (53). Other studies have shown potential benefits from antidepressants such as citalopram (54,55) and naltrexone (56).

It should be highlighted that no pharmacological agent has received FDA approval for the treatment of stimulant use disorders, and therefore, studies of the previously mentioned agents have provided only preliminary data for the clinical usefulness in the treatment of stimulant abuse and dependence. From that perspective, their clinical use in adolescents for the purpose of controlling symptoms of stimulant abuse is possible on a case-by-case basis and at the clinicians' discretion (off-label use). Lastly, studies of comorbid drug use with ADHD or depression have reported that pharmacotherapy used to control ADHD and mood symptoms had minimal effect on symptoms related to drug use (57). The extent to which these studies can be informative about the efficacious treatment of the stimulant-dependent population is undoubtedly limited, given the many unknowns about the pathophysiological mechanisms of psychiatric illness in general.

11.11 Behavioral treatments

There are several therapeutic modalities that have been shown to successfully manage and treat adolescents and young adults with illicit stimulant abuse and dependence. These include psychoeducation, motivational interviewing, brief interventions, cognitive behavioral therapy (CBT), group treatments, multisystemic treatments, and therapeutic communities. The utility of each of these modalities is related to the therapeutic goal that the clinician sets for any individual case. For instance, educating the patient and the family about SUDs and their pervasive effects on one's functioning can help set the stage for developing an effective therapeutic alliance. Motivational interviewing is a technique that aims to engage patients that are unwilling or incapable of recognizing the extent and the severity of their drug use and are resistant to treatment. The efficient application of this technique requires a considerable amount of skill and clinical experience; however, when mastered, it is an effective means of bringing about awareness of a patient's drug use and its related problems. One such skill is to carefully monitor patient's own statements and quickly point out any contradictions (i.e., patient claims that he/she has no alcohol problems but has been arrested for driving under the influence). The challenge is to employ this method in a nonthreatening and nonjudgmental manner in an effort to overcome resistance about problem drug use and evoke considerations about the need to seek help. This process is also referred to as transition from denial to contemplation.

If successful with overcoming this initial resistance, primary care physicians are faced with the challenging next step – what kind of treatment intervention(s) may be indicated, and who shall deliver them? In most cases, it is clinically prudent to set up flexible short-term goals such as frequent appointments and encouragement for patients and family to keep showing up. This approach is akin to brief intervention, which mainly aims to solidify engagement and establish compliance with whatever recommended treatment may come next. On the level of the individual, CBT could be administered to facilitate recognition of triggers for drug use and patterns of behaviors leading to it and design coping strategies to manage stress and other factors that may contribute to drug use or relapse. However, there is evidence suggesting that patients with SUDs may exhibit cognitive deficits associated with either comorbid ADHD or mood/anxiety disorder(s) or as a result of the effects of substances on the brain functions. These may be further linked to low treatment retention; therefore, retaining patients with cognitive deficits in CBT-based SUD treatment is difficult, and individualized treatment strategies may need to be developed (58).

Group treatment programs are useful in that many individuals gain empowerment through shared experiences. In this controlled setting, validation of personal experience, exchange of ideas for treatment, and the shedding of embarrassment and/or humiliation through destigmatization of illness are some of the many benefits. Broader family involvement can be achieved through the use of multisystemic treatments that include family members and a wider array of providers. In cases of persistent use and relapse, a therapeutic community model may need to be considered. This treatment modality requires that individuals may be placed in an inpatient hospital-type of setting. Additional, but less studied behavioral strategies include coaching and behavior modification. Coaching is a collaborative relationship between the patient and the clinician to develop strategies for managing drug-related problems such as avoiding exposure to drugs, peer associations, and management of peer pressure to use drugs. Behavior modification is a technique used in young adolescents where desired behaviors are positively reinforced to increase their frequency.

While individual clinicians are unable to offer the whole gamut of treatments available to patients who struggle with drug abuse and dependence and their families, it is the clinicians' responsibility to be knowledgeable about the array of treatment options as well as how and where these services can be accessed within the community. For the majority of cases, the treatment plan includes several modalities (i.e., individual cognitive behavioral sessions and peer and family groups) that require coordination of multiple providers. Therefore, after the initial phase of identification and engagement, primary care physicians may take a central role in this coordination effort. In some instances, individuals may be able to reach out to self-help groups, but for majority of cases, these will be ancillary rather than main treatment.

11.12 Clinical management of co-occurring ADHD and stimulant use disorders

The management of adolescents and young adults with co-occurring ADHD and stimulant use disorders is of paramount importance since nonmedical use of prescription stimulants has been on the rise (see chapters 10 and 16). Further, it is possible that some individuals may use nonprescription stimulants to self-medicate unrecognized symptoms of ADHD. A conservative approach for treating co-occurring ADHD and stimulant use disorders would be to initiate treatment with a nonstimulant pharmacotherapy. However, a more likely scenario would include treatment with stimulants that requires careful attention to the treatment boundaries, close monitoring, and frequent urine toxicology testing. It should be discussed explicitly with the patient that the use of stimulant medication carries an inherent risk of misuse or abuse. The patient and his or her family should be advised in advance about the potentially dangerous sequelae of abrupt discontinuation of stimulants in the event of stimulant treatment abuse and subsequent switching of pharmacological agents.

Repetitive requests to replace "missing," "lost," or "stolen" medication, as well as requests for dose increases when not clinically indicated, should raise concern for misuse. Emphasis should be placed on adherence to a prescribed medication regimen and reinforcement that medication should not be taken on an "as needed" or "catch-up" basis. Careful documentation of all prescriptions must be maintained in order to monitor the amount and frequency of the drug being prescribed. When prescribing stimulants, delayed-release preparations are preferred to avoid potential for nonoral abuse (i.e., extracting the substance and snorting or injecting it) and prevent abrupt changes in blood levels of the drug, which can reinforce maladaptive brain changes to the reward system.

Since the assessment of ADHD symptoms in young adults is almost entirely based on self-report, the potential for patients with SUDs attempting to mislead clinicians in an effort to obtain stimulants is always present. Therefore, assessment for malingering is another important component of managing patients with co-occurring ADHD and SUD. In such cases, efforts to obtain collateral data from family and other sources become very important to reliably establish the ADHD diagnosis. In patients diagnosed with ADHD, visits should be frequently scheduled with a plan to have medications brought to each visit. Despite all efforts to reduce the risk of diversion, misuse, or abuse of stimulants, it should be expected that a small percentage of patients with ADHD comorbid with SUDs will attempt to do so; for the majority of patients, however, psychostimulants can be used safely and effectively when careful monitoring during treatment is put in place.

11.13 Summary

Although there seems to be an overall decline in cocaine and methamphetamine abuse in all age groups in the United States, a substantial number of adolescents and young adults continue to use and abuse illicit stimulants. As such, identification of early warning signs can allow for timely medical, psychological, and programmatic interventions. Therefore, clinicians' ability to identify such warning signs is of great importance in primary care settings. Understanding how to communicate with the patient as well as the patient's family is an extremely powerful preventative strategy. Furthermore, understanding risk factors and comorbidities in patients who are abusing stimulants allows for appropriate risk management during clinical visits. Once stimulant abuse has been identified, clinicians need to also identify available treatment resources and make referrals to ensure proper management. Stimulant abuse, as well as drug abuse overall, is a multisystem-wide problem and a shared responsibility between various health care providers, the patient, the family of the patient, and any individuals who interact with the patient out of the home, at work, school, or other places where the individual interacts with others. This chapter has reviewed the current literature and has summarized the recommendations for diagnosis and management of illicit stimulant use, abuse, and dependence in adolescents and young adults that are applicable for physicians in primary care.

References

1. Hanna JM, Hornick CA. Use of coca leaf in southern Peru: Adaptation or addiction. Bull Narc 1977;29(1):63–74.
2. Spillane JF. Cocaine: From medical marvel to modern menace in the United States, 1884–1920. Baltimore, MD: The Johns Hopkins University Press, 2000.
3. Schoenberg BS. Coke's the one. South Med J 1988;81:69–74.
4. Gootenberg, P, ed. Cocaine: Global histories. London: Routledge, 1999.

5. Vearrier D, Greenberg MI, Miller SN, Okaneku JT, Haggerty DA. Methamphetamine: History, pathophysiology, adverse health effects, current trends, and hazards associated with the clandestine manufacture of methamphetamine. Dis Mon 2012;58(2):38–89.
6. Kelly BC, Parsons JT, Wells BE. Prevalence and predictors of club drug use among club going young adults in New York City. J Urban Health 2006;83(5):884–95.
7. Burgess JL, Barnhart S, Checkoway H. Investigating clandestine drug laboratories: Adverse medical effects in law enforcement personnel. Am J Ind Med 1996;30:488–94.
8. National Institutes of Drug Abuse. Research reports: Cocaine: Abuse and addiction. NIH Publication Number 10–4166. Printed May 1999; revised September 2010. Accessed January 8, 2013. URL: http://www.drugabuse.gov/publications/research-reports/cocaine-abuse-addiction
9. Substance Abuse and Mental Health Services Administration. Results from the 2010 National Survey on Drug Use and Health: Mental health findings. NSDUH Series H-42, HHS Publication No (SMA) 11–4667. Rockville, MD: Substance Abuse and Mental Health Services Administration, 2012.
10. Substance Abuse and Mental Health Services Administration. Cocaine use: 2002 and 2003. Research Triangle Park, NC: Substance Abuse Mental Health Services Administration, 2005.
11. National Center for Health Statistics. Health, United States, 2010: With special feature on death and dying. Hyattsville, MD: National Center for Health Statistics, 2011.
12. Johnston LD, O'Malley PM, Bachman JG, Schulenberg JE. Monitoring the future – National results on adolescent drug use: Overview of key findings, 2011. Ann Arbor: University Michigan Institute Social Research, 2012.
13. Rao RB, Hoffman RS. Cocaine and other sympathomimetics. In: Rosen's emergency medicine: Concepts and clinical practice, 6th ed. Philadelphia, PA: Mosby-Elsevier, 2006.
14. National Institute on Drug Abuse. 1. Epidemiologic trends in drug abuse: Advance report, Community Epidemiology Work Group. NIH Pub. No. 06–5878. Bethesda, MD: NIH, DHHS, 2006.
15. National Institute on Drug Abuse. 2. Epidemiologic trends in drug abuse. Vol. 1, Proceedings of the Community Epidemiology Work Group: Highlights and executive summary. NIH Pub. No. 06–5879. Bethesda, MD: NIH, DHHS, 2006.
16. National Institute on Drug Abuse. 3. Epidemiologic trends in drug abuse. Vol. 2, Proceedings of the Community Epidemiology Work Group. NIH Pub. No. 06–5880. Bethesda, MD: NIH, DHHS, 2006.
17. Substance Abuse and Mental Health Services Administration, Office of Applied Studies. Drug Abuse Warning Network, detailed tables: National estimates of drug-related emergency department visits 2004–2008. Accessed January 8, 2013. URL: https://dawninfo.samhsa.gov/data
18. Krueger RF. Personality traits in late adolescence predict mental disorders in early adulthood: A prospective-epidemiological study. J Pers 1999;67(1):39–65.
19. Bornovalova MA, Lejuez CW, Daughters SB, Zachary RM, Lynch TR. Impulsivity as a common process across borderline personality and substance use disorders. Clin Psychol Rev 2005;25(6): 790–812.
20. Kasperski SJ, Vincent KB, Caldeira KM, Garnier-Dykstra LM, O'Grady KE, Arria AM. College students' use of cocaine: Results from a longitudinal study. Addict Behav 2011;36(4):408–11.
21. Etten MLV, Neumark YD, Anthony JC. Male-female differences in the earliest stages of drug involvement. Addiction 1999;94:1413–9.
22. Freeman RC, Collier K, Parillo KM. Early life sexual abuse as a risk factor for crack cocaine use in a sample of community-recruited women at high risk for illicit drug use. Am J Drug Alcohol Abuse 2002;28(1):109–31.
23. Back SE, Brady KT, Waldrop AE, Yeatts SD, McRae AL, Spratt E. Early life trauma and sensitivity to current life stressors in individuals with and without cocaine dependence. Am J Drug Alcohol Abuse 2008;34:389–96.

24. Narvaez JC, Magalhaes PV, Tridade EK, Viera DC, Kauer-Sant'anna M, Gama CS, et al. Childhood trauma, impulsivity, and executive functioning in crack cocaine users. Compr Psychiatry 2012; 53(3):238–44.
25. Pantalone DW, Bimbi DS, Holder CA, Golub SA, Parsons JT. Consistency and change in club drug use by sexual minority men in New York City, 2002 to 2007. Am J Public Health 2010; 10(10):1892–5.
26. Kandel D. Stages in adolescent involvement in drug use. Science 1975;190(4217):912–4.
27. U.S. Department of Health and Human Services. Preventing tobacco use among youth and young adults: A report of the surgeon general. Atlanta, GA: DHHS, CDC, 2012.
28. Levine A, Huang Y, Drisaldi B, Griffin EA Jr, Pollak DD, Xu S, et al. Molecular mechanism for a gateway drug: Epigenetic changes initiated by nicotine prime gene expression by cocaine. Sci Transl Med 2011;3(107):107–9.
29. Collins SL, Izenwasser S. Chronic nicotine differentially alters cocaine-induced locomotor activity in adolescent vs. adult male and female rats. Neuropharmacology 2004;46(3):349–62.
30. Herrero MJ, Domingo-Salvany A, Torrens M, Brugal MT; ITINERE Investigators. Psychiatric comorbidity in young cocaine users: Induced versus independent disorders. Addiction 2008;103 (2):284–93.
31. Salo R, Flower K, Kielstein A, Leamon MH, Nordahl TE, Galloway GP. Psychiatric comorbidity in methamphetamine dependence. Psychiatr Res 2011;186(2–3):356–61.
32. Glasner-Edwards S, Marinelli-Casey P, Hillhouse M, Ang A, Mooney LJ, Rawson R. Methamphetamine treatment project corporate authors. J Nerv Ment Dis 2009;97(4):225–31.
33. Glasner-Edwards S, Mooney LJ, Marinelli-Casey P, Hillhouse M, Ang A, Rawson R. Methamphetamine treatment project corporate authors. Drug Alcohol Rev 2010;29(1):12–20.
34. Copeland AL, Sorensen JL. Differences between methamphetamine users and cocaine users in treatment. Drug Alcohol Depend 2001;62:91–5.
35. Behrman, AD. Luck of the draw: Common adulterants found in illicit drugs. J Emer Nurs 2010;36(2):99.
36. Cruickshank CC, Dyer KR. A review of clinical pharmacology of methamphetamine. Addiction 2009;104(7):1085–99.
37. Hoffman HS, Henry GC, Howland MA, Weisman RS, Weil L, Goldfrank LR. Association between life-threatening cocaine toxicity and plasma cholinesterase activity. Ann Emer Med 1992;21 (3):247–53.
38. Volkow ND, Wang GJ, Fowler JS, Telang F, Jayne M, Wong C. Stimulant-induced enhanced sexual desire as a potential contributing factor in HIV transmission. Am J Psychiatry 2007;164(1):157–60.
39. Howell LL, Kimmel HL. Monoamine transporters and psychostimulant addiction. Biochem Pharmacol 2008;75(1):196–217.
40. Volkow ND, Fowler JS, Wang GJ, Baler R, Telang F. Imaging dopamine's role in drug abuse and addiction. Neuropharmacology 2009;56(Suppl 1):3–8.
41. Spear LP. The adolescent brain and age-related behavioral manifestations. Neurosci Biobehav Rev 2000;24(4):417–63.
42. Bailey DN. Cocaethylene: A novel cocaine homolog. West J Med 1997;167(1):38–9.
43. American Psychiatric Association. Diagnostic and statistical manual of mental disorders, 4th ed., text rev. Washington, DC: APA, 2000.
44. Shetty V, Mooney LJ, Zigler CM, Belin TR, Murphy D, Rawson R. The relationship between methamphetamine use and increased dental disease. J Am Dent Assoc 2010;141(3):307–18.
45. Office of Applied Studies. Results from the 2004 National Survey on Drug Use and Health: National findings. DHHS Publication No. SMA 05-4062, NSDUH Series H-28. Rockville, MD: Substance Abuse Mental Health Services Administration, 2005.

46. Kalivas PW, Volkow ND. The neural basis of addiction: A pathology of motivation and choice. Am J Psychiatry 2005;162(8):1403–13.
47. Wang GJ, Smith L, Volkrow ND, Telang F, Logan J, Tomasi D, et al. Decreased dopamine activity predicts relapse in methamphetamine abusers. Mol Psychiatry 2012;19(9):918–25.
48. Herin DV, Rush CR, Grabowski J. Agonist-like pharmacotherapy for stimulant dependence: Preclinical, human laboratory, and clinical studies. Ann NY Acad Sci 2010;1187:76–100.
49. Rush CR, Stoops WW, Hays LR. Cocaine effects during d-amphetamine maintenance: A human laboratory analysis of safety, tolerability and efficacy. Drug Alcohol Depend 2009;99:261–71.
50. Shearer J, Wodak A, van Beek I, Mattick RP, Lewis J. Pilot randomized double blind placebo-controlled study of dexamphetamine for cocaine dependence. Addiction 2003;98(8):1137–41.
51. Mooney ME, Herin DV, Schmitz JM, Moukaddam N, Green CE, Grabowski J. Effects of oral methamphetamine on cocaine use: A randomized, double-blind, placebo-controlled trial. Drug Alcohol Depend 2009;101(1–2):34–41.
52. Volkow ND, Fowler JS, Logan J, Alexoff D, Zhu W, Telang F, et al. Effects of modafinil on dopamine and dopamine transporters in the male human brain: Clinical implications. JAMA 2009;301(11):1148–54.
53. Dackis CA, Kampman KM, Lynch KG, Pettinati HM, O'Brien CP. A double-blind, placebo-controlled trial of modafinil for cocaine dependence. Neuropsychopharmacology 2005;30(1):205–11.
54. Moeller FG, Schmitz JM, Steinberg JL, Green CM, Reist C, Lai LY, et al. Citalopram combined with behavioral therapy reduces cocaine use: A double-blind, placebo-controlled trial. Am J Drug Alcohol Abuse 2007;33(3):367–78.
55. Poling J, Oliveto A, Petry N, Sofuoglu M, Gonsai K, Gonzalez G, et al. Six-month trial of bupropion with contingency management for cocaine dependence in a methadone-maintained population. Arch Gen Psychiatry 200;63(2):219–28.
56. Jayaram-Lindström N, Konstenius M, Eksborg S, Beck O, Hammarberg A, Franck J. Naltrexone attenuates the subjective effects of amphetamine in patients with amphetamine dependence. Neuropsychopharmacology 2008;33(8):1856–63.
57. Warden D, Riggs PD, Min SJ, Mikulich-Gilbertson SK, Tamm L, Trello-Rishel K, et al. Major depression and treatment response in adolescents with ADHD and substance use disorder. Drug Alcohol Depend 2012;120(1–3):214–9.
58. Mariani J, Levin F. Treatment strategies for co-occurring ADHD and substance use disorders. Am J Addict 2007;16(Suppl 1):45–56.

12 Date rape drugs and hallucinogens

Colleen Dodich and Monika Siedlarz

Drug use is a widespread problem in the adolescent population, and hallucinogens, although having dropped in popularity, are still readily available to this age group. This chapter gives an overview of the main hallucinogens and date rape drugs that are abused in this population. The specific drug information discussed includes the history of the drug, alternate/street names, physical characteristics, route of ingestion, mechanism of action, psychological effects, adverse effects, duration of effects, dependence and withdrawal symptoms, long-term effects, and common derivatives. The epidemiological trends of these drugs are discussed, along with diagnostic parameters and clinical management. A table (table 12.1) at the end succinctly summarizes the main attributes of each drug discussed.

12.1 Introduction

Hallucinogens are a broad category of drugs generally thought to alter the user's view of reality by affecting sensory perception, mood, and cognition. These drugs can be both natural and synthetic in origin. When individuals are under the influence of these substances, they can have visual and auditory hallucinations and feel sensory stimuli that do not exist. The user can also experience extreme emotional lability. Different types of hallucinogens have been used throughout history in both ritualistic and religious activities. Initially, hallucinogens were naturally derived from plants, but in 1938, the first synthetic one, lysergic acid diethylamide (LSD), was synthesized by Swiss chemist Albert Hofmann (1906–2008) (1,2).

Although the use of LSD has been declining in recent years, it is still the prototypical hallucinogenic drug and has been the most closely studied. Since its initial creation, numerous other synthetic hallucinogens have been produced. These drugs are sometimes created for medical use, such as for anesthesia, but many times they are used in an illicit manner. The synthetic and naturally occurring hallucinogens are often used at clubs, raves, and parties and thus are also referred to as "club drugs" (1–3). Because of their psychotropic properties, some of these drugs are used to facilitate date rape and are thus termed "date rape drugs." Many of these hallucinogenic drugs have been banned in the United States because of the illicit manner in which they are being used. Yet, there are still some medications that are used in a very controlled manner within the medical community.

The classification of specific compounds into different categories (hallucinogens, club drugs, and date rape drugs) vary based on the source, and there can be overlap between categories. According to the National Institute on Drug Abuse (NIDA) (1), the specific drugs classified as hallucinogens include LSD, peyote cactus (mescaline), psilocybin, and phencyclidine (PCP) (15). *Salvia divinorum*, MDMA (3,4-methylenedioxy-N-methylamphetamine or 3,4-methylenedioxymethamphetamine), ketamine, and methamphetamine are often added to this category as well (16). The club drugs, according to NIDA, include GHB (γ-hydroxybutyric acid or gamma hydroxybutyrate), flunitrazepam, ketamine, MDMA (Ecstasy), methamphetamine, and LSD (17,18). The drugs commonly described as date rape drugs are GHB, flunitrazepam, and ketamine, although others listed previously have been implicated in cases of date rape as well (17).

12.2 Hallucinogens

12.2.1 LSD

LSD ("Blotter Acid," "Acid," "Dots," "Pane," "Zen," "Mellow Yellow," "Window Pane") was the first synthetic hallucinogen and was created initially for medical applications. Its hallucinogenic properties were accidently discovered later. Abuse was widespread in the 1960s but is currently declining. All LSD manufacturing in the United States is illegal because it has no accepted medical use (2,4).

Initially, LSD is clear or white in appearance and is odorless. When the drug degrades, it discolors. LSD is initially produced in a crystalline form and can be taken orally as a pill or liquid. In liquid form, it is commonly added to blotter paper in different colors and shapes, with each shape representing its own dose. Color is often added to mask the purity and age of the drug. The typical recreational dose is 25–80 mcg but can range up to 250 mcg as tolerance develops (2).

The exact mechanism of action is unknown for LSD, but it is believed to involve the interaction of numerous neurotransmitters including serotonin (5-HT), glutamate, and dopamine. Its effects are most prominent in the cerebral cortex and locus ceruleus (2,7). The cerebral cortex is the area involved in mood, cognition, and perception. The locus ceruleus receives sensory signals and is the "novelty detector" for external stimuli. LSD is considered one of the most potent mood and perception-altering drugs in existence. It can cause a heightened sensory input, time distortion, euphoria, synesthesia (blending of senses, such as hearing colors or seeing sounds), out of body experiences, visual illusions, and expansiveness. These effects are called "trips" and may cause panic. Most people remain oriented and know that their experiences are drug induced.

Adverse effects of LSD include sympathomimetic effects such as mydriasis, tachycardia, hypertension, piloerection, diaphoresis, and hyperthermia. It can also cause dizziness, loss of appetite, nausea, numbness, and tremors. Users may have "bad trips" where they have feelings of anxiety, despair, and even terrifying thoughts or nightmares. Severe adverse effects such as cardiovascular collapse and hyperthermia are not common but can be seen in high doses and inexperienced users. Life-threatening toxicity is sometimes seen at the highest doses, greater than 400 mcg. Death is more commonly a result of impaired judgment while under the influence. Users may feel effects from the drug within 30–90 minutes, with the duration of action lasting 6–12 hours for a usual recreational dose (2,7).

LSD users develop tolerance quickly and need increased doses after repeated use to get the desired effect. Tolerance is short-lived and is lost if the user stops for several days. Most LSD users decrease or stop using over time. LSD is not considered an addictive drug because it does not produce compulsive drug-seeking behavior. There is no evidence of physical withdrawal symptoms.

In the long term, LSD can lead to psychosis, a distortion or disorganization of a person's capacity to recognize reality or think rationally. This may persist for years after the "trip" has ended. LSD can also cause hallucinogen persisting perception disorder, or "flashbacks" (1,4). These are spontaneous, repeated, sometimes continuous sensory distortions originally produced by the LSD. They can be persistent and unchanged for years after drug use is stopped. There is no treatment for these long-term effects. Derivatives of LSD include several morning glory species (*Ipomoea violacea* and *Rivea corymbosa*) and Hawaiian baby woodrose.

12.2.2 Mescaline (2,3,5-trimethoxy-phenethylamaine)

Mescaline ("Buttons," "Cactus," "Sesc," "Peyoto") occurs naturally in the peyote cactus (*Lophophora williamsii*), a small, spineless cactus found in the Southwest United States and northern Mexico. It may be used legally by the members of the Native American Church (2). Mescaline was first isolated and identified in 1897 and was first synthesized in 1919 (2,4).

The top of the cactus is referred to as the crown and consists of disc-shaped buttons that are cut off and used for pharmacological effects. Mescaline is ingested as dried or fresh buttons, and the buttons can be crushed and smoked or brewed into a tea. They may also be ground into a powder, which can then be put into gelatin capsules for swallowing. The typical recreational dose is 6–12 buttons, and the average button contains 25 mg mescaline (2,4).

Mescaline belongs to a family of compounds known as phenethylamines. The chemical structure is similar to dopamine and norepinephrine; thus it interacts with their actions in the brain. The psychological effects of mescaline are similar to LSD, psilocycbin, and PCP, but not as potent. It causes varying degrees of illusions and hallucinations, as well as an altered perception of space and time and body image. Users may experience euphoria followed by feelings of anxiety. Consumption may lead to nausea, vomiting, dilation of the pupils, increased heart rate, increased blood pressure, a rise in body temperature that causes heavy perspiration, headaches, muscle weakness, and impaired motor coordination. There have been no verified human deaths from mescaline. It usually begins to work 1–2 hours after ingestion and the effects last 12–18 hours depending on the amount taken (2,7).

Mescaline has a high potential for abuse, but it carries no risk of physical dependence, and no recognizable withdrawal symptoms have been documented (15). Tolerance does develop, though, and this tolerance builds with repeated use over time. It can cause cross-tolerance with other serotonergic psychedelics such as LSD and psilocybin. Derivatives of mescaline include difluoromescaline and trifluoromescaline.

12.2.3 Psilocybin (and closely related psilocyn)

Psilocybin ("Magic Mushrooms," "Mushrooms," "Shrooms," "Boomers," "Caps," "Cubes," "God's Flesh," "Fungus Delight") is found in dozens of species of mushrooms, including members of the genus *Psilocybe*. These mushrooms grow in the Pacific Northwest and southern regions of the United States, as well as in Mexico and Central America. Central and South American Indians have considered the mushrooms "god's flesh," and thus they are sacred. They have been used in social and religious rituals. Use of this drug became more popular in the mid-1950s and was made illegal by 1968 due to abuse (8). It has been studied for the treatment of cancer-related anxiety, although currently there is no accepted medical use in the United States.

Psilocybin can be found as fresh or dried mushrooms. Fresh mushrooms have white or white/gray stems, and the caps are light brown or white in the center with dark brown edges. Psilocybin can be synthesized, but it is expensive and rarely done. When available, synthetic psilocybin is a white crystalline powder. The mushrooms are ingested orally and may be brewed as a tea or added to other foods to mask their bitter flavor. The age and preservation of the mushroom extract is highly unpredictable. There are varying species of "magic" mushrooms that contain varying amounts of the extract and other chemicals. The potency varies, but most have 0.2% to 0.4% psilocybin and only trace amounts of psilocin. The typical ingested dose is 20–30 mg of fresh mushrooms or 1–2 g of dried mushroom powder (2,4).

Psilocybin is structurally related to serotonin and thus disrupts its physiological action in the central nervous system (CNS). Once in the body, psilocybin becomes unstable and converts to psilocin, which is 1.4 times as potent and is thought to be the source of physical and psychological effects (7). Psilocybin is similar to LSD, mescaline, and peyote in its psychotropic effects. The effects of consuming preparations of dried or brewed mushrooms are not predicable, largely due to the variation in age and preservation of the extract. Hallucinations and the inability to discern fantasy from reality are common effects. Ingestion also causes heightened sensory experiences and perceptual distortions, as well as synesthesia. Psilocybin also causes difficulty concentrating, focusing, and thinking with impaired judgment.

Panic and psychosis occur after ingesting large doses. The onset of action is 20 minutes to 2 hours, and the effects last 4–6 hours (2,7).

Adverse effects of psilocybin include prominent gastrointestinal (GI) symptoms such as nausea, vomiting, abdominal cramps, and diarrhea. It can also cause muscle relaxation, weakness, and twitching, as well as dilation of pupils and emotional disturbances. Yawning, drowsiness, dizziness, and lightheadedness are also common. Serotonin syndrome (increased temperature, altered mental status, and potentially death) can occur if overdosed or with concomitant use of selective serotonin reuptake inhibitors (SSRIs) (2). An overdose can cause a longer, more intense episode of intoxication, psychosis, and possible death. Tolerance occurs with regular and repeated use of psilocybin. Cross-tolerance occurs with other drugs such as LSD and mescaline. There are no reports of psychological or physical addiction, and use does not lead to dependence. For several days following the use of mushrooms, users may experience a period of psychological withdrawal and have difficulty discerning reality. Persons with mental illness may be triggered into conditions such as schizophrenia, mania, or depression (2,4).

Derivatives include other tryptamines such as alpha-methyltryptamine (AMT), N, N-dimethyltryptamine (DMT), and 5-methoxydimethyltryptamine (5-Me-DIPT). AMT is a synthetic tryptamine developed as an antidepressant in the 1960s. DMT is naturally occurring, short-acting, and usually smoked but can be snorted or ingested. 5-MeO-DIPT ("Foxy" or "Foxy Methoxy") was synthesized in 1980.

12.2.4 *Salvia divinorum*

Salvia ("Maria Pastora," "Sylly-D," "Salvia") is marketed as a "safe" hallucinogen. Although it is not a controlled substance in the United States but rather listed as a "Drug of Concern," it is classified as controlled in Australia and several European countries (9,10). It is native to the Sierra Mazaleca region of Oaxaca, Mexico, and used there by the Mazatec Indians for ritual divination. Its use was first recorded in 1938.

Salvia is a perennial herb of the mint family and is sold on the Internet as whole plants, leaves, and extracts. The plant has spade-shaped, variegated green leaves; hollow, square-shaped stems; and white flowers with purple calyces. It grows more than 3 feet high. Fresh leaves are chewed, and dried leaves are smoked or vaporized. The typical recreational dose is 10–20 fresh leaves or 2–5 dried leaves, and active doses are as low as 200 μg (2).

Salvia is a diterpene alkaloid and kappa opioid agonist. Salvinorin A is believed to be the ingredient responsible for the psychoactive effects of *Salvia divinorum* (7). Psychotropic effects include a sense of calm, elevated mood, introspection, and synesthesia. Perceptions of bright lights, vivid colors, shapes, and body movements as well as body or object distortions are experienced with use. Salvia use may also cause fear and panic, uncontrollable laughter, and a sense of overlapping realities and hallucinations.

Adverse effects of the drug include sympathomimetic symptoms, which are usually mild. It may cause a loss of coordination, dizziness, and slurred speech, as well as nausea, decreased heart rate, and chills. The duration of these effects is 1–2 hours, or less when smoked. It is not considered a dependence-causing drug or a social/party drug. Withdrawal from the drug causes loss of coordination, dizziness, and slurred speech. Salvia can have deleterious effects on learning and memory, but generally long-term effects have not been investigated systematically. The derivatives of this drug include herkinorin and 2-methoxymethyl Salvinorin B.

12.2.5 PCP

PCP ("Angel Dust," "Ozone," "Rocket Fuel," "Love Boat," "Hog," "Embalming Fluid," "Superweed") is a dissociative anesthetic that was developed in the 1950s as a surgical anesthetic. It was used in veterinary medicine but was never approved for human use due to its serious adverse effects. It began to be widely abused in the 1960s and 1970s and is currently illegal in the United States (1,4).

PCP is a white crystalline powder, which is soluble in water or alcohol (see chapter 19). The powdered form of the drug is often sprinkled on marijuana or tobacco and smoked, although it can be snorted as well. In addition, it can be swallowed in tablet form or injected. The typical recreational dose is 1–3 mg when injected or smoked and 2–6 mg when ingested (2,4).

PCP is a noncompetitive antagonist of N-methyl-D-aspartate (NMDA) receptor complexes, which are receptors for glutamate in the brain. It also alters actions of dopamine receptors (7). It causes a sense of invulnerability and exaggerated strength, and at low doses, it has a dissociative effect. The drug can produce amnesia and analgesia, and at moderate doses, it produces a distortion of sound and vision. High doses give disorientation, severe agitation, auditory hallucinations, and violent behavior.

Violent behavior can lead to disorientation and suicidal ideation (1,2). Shallow, rapid breathing, hypertension, hyperthermia, and tachycardia can be seen at lower doses. Higher doses (10 mg or more) may have more severe changes in blood pressure, heart rate, and respiration and can also cause nystagmus (vertical and horizontal), nausea, blurred vision, dizziness, and decreased awareness of pain. Muscle contractions, bizarre postures, and uncoordinated movements can also be present at these higher doses. Very high doses can cause convulsions, catatonic stupor, and death. Most fatalities are due to injuries and trauma while under the influence of PCP (2,4).

The drug has a long delay between ingestion and effects when taken in pill form. When it is taken in powdered form, the onset is more rapid. Total effects of the drug can last 4–6 hours. Repeated use can lead to addiction, and prolonged use can cause withdrawal symptoms such as depression, anxiety, hypersomnia, poor memory, confused thought, increased cravings, violent behavior, hallucinations, and delusions. Long-term effects include memory loss and depression, which may last for as long as a year after a chronic user stops use. Derivatives of PCP include BTCP (1-bensothiophenyl cyclohexylpiperidine) and benzomorphan pentazocine (Talwin).

12.2.6 Ketamine

Ketamine ("Jet," "Jet K," "K," "Special K," "cat Valium," "Bump," "Green," "Super C," "Vitamin K," "Special La Coke," "Super Acid") is a dissociative anesthetic and CNS depressant that was developed in the 1960s to replace PCP (see chapter 19). The U.S. military used ketamine as a field anesthetic during the Vietnam War, and the drug gradually gained popularity for use in brief surgical procedures as both an induction and maintenance agent for general anesthesia. By the 1970s, ketamine became a widely used recreational drug. Currently, it can only be legally used in human anesthesia and veterinary medicine (1,6). Due to its tasteless and odorless characteristics, it is easily used as a date rape drug.

Ketamine comes in clear liquid and a white or off-white powder. It is typically packaged in small glass vials, small plastic bags, capsules, and paper, glassine, or aluminum foil folds. Most commonly, ketamine is used intranasally or injected intramuscularly (IM). It can also be used orally, subcutaneously, and intravenously (IV), as well as smoked in marijuana or tobacco cigarettes. Ketamine can be found by itself but is often used in combination with MDMA, amphetamine, methamphetamine, or cocaine. The typical recreational dose depends on method of usage: 75–125 mg IM or subcutaneously, 60–250 mg intranasally, 50–100 mg IV, and 200–300 mg orally (1,2).

Ketamine has a similar mechanism of action to PCP but is less potent. It acts on the NMDA receptor antagonist, arylcycloalkylamine (1,7). Ketamine distorts perceptions of sight and sound and produces a feeling of detachment from the environment. It has been used to facilitate sexual assault due to these characteristics. At low doses, the effects include impaired attention, learning ability, and memory; at higher doses, it can cause dream-like states and hallucinations. At even higher doses, delirium and amnesia can ensue (6). Typically, the effects of the drug last 30–60 minutes. Slang terminology referring to ketamine includes "K-land," which describes a mellow and colorful experience; "K-hole," which refers to the out-of-body, near-death experience; "Baby food," where users sink into a blissful infantile inertia; and "God," as some users are convinced that they have met their maker.

Adversely, ketamine can cause anxiety, chest pain, palpitations, tachycardia, extreme salivation, agitation, depression, cognitive difficulties, and unconsciousness. At high doses, it can lead to impaired motor function, high blood pressure, and potentially fatal respiratory problems. There have been reports of ketamine binging. Ketamine users can develop signs of tolerance and cravings for the drug. In chronic users that inject the drug, close to permanent tolerance can develop so that after months of use they are unable to experience the psychedelic effects. It is considered to have moderate to low physical but high psychological dependence.

Withdrawal leads to tension, twitchiness, poor attention span, and restlessness, although the drug does not appear to produce physical withdrawal symptoms in chronic users (1,6). The psychological dependence may produce depression, irritability, and insomnia. Long-term use may cause depression, irritability, and insomnia. Derivatives of this drug include methoxetamine, thialysine, lanthionine, cystathionine, and cysteine.

12.2.7 MDMA

MDMA ("Ecstasy," "E," "XTC," "Adam," "Clarity," "Stacy," "Lover's speed," "Essence," "Beans," "Disco Biscuit," "Eve," "Go," "Hug Drug," "Peace") is a stimulant with no accepted medical use in the United States. A German pharmaceutical company first produced it in 1912. The drug was utilized in psychotherapy in the United States until 1988, when it was made illegal due to illicit use and its popularity at "raves" (5,8). It is a synthetic chemical made in labs and often smuggled into the United States from Canada and the Netherlands. A small number of MDMA labs have been identified in the United States.

MDMA is sold as a capsule, tablet, or liquid and sometimes is found in a white or off-white powder (see chapter 11). Often the tablets are sold with logos, creating brand names for users to seek out. The colorful pills are often hidden among colorful candies. Many tablets contain a number of other drug combinations that can be harmful such as methamphetamine, ketamine, cocaine, dextromethorphan (DXM), ephedrine, and caffeine. MDMA is often taken orally or snorted and is rarely injected. MDMA abusers usually take it by "stacking" (taking three or more tablets at once) or by "piggybacking" (taking a series of tablets over a short period of time). One trend is "candy flipping," which is the coabuse of MDA (methylenedioxyamphetamine or 3,4-methylenedioxyamphetamine) and LSD. It is rarely used alone and thus has a high potential for harm. The typical recreational dose is 50–200 mg capsules (2,5).

The drug is a serotonergic amphetamine and acts on serotonin pathways in the brain. It has a chemical structure similar to both the hallucinogen mescaline and the stimulant methamphetamine (2,7). MDMA causes feelings of euphoria, empathy, excitement, and well-being. It produces an energizing effect, distorts time and perception, and enhances enjoyment of tactile experience. Adolescents use it to reduce inhibitions and promote feelings of closeness and sexuality. It is often used as a sexual enhancer and is sometimes considered a date rape drug due to aphrodisiac effects. Reports of a new combination of Ecstasy and Viagra is being used and referred to as "sextasy" or "trail mix" (5,11).

Unwanted psychological effects include confusion, anxiety, depression, paranoia, sleep problems, and drug craving. Physically, individuals may exhibit CNS agitation, hypertension, tachycardia, and possibly hyperthermia. Increased motor activity, alertness, muscle tension, tremors, involuntary teeth clenching, muscle cramps, nausea, faintness, chills, sweating, and blurred vision may also occur. MDMA intoxication can cause severe hypernatremia, seizures, obtundation, prolonged QT interval, and coma. Serotonin syndrome can occur with concomitant use of other SSRIs. Other drugs similar to MDMA, such as MDA or paramethoxyamphetamine (PMA), are often sold under the name of Ecstasy. This can lead to overdose and death when the user takes additional doses to obtain the desired effect. Fatalities after a pure MDMA dose of 300 mg have been noted. The onset of action is within 30–45 minutes of ingestion with effects lasting 4–6 hours. Some users may experience effects weeks after ingestion (5,12).

MDMA is considered to be addictive and can cause dependence, tolerance, and withdrawal symptoms. Depression is a common after-effect. Fatigue, loss of appetite, depressed feelings, and problems with concentration are also common in withdrawal from the drug. Chronic use of MDMA in typical recreational doses can lead to a paranoid psychosis that is clinically indistinguishable from schizophrenia (16,19). Usually, it is reversible after a prolonged drug-free state. MDMA use can lead to long-term problems with memory and learning and can cause damage that reduces a person's ability to feel pleasure. There are four precursors, which can be used in the manufacturing of MDMA and related drugs: safrole, isosafrole, piperonal, and 3,4-methylenedioxyphenyl-2-propanone (PMK). There are a number of homologous compounds with broadly similar effects such as MDA and methylbenzodioxolylbutanamine (MBDB) (16,24).

12.2.8 Methamphetamine

Methamphetamine ("Meth," "Speed," "Crank," "Crystal Meth," "Ice," "Chalk," "Glass") is a stimulant derived from amphetamine that was first created in Japan in 1919 and was originally used as a nasal decongestant and as a bronchial inhaler. It has also been used in the treatment of obesity. It first came to the United States in the 1930s, and its use surged in the 1950s and 1960s. The drug was outlawed in the 1970s due to its high potential for abuse. It is available via prescription for limited medical use, such as in attention-deficit/hyperactivity disorder and severe exogenous obesity (as referenced in the package insert of desoxyn). Most of the methamphetamine that is abused in the United States comes from domestic or foreign superlabs, although some is produced in small illegal labs where production may endanger the people in the labs, their neighbors, and the environment (see chapter 11).

Methamphetamine is a white, odorless, bitter-tasting crystalline powder that easily dissolves in water or alcohol. The crystal can be processed into a rock ("ice") or made into a liquid form for injection. It can be inhaled, taken orally, injected IV, or smoked. It is available in 5, 10, and 15 mg tablets when used in prescription form. At 10–30 mg of methamphetamine, the user begins to have feelings of euphoria. Drug users tend to use more than 60 mg doses (13,14).

Methamphetamine increases the release and blocks reuptake of dopamine in the brain (14). It is known to release serotonin as well. The drug affects parts of the brain involved with reward, motivation, pleasure, and motor function. It causes an intense euphoria or a "rush." Chronic users can display psychotic features including paranoia, visual and auditory hallucinations, and delusions. Psychosis can be similar to schizophrenia and is characterized by picking at the skin, paranoia, self-absorption, auditory and visual hallucinations, and sometimes episodes of violence. It alters judgment and inhibition and can lead people to engage in unsafe behaviors. The most dangerous stage of abuse is when the abuser has not slept in 3–15 days and is irritable and paranoid. This is referred to as "tweaking," and the user is known as a "tweaker" (14). Methamphetamine has a rapid onset with a long duration of about 12 hours. There is an initial intense rush that lasts 5–30 minutes with continued longer-lasting effects. The dextro form of methamphetamine, referred to as "ice," is smoked and has a rapid onset and effects that last 6–24 hours. Similar drugs that metabolize to amphetamine and methamphetamine include benzphetamine, furfenorex, famprofazone, and selegiline.

Physiological effects of this drug include severe agitation, CNS stimulation, tachycardia, hypertension, hyperthermia, dilated pupils, and diaphoresis. The drug causes increased wakefulness, increased physical activity, decreased appetite, increased respiration, rapid heart rate, irregular heartbeat, increased pressure, and hyperthermia. Some adverse effects can be attributed to contaminants in the meth such as lead and organic solvents. Treatment may require chelation therapy for lead effects such as anemia, encephalopathy, hepatitis, and myalgias (13,14). Chronic use leads to structural and functional changes in the brain that destroy cells that contain dopamine and serotonin, which over time can result in symptoms like those of Parkinson's disease.

Methamphetamine has a high potential for abuse, which may cause insomnia, anxiety, violent behavior or psychotic behavior, poor hygiene, pallor, and sores on the body from picking at "crank bugs" from tactile hallucinations (14). Cracked teeth due to extreme jaw clenching during a high are common. With an acute withdrawal after persistent abuse of the drug, the brain may have altered neurochemistry, and withdrawal symptoms such as depression may result (15). Fatigue, depression, apathy, long periods of sleep, irritability, and disorientation can also occur. The acute withdrawal symptoms usually peak in a few days and may last up to 2 weeks. A subacute withdrawal phase may follow that can last up to 3 weeks. Suicidal ideation and lucid dreams can also be seen (15).

Chronic abuse changes brain function. It causes reduced motor skills and impaired verbal learning. There are structural and functional changes in the locations of the brain associated with emotion and learning (14,15). Long-term use can lead to extreme weight loss, severe dental problems ("meth mouth"), anxiety, confusion, insomnia, mood disturbances, and violent behavior. Transmission of HIV and hepatitis B and C can be consequences of methamphetamine abuse. Methamphetamine abusers who are HIV positive have greater neuronal injury from HIV and increased cognitive impairment compared to individuals with HIV who do not use methamphetamines (16). Other long-term effects include high blood pressure, psychotic behavior, cracked teeth, sores, skin infections, acne, strokes, lung disease, heart infections, kidney failure, liver damage, and death often by suicide (12,14).

12.3 Date rape drugs

12.3.1 GHB

GHB ("Easy Lay," "G," "Georgia Home Boy," "Goop," "Grievous Bodily Harm," "Liquid Ecstasy," "Liquid X," "Scoop") is a CNS depressant and γ-aminobutyric acid (GABA) receptor agonist. The generic name for GHB is sodium oxybate, which is marketed as Xyrem and is FDA approved for narcolepsy, although strictly controlled (17). Gamma butyrolactone (GBL) and 1,4-butanediol (BD), which are metabolites of GABA, are available legally as industrial solvents used to produce polyurethane, pesticides, and elastic fibers. GHB and its metabolites have also been inappropriately and illicitly marketed for a wide variety of uses including fat loss, reversal of baldness, improved eyesight, to combat aging, depression, drug addiction, and insomnia. GBL and BD are also found in fish tank cleaners, ink stain remover, ink cartridge cleaners, and nail enamel remover. GHB became popular among teens and young adults at dance clubs and raves in the 1990s and has gained notoriety as a date rape drug. The drug is produced illegally in domestic and foreign clandestine labs. Xyrem has potential for diversion and abuse like any other pharmaceutical containing a controlled substance.

The drug comes in a liquid or white powder that dissolves in liquid. The liquid is colorless and odorless with a slight salty taste. GHB is taken orally and often used with a combination of other drugs, primarily alcohol as well as other depressants, stimulants, hallucinogens, and marijuana. GHB has a very narrow safety margin, and it is easy to overdose. The typical dose taken is 1–5 g, although usually it is difficult to decipher the dosage taken (6).

GHB is a metabolite of the inhibitory neurotransmitter GABA. It has two acting sites in the brain: the GABA-B receptor and a specific GHB binding site. It is not detected in routine hospital toxicology screens. Definitive confirmation requires analysis using gas chromatography/mass spectrometry, which may require 7–14 days and therefore does not contribute to the diagnosis or management of acute toxicity.

The drug causes euphoria and calming effects and is believed to build muscles and cause weight loss (6). It is known to cause amnesia, inhibition, increased libido, suggestibility, passivity, decreased anxiety, and increased confusion. For these reasons, it is used as a date rape drug. GHB can also produce visual hallucinations and, paradoxically, excited and aggressive behavior. Adversely, GHB causes CNS depression, hypotension, bradycardia, decreased respiratory rate, agitation, amnesia, seizures, ataxia, loss of muscle control, nausea, hypothermia, and coma, and it may be lethal.

The drug has an abrupt onset of effects within 15–30 minutes and lasts 3–6 hours. Regular use of GHB can lead to addiction and withdrawal. Withdrawal symptoms include insomnia, anxiety, tremors, sweating, increased heart rate and blood pressure, with occasional psychotic thoughts. Overdose is easy and can cause coma, seizures, and death. GBL, BD, barbiturates, and methaqualone also produce effects similar to GHB (6,17).

12.3.2 Flunitrazepam (Rohypnol)

Flunitrazepam, a benzodiazepine with the trade name Rohypnol ("Roofies," "Rophy," "Circles," "Mexican valium," "Rib," "Roach-2," "Roopies," "Rope," "Ropies," "Ruffies Drug"), is used in the short-term treatment of insomnia and as a sedative hypnotic and preanesthetic medication. It has physiological effects similar to diazepam. It is produced and sold legally by prescription in Europe and Latin America. The drug is usually smuggled into the United States as it is neither manufactured nor distributed in the United States for medical use. It began gaining popularity in the United States in the early 1990s and was banned.

Flunitrazepam is an odorless, colorless, and tasteless liquid that can be mixed with alcohol and other beverages. It also comes in an oral pill form of white tablets and recently has been manufactured as an olive-green tablet with speckled blue core that when dissolved in light colored drinks will turn the liquid blue. The generic forms do not contain the dye. The drug can also be ground up and snorted. The typical recreational dose is 1–2 mg tablets (6).

The drug acts on the GABA-A receptor and has sedative, hypnotic, antianxiety, and muscle relaxant effects. It causes memory impairment (anterograde amnesia), visual disturbances, inhibition, and impaired judgment and has a euphoric effect. It also leads to decreased reaction time, impaired mental functioning and judgment, confusion, aggression, and excitability. The physical effects of flunitrazepam include hypotension, drowsiness, dizziness, confusion, urinary retention, agitation, GI disturbances, and aggressive behavior. It can be lethal when mixed with alcohol or other CNS depressants, which will cause severe muscle relaxation, slurred speech, loss of motor coordination, weakness, headache, and respiratory depression. Effects of the drug begin within 30 minutes, peak at 2 hours, and may persist 8 hours or more (6,12).

Flunitrazepam can cause dependence and is often used with alcohol and cocaine. It produces tolerance, physical dependence, and addiction. Withdrawal symptoms include headache, muscle pain, anxiety, restlessness, confusion, irritability, numbness, tingling of the extremities, loss of identity, hallucinations, delirium, convulsions, shock, and cardiovascular symptoms. Withdrawal seizures can occur a week or more after cessation. The drug must be tapered to avoid withdrawal. At high doses, flunitrazepam can cause severe sedation, unconsciousness, slow heart rate, and suppression of respiration, which may be sufficient to result in death. Drugs that cause similar effects are GHB and other benzodiazepines such as alprazolam, clonazepam, and diazepam.

12.4 Epidemiology

Hallucinogens, and specifically LSD, peaked in the 1960s and 1970s as popular recreational drugs. Since that time, popularity and usage have been on the decline. According to Monitoring the Future, a longitudinal study that, among other things, tracks the prevalence of drug use and abuse in high school students in the United States, funded in part by the NIDA (8,18), recent use of hallucinogens has been relatively stable.

In the early 1990s, the use of hallucinogens by high school students was between 6.1% and 7.7%. There was a slight increase in hallucinogen usage in the late 1990s, and the prevalence peaked at 10.2% in 1997 (18). Since that time, the prevalence of use of hallucinogens in the high school population has been slowly decreasing. Between the years 2005 and 2011, the prevalence has been varying between 5.3% and 5.9% (8). Also of note, the usage of LSD in particular has been on a consistent decline. In the 1990s, the prevalence peaked at 9.1% for high school students, and since then, there has been a steady decline in its use. Since 2005–2011, the prevalence of LSD usage in high school students has been ranging between 2.5% and 2.8% (3,8,19). This is thought to be due in part to the perceived risk of the drug but may also be due in part to a decline in availability. There has been, however, a slight increase in the usage of other hallucinogens, such as MDMA and other club drugs. The prevalence of MDMA use in teenagers between 2005 and 2011 was between 4.0% and 5.5%. The prevalence of hallucinogen use, other than LSD, between the years of 2005 and 2011 has been between 4.7% and 5.4% (8,20). It appears that since the early 2000s, the use of LSD has been supplanted by the use of club drugs and naturally occurring hallucinogens, such as psilocybin and *Salvia divinorum*. This is thought to be due in part to easier availability of the latter and also the perceived safety of more natural hallucinogens (8,19).

In a National Survey on Drug Use and Health (20) regarding the patterns of initiation and use of hallucinogens in the years 2004 and 2005, it was shown that the two most common hallucinogens abused were psilocybin and MDMA. The data in this study showed that of individuals who had recently tried hallucinogens for the first time, 52.3% used psilocybin mushrooms and 42.9% used MDMA. MDMA was more likely to be used by females, while psilocybin was preferred by males. It also concluded that LSD and PCP usage was on the decline. In the same study, first-time users were much less likely to start with LSD or PCP, and the largest age group to initiate hallucinogen use during that time frame was 18- to 25-year-olds at 6.2%, followed by 12- to 17-year-olds at 2.8%. In a follow-up study from data collected in 2006 (3), there was an increase in Ecstasy and "natural herbal hallucinogen" usage among young people, consistent with the Monitoring the Future study usage (21,22).

In another National Household Survey on Drug Abuse (NHSDA) report, racial and ethnic differences were investigated in regard to hallucinogen use in the year 2001 (9). In this study, it was found that blacks were less likely than whites, Hispanics, or Asians to have tried any hallucinogen in their lifetime. White and Asian youths had similar rates of hallucinogen use, yet whites were more likely to have tried PCP or psilocybin at least once. Blacks and Hispanics were more likely, in this study, to perceive a greater risk in using LSD, and white youth perceived LSD to be much easier to obtain than any other racial group. This may contribute to the racial differences in hallucinogen usage withdrawal (25–27).

12.5 Diagnosis

In many cases, individuals who are intoxicated with a hallucinogen are aware that their symptoms are drug-induced and should be able to give that history, if they so choose. They are generally oriented and can speak clearly. If the individual is overly confused or has overt psychosis, severe agitation, or markedly abnormal vital signs, this could be a sign of different pathology or a severe overdose. Substances that may cause the previously discussed symptoms along with hallucinations include stimulants, such as amphetamines, methamphetamines, and cocaine. Stimulant-caused hallucinations are generally auditory, while hallucinations due to hallucinogens are generally visual. Other toxicological differentials to keep in mind include anticholinergic delirium, neuroleptic malignant syndrome, serotonin syndrome, and sedative-hypnotic or ethanol withdrawal.

Differential diagnoses to keep in mind when dealing with an individual with altered mental status include hypoglycemia, hypoxia, head trauma with or without an intracranial bleed, thyroid storm, a psychiatric illness such as schizophrenia, or an infection, such as sepsis, encephalitis, or meningitis.

If the individual is not having severe symptoms and is able to give the history of hallucinogen intoxication, routine lab work and imaging is usually not necessary.

Common hallucinogens do not routinely come up on drug screens, so these are only necessary if concurrent drug use and abuse is suspected. If there is no clear history of hallucinogen abuse or the individual's symptoms are severe or of an unclear etiology, it is necessary to further evaluate.

Routine lab work for a person with altered mental status or hallucinations should include a fingerstick glucose level to ensure that hypoglycemia is not a cause of the symptoms. A pregnancy test should be performed in women of childbearing age. Acetaminophen levels and salicylate levels should be drawn to ensure that there were no serious coingestions. A urine drug screen may also be done to assess for concurrent drug ingestions. Also, an electrocardiogram (ECG) is important to rule out any drug ingestion that would affect cardiac function.

Other testing should be obtained based on the history of clinical findings. Although severe agitation could be indicative of PCP intoxication, the individual may also be at risk of rhabdomyolysis from muscle contractions and should be evaluated as such. If this is a possibility, electrolytes, a renal panel, a creatine kinase, and a urine myoglobin should be obtained. If the patient has fever in addition to altered mental status, an infection must be considered. A complete blood count and specific cultures, including cerebrospinal fluid cultures, may be indicated. If there are concerns of head trauma or any sort of intracranial process, imaging of the head, such as computerized tomography or magnetic resonance imaging, should be obtained. Other testing will be tailored to the clinical picture presented by the patient.

12.6 Management principles

For most individuals undergoing hallucinogen intoxication, the main management is supportive care. Usually, the symptoms are self-limited and not severe, so the person only needs to be monitored for any complications. It is recommended that the patient be placed in a quiet, calm room with minimal stimulation. Since hallucinogens are known to distort sensory input, it is necessary to diminish this as much as possible. Usually, vital signs are normal in a person who is acutely intoxicated with hallucinogens, but serial vital signs measurements should be monitored. Initially, they can be monitored every 15 minutes, which can be lengthened as symptoms start to resolve. If there are any abnormalities with vital signs, a cardiac monitor should be added and IV access obtained, as medications and fluids may be needed. If the patient's symptoms are more severe, initial management must be geared to stabilizing the patient. As with all other emergent situations, it is necessary to guarantee the patient's airway, breathing, and circulation.

Although rare in hallucinogen intoxications, if the patient is hyperthermic, this must be treated emergently. Hyperthermia is defined as a core temperature greater than 41.1°C. Antipyretics are not key to therapy in this case because the hyperthermia is most likely due to increased muscle activity with agitation (2,28). It is important to sedate the person, initially with benzodiazepines, although paralytics may be needed if symptoms are very severe. Cooling blankets and IV hydration can also be used to aid in the management of hyperthermia.

If agitation is the main clinical finding, and it is not being well managed with routine supportive care and a quiet, low stimulation environment, further management must be considered. The first line of treatment for agitation from suspected hallucinogen intoxication is with benzodiazepines. Examples of benzodiazepines used include midazolam, lorazepam, and diazepam. It is important to give these via IV infusion because it is easier to titrate the medication dose. If IV access is difficult to achieve, due to severe agitation, it is possible to give the first dose of benzodiazepines IM and once initial sedation is achieved, IV access can be obtained and the subsequent doses can be given IV (2).

If adjunctive therapy is needed, neuroleptic medications may be used. These are usually added when agitation and psychotic symptoms continue to persist, even with aggressive use of benzodiazepines. They are also used when agitation has improved but a psychotic clinical picture continues. The main recommended neuroleptic medication is Haloperidol, which should be given via IV injection (28). The lowest dose possible should be titrated. It is important to obtain an ECG before starting this medication. It is important to closely monitor a patient on a neuroleptic medication, as some of the adverse effects of the medication can closely mimic the complications of the drug intoxication.

There are no known antidotes for hallucinogen intoxication, although if there is suspicion of a coingestion, other medications may be evaluated for antidotes. Urine acidification was once used in hallucinogen intoxication but is no longer recommended. GI decontamination is not routinely recommended either, as hallucinogens rarely cause serious medical problems and are rapidly absorbed into a person's system. Exceptions to this would be the suspicion of concurrent drug ingestions that could benefit from decontamination or if it is known that the oral ingestion was a very large quantity that was taken less than 1 hour prior to treatment. Also, it is important to protect the airway of any patient who has an altered mental status.

Patients can usually be discharged, either home or to law enforcement, when their psychotic symptoms have resolved and their vital signs are consistently stable. The timing of this depends on the substance that was used.

12.7 Conclusions

As outlined in this chapter, hallucinogens are a broad category of drugs that can produce a wide variety of physical and psychotropic effects. They can be synthetic or naturally obtained. Although some of these medications have legitimate medical indications, most of them do not and are used illicitly. These drugs can be used to produce auditory and visual hallucinations and euphoria, as well as to facilitate rape.

Table 12.1: Drugs of abuse used alone and in combination for date rape and other properties and their dangers

Drug category	Also categorized as:	Drugs	Looks like, smells like, tastes like	Recreational dose	Dangers
Hallucinogens		LSD	Clear, white that becomes clear in liquid, odorless	25–80 mcg, up to 250 mcg	Commonly colored; user doesn't know purity
	Phenylethylamine	Mescaline	Disc-shaped buttons of cactus	6–12 buttons (200–400 mg)	
	Tryptamine	Psilocybin	Mushroom	10–50 mg	Poisoning from misidentification; serotonin syndrome
		Salvia divinorum	Mint family leaf	200 μg	
	Stimulant, depressant	Marijuana	Green/brown dry mix	10 mcg/kg	"Gateway drug"; amotivational syndrome
	Stimulant	Bath salts	White crystals, white powder	5–20 mg, upto 50 mg	Unknown safety; not controlled currently
Anesthetics		PCP	White powder	1–3 mg IV, 2–6 mg ingested	High fatalities from injuries/trauma
	Depressant	Ketamine	Clear liquid, white powder, odorless, tasteless	75–125 mg IM, 50–100 mg IV, 300 mg orally, 60–250 mg snorted	Date rape drug; "dissociative anesthetic" Often used with MDMA, amphetamine, methamphetamine, or cocaine
Stimulants	Amphetamine	MDMA	Colorful tablets, white powder	50–200 mg	Hidden among colorful candies; used with methamphetamine, ketamine, cocaine, DXM, ephedrine, and caffeine; date rape drug when used in combination
	Amphetamine	MDA	Colorful tablets sold as MDMA	60–160 mg	Sold as Ecstasy; dramatic hyperthermia leading to death

(*Continued*)

Table 12.1: Drugs of abuse used alone and in combination for date rape and other properties and their dangers (*Continued*)

Drug category	Also categorized as:	Drugs	Looks like, smells like, tastes like	Recreational dose	Dangers
	Amphetamine	MDEA (methylenedioxyethyl amphetamine or 3,4-methylenedioxy-N-ethylamphetamine)	Sold as MDMA	60–175 mg per tab (1–3 tabs)	Sold as Ecstasy; dramatic hyperthermia leading to death
	Amphetamine	PMA	Sold as MDMA	50 mg and up	Sold as Ecstasy; people overdose by taking too much while trying to gain effects
	Stimulant	Methamphetamine	White, odorless, bitter-tasting powder	>60 mg	Serotonin syndrome
		Cocaine	White powder	35–100 mg snorted, 120 mg IV	"Cut" with sugars and local anesthetics to increase dealer's profits; tolerance develops within hours – very addictive
Other	GABA receptor analogue, CNS depressant	GHB	Liquid; white powder dissolves into colorless/odorless solution	1–5 g	Date rape drug
	Benzodiazepine, CNS depressant	Flunitrazepam	Colorless, odorless, tasteless liquid	1–2 mg	Date rape drug (category itself)
	Cough suppressant, sedative	DXM	Cough syrup, tablets, capsules, powder	100–200 mg, up to 1,500 mg	Lethal when mixed with alcohol or other drugs

Although hallucinogen use has recently been on the decline, it is still a problem in the adolescent population. It is especially important to note that natural hallucinogens have become more popular because of an incorrect perception of safety and because they are also readily available via Internet vendors.

When an adolescent presents with altered mental status, hallucinogen abuse must always be on the differential. Although the youngster may disclose the use of one of these drugs, fear of repercussion may lead to covering up. Even after disclosure, it is prudent to investigate other concomitant drug use to determine if additional management is needed beyond the usual monitoring provided for hallucinogen intoxication. Morbidity and mortality resulting from hallucinogen use except for severe overdose is due to the actions facilitated by the influence of the drug rather than due to the drug itself.

References

1. National Institute on Drug Abuse. Hallucinogens and dissociative drugs, including LSD, PCP, ketamine, dextromethorphan. Rockville, MD: DHHS, 01–4209, 2001.
2. Delgado, J. Intoxication from LSD and other common hallucinogens. In: Basow, DS, ed. UpToDate. Waltham, MA: UpToDate, 2012. Updated 2011, June 15; cited 2013, May 22.
3. Substance Abuse and Mental Health Services Administration, Office of Applied Studies. The NSDUH report: Use of specific hallucinogens: 2006. Rockville, MD: Substance Abuse Mental Health Services Administration, 2008.
4. National Institute on Drug Abuse. Drug Facts: Hallucinogens – LSD, peyote, psilocybin, and PCP. Rockville, MD: DHHS, 2009.
5. National Institute on Drug Abuse. DrugFacts: MDMA (Ecstasy). Rockville, MD: DHHS, 2010.
6. National Institute on Drug Abuse. DrugFacts: Club drugs: GHB, ketamine and Rohypnol. Rockville, MD: DHHS, 2010.
7. Abraham HD, Aldridge AM, Gogia P. The psychopharmacology of hallucinogens. Neuropsychophrmacology 1996;14:285–98.
8. Johnston LD, O'Malley PM, Bachman JG, Schulenberg JE. Monitoring the Future national survey results on drug use, 1975–2011. Vol. 1, Secondary school students. Ann Arbor: Institute Social Research, University of Michigan, 2012.
9. Dennehy CE, Tsourounis C, Miller AE. Evaluation of herbal dietary supplements marketed on the Internet for recreational use. Ann Pharmacotherapy 2005;39:1634–9.
10. Hoover V, Marlowe DB, Patapis NS, et al. Internet access to Salvia divinorum: Implications for policy, prevention and treatment. J Subst Abuse Treat 2008;35:22.
11. European Monitoring Centre for Drugs and Drug Addiction. Last updated October 12, 2012. Accessed October 12, 2012. URL: www.emcdda.europa.eu
12. CESAR: Center for Drug Abuse Research. Updated September 24, 2012. Accessed October 12, 2012. URL: http://www.cesar.umd.edu/
13. Christophersen AS. Amphetamine designer drugs: An overview and epidemiology. Toxicol Lett 2000;112–113:127–31.
14. National Institute on Drug Abuse. Drug Facts: Club drugs: Methamphetamine. Rockville, MD: DHHS, 2010.
15. Mancino MJ, Gentry BW, Feldman Z, et al. Characterizing methamphetamine withdrawal in recently abstinent methamphetamine users: A pilot field study. Am J Drug Alcohol Abuse 2011;37:131.

16. Langford D, Adame A, Grigorian A, et al. Patterns of selective neuronal damage in methamphetamine-user AIDS patients. J Acquir Immune Defic Syndr J 2003;34(5):467–74.
17. Brown University Health Education. Alcohol, tobacco and other drugs: General information. Accessed October 12, 2012. URL: http://brown.edu/Student_Services/Health_Services/Health_Education/alcohol,_tobacco,_&_other_drugs/
18. Greydanus DE, Patel DR, Omar HA, Feucht C, Merrick J. Adolescent medicine: Pharmacotherapeutics in general, mental and sexual health. Berlin: Walter de Gruyter, 2012:181–97.
19. Substance Abuse and Mental Health Services Administration, Office of Applied Studies. The NSDUH report: Perceptions of risk from substance abuse among adolescents. Rockville, MD: Substance Abuse and Mental Health Services Administration, 2009.
20. Substance Abuse and Mental Health Services Administration, Office of Applied Studies. The NSDUH report: Patterns of hallucinogen use and initiation: 2004 and 2005. Rockville, MD: Substance Abuse and Mental Health Services Administration, 2007.
21. Richardson WH III, Slone CM, Michels JE. Herbal drugs of abuse: An emerging problem. Emerg Med Clin North Am 2007;25:435.
22. Halpern JH. Hallucinogens and dissociative agents naturally growing in the United States. Pharmacol Ther 2004;102:131.
23. Substance Abuse and Mental Health Services Administration, Office of Applied Studies. The NHSDA report: Racial and ethnic differences in youth hallucinogen use. Rockville, MD: Substance Abuse and Mental Health Services Administration, 2003.
24. Wallace JM, Bachman JG, O'Mailey PM, Johnston LD, Schulenberg JE, Cooper SM. Tobacco, alcohol and illicit drugs: Racial and ethnic differences among US high school seniors, 1976–2000. Public Health Rep 2002;117(Suppl 1):67–75.
25. Strasburger VC, Greydanus DE. AM:STARS: At-risk adolescents: An update for the new century. Adolesc Med 2000;11:79–101.
26. Boyer EW, Shannon M. The serotonin syndrome. N Engl J Med 2005; 352:1112.
27. Joffe A, Blythe MJ. Adolescent Medicine: State of the Art Reviews: Handbook of adolescent medicine, 2nd ed. Elk Grove Village, IL: American Academy Pediatrics. Adolesc Med 2009;20(2): 758–87.
28. Baumann MH, et al. The designer methcathinone analogs, mephedrone and methylonea re substrates for monoamine transporters in brain tissue. Neuropsychopharmacology 2012;37:1192–203.
29. Callaway CW, Clark RF. Hyperthermia in psychostimulant overdose. Ann Emerg Med 1994;24:68.

13 The role of the pediatrician and primary care clinician

Ray Chih-Jui Hsiao, Kristin A. Miselis, and Christopher K. Varley

Pediatricians and primary care clinicians have important roles to play in identifying, screening, and referring adolescents and young adults with substance use disorders for in-depth assessment or treatment and in delivering brief interventions in patients with milder substance-related problems. By following established protocols for substance use screening, brief intervention, and referral to treatment (SBIRT) in the primary care setting, pediatricians and primary care clinicians can be effective at promoting good health outcomes throughout their patient's recovery process.

13.1 Introduction

Adolescence and young adulthood are two developmental periods during which patients are more likely to engage in drug and alcohol experimentation and use (1,2). Nearly half of high school seniors in the United States report having tried at least one illicit drug in their lifetime, and almost three-quarters have tried alcohol (3). Although many of these adolescents will not go on to develop drug or alcohol dependence, a substantial portion encounters significant medical, social, and psychological problems related to their use. According to the 2010 National Survey on Drug Use and Health, 19.8% of young adults between ages 18 and 25 were abusing or dependent on substances in the past year, a rate that is more than double the rate of 7.3% for adolescents aged 12–17 (4) (see chapter 16).

Early use also increases the risk for later developing a substance use disorder (i.e., substance abuse or dependence). In adults who had their first drink before the age of 14, 15.1% went on to be diagnosed with substance abuse or dependence as compared to only 2.7% of adults who had their first drink after the age of 21 (4) (see chapter 9). Adolescence is the primary age of onset for drug abuse and dependence, which reaches peak prevalence around the age of 19 (1). The onset of substance use disorders after the age of 25 is rare. Therefore, addressing substance misuse and substance use disorders in adolescents and young adults is critical in promoting long-term health and wellness.

Despite the high rate of substance use disorders in adolescents and young adults, they are often underrecognized in the clinical setting including primary care offices (5–8) (see chapter 9). Furthermore, even when properly identified, most adults with substance use disorders do not receive needed treatment, and the mean age of treatment onset is around 27 (1,4). Adolescents with identified substance abuse or dependence are even less likely to receive treatment. In one U.S. national study, only 15.2% of adolescents identified as having substance abuse or dependence received disorder-specific treatment (9). Adolescents and young adults may not be interested in pursuing treatment on their own, they may not be aware of their treatment options, and they may not have very many treatment options available to them (4). Although access and contact with specialized treatment providers may be limited, most adolescents and young adults do have access to and visit a pediatrician or primary care clinician. The pediatrician and primary care clinician are therefore in the position to play an essential role in the prevention, detection, and management of substance use disorders in adolescents and young adults.

Although the importance of pediatricians and primary care clinicians in addressing substance use in adolescents and young adults is widely recognized, there are few practice guidelines that have been developed by leading U.S. national professional organizations that define the exact role of the primary care clinician in substance-abusing young adults. The American Academy of Pediatrics (AAP) does have a detailed policy statement from 2005 defining the role of the pediatrician in this population (10) and recently issued a policy statement recommending an algorithm-based approach to universal substance use SBIRT as a way of augmenting current assessment and treatment approaches in managing substance use and abuse in adolescents (11). A similar SBIRT framework has also been recommended by the Substance Abuse and Mental Health Services Administration (SAMHSA) as part of routine health care for adults (12,13).

Therefore, in this chapter addressing the role of the pediatrician and primary care clinician in substance-abusing adolescents and young adults, the discussion will focus on the SBIRT approach and other management issues confronting the pediatrician and primary care clinician with substance-abusing patients such as safety, consent, and confidentiality in general and specifically for adolescents. A full discussion and systematic review of SBIRT is beyond the scope of this chapter, and interested readers are referred to the references provided for a more detailed discussion on the implementation of SBIRT in clinical practice (11,12).

Furthermore, although there are clear distinctions between adolescents and young adults based on available SBIRT literature, the description in this chapter will focus on SBIRT general principles and application to both adolescents and young adults with the primary discussion on the framework suggested by the AAP while highlighting relevant findings from the adult literature (12–14). The assessment and treatment of substance abuse in adolescents and young adults are covered elsewhere in this book.

13.2 Screening and assessment

Pediatric and adult primary care visits provide important opportunities for the early identification of problematic drug and alcohol use that should not be missed (see chapters 4 and 9). Table 13.1 outlines the spectrum of substance use with matching recommended goals for office intervention.

Table 13.1: Substance use spectrum and goals for office intervention for adolescents and young adults

Stage	Description	Office intervention
Abstinence	The time before an individual has ever used drugs or alcohol (more than a few sips)	Prevent or delay initiation of substance use through positive reinforcement and patient/parent education
Experimentation	The first 1–2 times that a substance is used and the patient wants to know how intoxication from using a certain drug(s) feels	Promote patient strengths; encourage abstinence and cessation through brief, clear medical advice and educational counseling
Limited use	Use together with ≥1 friends in relatively low-risk situations and without related problems: use typically occurs at predictable times such as on weekends (for adolescents) or at work-related functions or social gatherings (for young adults)	Promote patient strengths; further encourage cessation through brief, clear medical advice and educational counseling
Problematic use	Use in a high-risk situation, such as when driving or babysitting; use associated with a problem such as a fight, arrest, school suspension, or loss of employment/inability to gain employment; or use for emotional regulation such as to relieve stress or depression	As stated previously, plus initiate office visits or referral for brief intervention to enhance motivation to make behavioral changes; provide close patient follow-up; consider breaking confidentiality for adolescents
Abuse	Drug use associated with recurrent problems or that interferes with functioning, as defined in the *DSM-IV-TR*	Continue as stated previously, plus enhance motivation to make behavioral changes by exploring ambivalence and triggering preparation for action; monitor closely for progression to alcohol and other drug addiction; refer for comprehensive assessment and treatment; consider breaking confidentiality
Addiction (dependence)	Loss of control or compulsive drug use, as defined in the *DSM-IV-TR* as "dependence"	As stated previously, plus enhance motivation to accept referral to subspecialty treatment if necessary; consider breaking confidentiality; encourage involvement of close family members whenever possible including parents or spouses

Adapted from: Committee on Substance Abuse, Levy SJ, Kokotailo PK. Substance use screening, brief intervention, and referral to treatment for pediatricians. Pediatrics 2011;128(5):e1331.

DSM-IV-TR indicates *Diagnostic and Statistical Manual of Mental Disorders*, fourth edition, text revision (15).

The U.S. Preventive Services Task Force (USPSTF) recommends screening and behavioral counseling interventions to reduce alcohol misuse in adults in primary care settings (16). Although the USPSTF has found insufficient evidence to recommend screening and brief intervention in the primary care setting for alcohol misuse in adolescents and other drug use in adolescents and young adults (16,17), more recent recommendations from the AAP and SAMHSA suggest that screening and brief intervention for alcohol and drug use can be beneficial in adolescents and young adults (11–13). However, there are a number of barriers to drug and alcohol screening in primary care including time constraints, lack of knowledge about how to manage a positive screen, and lack of available treatment resources (18). In addition, physicians may not have the opportunity to speak confidentially with their patients about sensitive health risk behaviors and may not be familiar with appropriate screening tools.

Unfortunately, if primary care clinicians do not screen for problematic alcohol and drug use, those patients with existing or developing substance use disorders miss the opportunity for treatment. That can be up to 15% of adolescents presenting for both sick and well-child care visits (8). Without screening and intervention, those adolescents are at high risk for developing dangerous and impairing addictions that can be incredibly costly to the health care system. Although it may require additional resources as well as more frequent visits with select patients, if primary care clinics can adapt the recommended SBIRT approach, they can help prevent the substantial negative personal and societal impact of addictive disorders.

13.3 Confidentiality and consent

In order to incorporate an effective screening tool into primary care visits, it is necessary to outline a clear clinic confidentiality policy that is communicated to adolescents and young adults (and parents in the case of adolescents) prior to administering the screen (see chapter 9). It is widely accepted practice to provide adolescents with confidential health care in order to increase the likelihood that they will honestly disclose information about high risk behaviors. Adolescents may be afraid to share personal information that they worry could be disclosed to their parents or other health care professionals (6,19–21). Some will even forgo care due to these fears (6,21). Federal law and regulations protect the confidentiality of patient information for both adolescents and adults receiving substance use prevention and substance use disorder treatment services as outlined in Code of Federal Regulations Title 42 Part 2 (42 U.S.C. 290dd-2, 42 CFR Part 2) (22). This law applies to all programs that receive direct or indirect federal funds and specifically prohibits parental notification without patient consent.

Exceptions to this rule are permitted if an adolescent lacks capacity to make a rational choice about parental notification or the adolescent's physical well-being is seriously threatened and this threat would be alleviated by disclosing information about their substance use to their parents (23). States also have laws that allow adolescents to consent for their own care of specific conditions including substance abuse, meaning that the consenting adolescent would have the right to refuse the provider permission to speak with their parents. The minimum age at which an adolescent may consent to a particular service varies between states and ranges from 12 to 16 (24). In institutions that must abide by state and federal law, the law that best protects confidentiality should be applied.

Although adolescents and young adults have the right to consent to their own treatment, it is always important to remember to assess whether or not they have the capacity to do so. Acute intoxication as well as chronic drug or alcohol use can lead to cognitive impairments. In order to have the capacity to consent to treatment and/or refuse to consent to release of information, adolescents and young adults must demonstrate the ability to communicate a choice, comprehend information, reason about options, risks and benefits, and appreciate the effect of their choices on their life course and values (25).

As noted previously, if a patient does not have the capacity to consent to treatment, it may be necessary to break confidentiality and inform a family member who has the right to consent to treatment for that person (e.g., parent, spouse, etc.). Tomas Silber refers to this as "justified paternalism" (26). He defines the circumstances under which violations of confidentiality should be considered as those in which there is a clear risk of harm to the patient that could be prevented by violating their confidentiality and that the benefit of preventing harm clearly outweighs the risk of violating the patient's privacy (26).

It is imperative to discuss the limitations of confidentiality with adolescents and young adults presenting for treatment. This will hopefully temper the anger and sense of betrayal that can sometimes occur when a patient's confidentiality must be broken due to safety concerns. Clear exceptions to confidential care include mandated reporting of child abuse, suicidal intent, and the duty to warn with respect to patients with a specific, reported plan to hurt or kill someone else.

The discussion about confidential care can also be used as a platform to encourage adolescents and young adults to include their parents or other supportive family members in their care. Substance abuse treatment is more likely to be successful if patients have social supports who can participate in their treatment (27,28). The emphasis on protecting the confidentiality of treatment should therefore not interfere with the recommendation to actively include supportive family members in the treatment process. Although some adolescents may not want their parents to know, many, especially younger adolescents, may actually prefer to have their parents involved (19).

Lastly, any clinician who offers confidential treatment must ensure that patient information is, in fact, kept confidential. Parents have the right to access their child's medical records. Information on substance abuse treatment may, therefore, need to be kept in a separate chart or protected in accordance with 42 CFR Part 2 (22). If adolescents or young adults are seeking treatment under their parents' insurance, their parents may also get insurance statements that identify the type of treatment the patient is receiving. If this is unavoidable in a particular circumstance, the patient should be made aware of the situation.

In summary, primary care offices that serve adolescents and young adults with substance use disorders should be familiar with both federal and state laws that apply to their practice, should have a clearly outlined confidentiality policy that is explained to patients and relevant family members, and should have a way of securing patient medical records so that patients cannot be identified as seeking out screening or treatment for a substance use disorder without specifically giving their consent.

13.4 Safety

Substance abuse can be very dangerous for adolescents and young adults. Problem alcohol use by adolescents is associated with an elevated risk of violent victimization (29). Alcohol use by younger female adolescents and risky drinking behaviors such as binge drinking are also risk factors for sexual victimization of female adolescents (30). Drug and alcohol use and abuse also have a number of direct and indirect health risks including impacts on cognitive functioning, memory and learning, sexually transmitted and blood-borne illness, motor vehicle accidents, and drug or alcohol overdose. Substance-abusing youth are also much more likely to have comorbid mental illness (28). Substance abuse alone is a risk factor for self-injurious behaviors and suicide (28). Adolescents and young adults with comorbid mental illnesses associated with suicide can have a very elevated risk for self-harm. Given the risks and psychiatric comorbidities associated with substance use, primary care providers should include a safety assessment for those patients who screen positive for high-risk substance use.

Young people should be asked directly during individual interviews about past and current suicidal thoughts and behaviors in order to determine the need for further evaluation or referral for more restrictive treatment. Whether gathering information from a clinical interview or screening questionnaire (see table 13.2), there are two primary goals in doing a risk assessment: determine whether or not suicidal ideation or behaviors exist, and then assess the risk that the patient will act on their thoughts (31). Past suicide attempts are the strongest predictor of current suicidal ideation and behaviors (32). In terms of determining imminent risk, the intent of the patient and their perception of whether or not they can keep themselves safe are important. Access to lethal means and the degree of supervision at home should also be taken into account. Lastly, ongoing environmental factors that contribute to the acute risk should also be evaluated.

Table 13.2 Screening instruments for suicidal ideation

Scale	Characteristics	Availability	References
Suicidal Ideation Questionnaire (SIQ)	• Self-administered • 30-item format for adolescents in grades 10–12 • 15-item format (SIQ-JR) for adolescents in grades 7–9	Psychological Assessment Resources Inc.: http://www4.parinc.com	Pinto A, Willsman MA, McCoy KJM. Suicidal ideation in adolescents: Psychometric properties of the Suicidal Ideation Questionnaire in a clinical sample. Psychol Assess 1997;9:63–6. Reynolds WM. Suicidal Ideation Questionnaire: Professional manual. Odessa, FL: Psychological Assessment Resources, 1988.
Beck Scale for Suicide Ideation (BSS)	• Self-administered • 21 items with 5 screening items • Identify the presence and severity of suicidal ideation	Pearson: http://www.pearsonassessments.com	Beck AT, Steer RA, Ranieri WF. Scale for Suicide Ideation: psychometric properties of a self-report version. J Clin Psychol 1988;44:499–505. Beck AT, Steer R: Manual for the Beck Scale for Suicide Ideation. San Antonio, TX: Psychological Corporation, 1991.
Suicide Attempt Self-Injury Interview (SASII)	• Structured, comprehensive interview • Measures multiple factors associated with suicide attempts and nonsuicidal self-injury • 6 screening items, 9 open-ended questions for interviewer coding, and 22 items and associated subitems • Measures intent	University of Washington Behavioral Research and Therapy Clinics: http://depts.washington.edu/brtc	Linehan MM, Comtois KA, Brown MZ, Heard HL, Wagner A. Suicide Attempt Self-Injury Interview (SASII): Development, reliability, and validity of a scale to assess suicide attempts and intentional self-injury. Psychol Assess 2006;18:303–12.

(*Continued*)

Table 13.2 Screening instruments for suicidal ideation (*Continued*)

Scale	Characteristics	Availability	References
Columbia Suicide Screen (CSS)	• Brief • Self-administered • Measures intent	Contact: Dr. Shaffer Department of Child Psychiatry New York State Psychiatric Institute Columbia University 1051 Riverside Drive, Unit 78 New York, NY 10032 shafferd@childpsych.columbia.edu	Shaffer D, Scott M, Wilcox H, Maslow C, Hicks R, Lucas CP, et al. The Columbia Suicide Screen: Validity and reliability of a screen for youth suicide and depression. J Am Acad Child Adolesc Psychiatry 2004;43:71–9.
Brief Reasons for Living Inventory for Adolescents (BRFL-A)	• Brief • Self-administered • 14 items • Assesses protective factors	University of Washington Behavioral Research and Therapy Clinics: https://depts.washington.edu/brtc	Osman A, Kopper BA, Barrios FX, Osman JR, Besett T, Linehan MM. The Brief Reasons for Living Inventory for Adolescents. J Abnorm Child Psychol 1996;24:433–43.
Beck Hopelessness Scale (BHS)	• Self-administered • 20 true-false items • Assesses thoughts and beliefs about the future	Pearson: http://www.pearsonassessments.com	Beck AT, Brown G, Steer RA. Prediction of eventual suicide in psychiatric inpatients by clinical ratings of hopelessness. J Consult Clin Psychol 1989;57:309–10. Beck AT, Steer R: Beck Hopelessness Scale manual. San Antonio, TX: Psychological Corporation, 1988.

Although it is very important to identify youth with a high risk for suicide and refer them for psychiatric hospitalization, not all suicidal youth warrant inpatient treatment. It is therefore helpful to have staff available in the clinic who can put together a safety plan for suicidal youth with a low risk of self-harm.

13.5 Screening tools and algorithm in adolescents

Screening tools are generally designed to identify patients with an elevated risk of having a substance use disorder. Follow-up assessment for those patients who screen positive is necessary in order to determine the level of intervention that an individual patient might need by distinguishing experimentation, use, abuse and dependence.

For adolescents aged 14–18, the National Institute on Alcohol Abuse and Alcoholism recommends two questions for the initial screening of alcohol misuse (33):

- "In the past year, on how many days have you had more than a few sips of beer, wine, or any drink containing alcohol?"
- "If your friends drink, how many drinks do they usually drink on an occasion?"

Any days drinking and any friends drinking more than three to four drinks (two for girls) in a day suggest the need for further assessment and advice.

For screening of both alcohol and other drug abuse in adolescents, the "CRAFFT" screen is the most widely used and validated instrument and is recommended by the AAP (10,11,34–36). "CRAFFT" is an acronym for the six questions that make up the screen:

- Have you ever ridden in a **Car** driven by someone (including yourself) who was "high" or had been using alcohol or drugs?
- Do you ever use alcohol or drugs to **Relax**, feel better about yourself, or fit in?
- Do you ever use alcohol or drugs while you are by yourself, **Alone**?
- Do you ever **Forget** things you did while using alcohol or drugs?
- Do your family or **Friends** ever tell you that you should cut down on your drinking or drug use?
- Have you ever gotten into **Trouble** while you were using alcohol or drugs?

The CRAFFT is verbally administered, simple to score, and easy to remember, making it well-suited for use during primary care visits. According to AAP recommendations, it should be preceded by three questions about specific substance use during the past 12 months. The AAP-Recommended SBIRT algorithm (figure 13.1) is summarized the in the subsequent paragraphs (11).

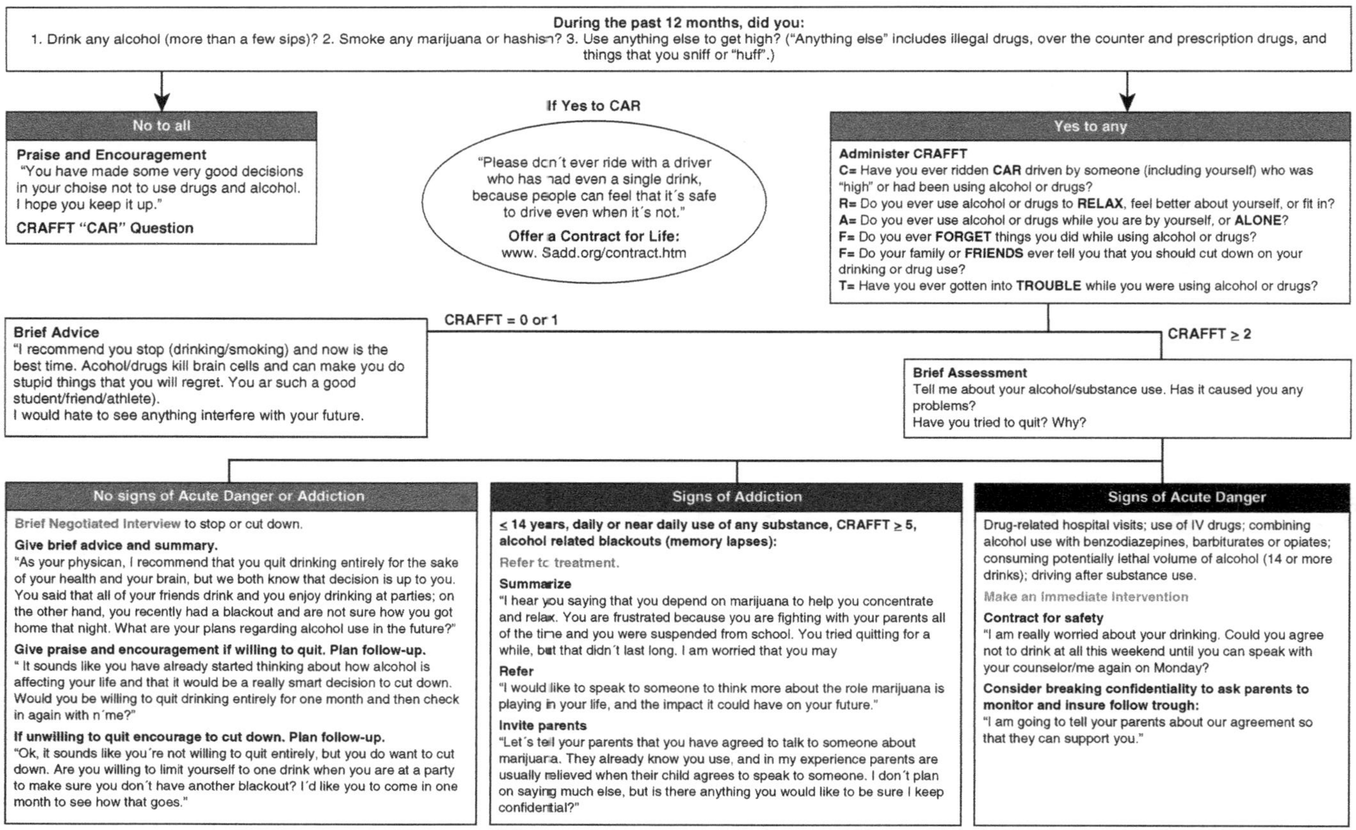

Figure 13.1: Adolescent SBIRT opening questions (© Children´s Hospital Boston 2011)

If adolescents deny drinking any alcohol, using marijuana or hashish, or using any substance to get high, they should be praised and encouraged for their good decision making and screened for ever having ridden in a car with someone under the influence of drugs or alcohol (C in CRAFFT). Adolescents who endorse having ridden in a car driven by someone who had been using drugs or alcohol should be counseled about the dangers associated with this behavior and specifically advised *not* to do so in the future. The adolescent should be requested to commit to a safety plan to avoid future driving risks. If the adolescent refuses to agree to the safety plan, a breach of confidentiality should be considered given the high risk of morbidity and mortality associated with driving under the influence.

All adolescents who answer "yes" to having used any drugs or alcohol during the past year should be administered the entire CRAFFT screen. A CRAFFT score of 2 or greater is considered to be a positive screen. This is an indicator of risk and not a diagnosis of either abuse or dependence. Adolescents who screen positive on the CRAFFT warrant a more in-depth evaluation for substance use. Adolescents who screen negative on the CRAFFT but report past-year use of drugs and/or alcohol should be clearly advised to stop using and educated about the health risks of use. Recognition of the adolescent's positive attributes and highlighting the connection between how substance use interferes with the adolescent's current goals can help motivate the patient to follow through on the recommendation.

Adolescents who screen positive on the CRAFFT should be asked follow-up questions about the details of their use, problems related to their use, and their willingness to change their behavior. A full substance use assessment may need to be divided over more than one primary care visit. Screening for signs of addiction or acute danger should be prioritized. Drug-related hospital visits, intravenous drug use, use of alcohol and sedatives together, and consuming potentially lethal amounts of alcohol or engaging in dangerous behaviors while intoxicated are all signs of acute danger. Their presence indicates the need for immediate intervention. Ask the adolescent to commit to not using until their follow-up appointment. Encourage them to let their parents know so they can be supportive of the agreement. Consider the need to break confidentiality in order to ensure safety and compliance with follow-up and treatment.

Indicators of possible addiction include a CRAFFT score greater than 2 in an adolescent under the age of 14, a CRAFFT score greater than 5 in older adolescents, daily or near-daily use of any substance, and alcohol-related blackouts. Adolescents with signs of addiction should be referred for a more detailed assessment and treatment. Pediatricians and primary care clinicians should encourage these adolescents to include their parents in treatment discussions in order to ensure follow-up.

Adolescents who screen positive on the CRAFFT and have no signs of acute danger or addiction should be engaged in a brief negotiated interview that includes a recommendation to quit using, a summary of the adolescent's reported use behaviors, and eliciting the adolescent's current intention with respect to their use.

Utilizing the principles of motivational interviewing (37), a brief negotiated interview is a negotiation that attempts to reduce substance use and related problems by focusing on the negative aspects of substance use as reported by the adolescent. Adolescents who are willing to quit should be praised and encouraged. Adolescents who are unwilling to quit should be encouraged to cut down and scheduled for follow-up.

13.6 Screening tools in young adults

Unlike the adolescent literature, the adult literature does not have a single, widely validated screening instrument like the CRAFFT for substance use (see chapter 9). For screening of alcohol misuse in adults, the Alcohol Use Disorders Identification Test (AUDIT) (38) is the most studied screening tool in primary care settings (16) and was used in a large multisite international randomized trial of brief intervention in primary care (39). With 10 items, it takes about 2 minutes to complete but does require additional time for scoring. With a score that can range from 0 to 40, a score of 8 or greater is generally considered a positive test for alcohol misuse. A score of 20 or greater suggests the presence of alcohol dependence (40). A briefer version of the AUDIT is available in the form of the AUDIT-C (41), a screening test comprised of 3 items on excess consumption from the AUDIT:

- "How often do you have a drink containing alcohol?"
- "How many drinks containing alcohol do you have on a typical day when you are drinking?"
- "How often do you have six or more drinks on occasion?"

The AUDIT-C has been validated in the primary care setting (42) and is scored on a scale of 0–12 with a score of 4 or more considered positive in men and a score of 3 or more considered positive in women.

Although the AUDIT-C is shorter than the AUDIT, it still requires scoring. Therefore, researchers have been exploring brief single-item screening tools that don't require scoring and are easily remembered. One such question has been validated in a primary care setting (43) – following the standard initial question of "Do you sometimes drink beer, wine or other alcoholic beverages?" the subsequent screening question is asked:

- "How many times in the past year have you had five (four for women) or more drinks in a day?"

The test is scored as positive when the response is greater than zero or when the patient is unsure of the correct number.

The 4-item CAGE (cut down, annoyed, guilty, eye opener) test (44) is the most popular screening test for detecting alcohol abuse or dependence in primary care and can be used as a quick follow-up to patients who were positive on the single screening question test. The CAGE questions are as follows:

- "Have you ever felt you should **Cut** down on your drinking?"
- "Have people **Annoyed** you by criticizing your drinking?"
- "Have you ever felt bad or **Guilty** about your drinking?"
- "Have you ever taken a drink first thing in the morning (**Eye opener**) to steady your nerves or get rid of a hangover?"

A single affirmative response is considered a positive screening test, and two affirmative responses are strongly suggestive of alcohol abuse and dependence with greater than 75% sensitivity and specificity (27,45).

For screening of illicit drug use in adults, the USPSTF found fair to good evidence for the Alcohol, Smoking and Substance Involvement Screening Test (ASSIST) (46); CAGE-AID (adapted to include drugs) (47); and the Drug Abuse Screen Test (DAST) (48) in detecting drug misuse (17). However, there's insufficient evidence to assess the clinical utility of these instruments in the primary care setting (47). The ASSIST can be very helpful in determining the severity of substance use, but its length (up to 80 items depending on the number of substances used) prevents its broad application in most primary care clinics. The DAST is a briefer 10-item instrument that also assesses for severity of drug use, and the CAGE-AID is an expanded version of the CAGE questions that also include drugs after the respondent answers "yes" to the question of "Do you drink alcohol?" or "Have you ever experimented with drugs?" A more recent study showed that a single-item screening test can serve as an alternative to those longer screening instruments in the primary care setting (49). The question is the following:

- "How many times in the past year have you used an illegal drug or used a prescription medication for nonmedical reasons?"

If asked to clarify the meaning of "nonmedical reasons," add "for instance because of the experience or feeling it caused." A response of greater than zero is a positive test and is 100% sensitive and 74% specific for a drug use disorder (49).

13.7 Summary

In most primary care office settings, a single-item screening question can be a helpful starting point for screening followed by more detailed instruments such as the CRAFFT in adolescents and AUDIT-C or DAST in young adults. For primary care offices that have more resources (e.g., time for administering and staff support for scoring), the AUDIT and ASSIST may be considered to help guide treatment. A brief assessment following a screening is warranted to determine the next steps. For patients who are not using substances, validation should be offered for positive health decisions. For patients who are misusing substances, brief intervention should be considered along with potential referral for further assessment and treatment. For patients who are demonstrating problems with substance abuse or dependence, referral for treatment and a more in-depth assessment by an addiction or mental health professional should be the primary task following the screening with the brief intervention focused on facilitating engagement in treatment. With the exception of the ASSIST, screening tools described in this section are available through the following SAMHSA website (http://www.integration.samhsa.gov/clinical-practice/screening-tools).

13.8 Brief intervention

One of the goals for screening adolescents and young adults for substance use in primary care clinics is to determine the need for referral for treatment. Patients with complicated psychiatric comorbidities and extensive, high-risk substance use may require more intensive and specialized care. However, this care is not always available, and there is good evidence that brief interventions conducted during primary care visits can lead to a significant reduction in use and better health outcomes.

Brief interventions involve a screening-outcome-responsive counseling that varies in length (10–30 minutes) and frequency (one or more session) with the goal of reducing substance use and substance-related behaviors (see chapter 5). It has consistently been shown to be helpful in reducing alcohol consumption 6 to 12 months later in primary care patients who are misusing alcohol (16,50,51), and there's emerging evidence to support its use in patients who are using illicit drugs (13). Although several models of brief intervention that have been tested in adolescents and adults include relatively unstructured adaptations of motivational interviewing, the current recommended interventions tend to be more structured and algorithmic as outlined previously in the previous section and contain several key components (11,12):

1. Give feedback about screening results, impairment, and risks while clarifying the findings. The clinician often expresses concern during the feedback, and the findings can include physical or laboratory findings as well as results of screening or assessment and evidence of adverse consequences. The feedback is usually followed by an open-ended question assessing the patient's own perception of the feedback and substance use pattern.

2. Inform the patient about safe consumption limits and offer advice about change after seeking patient permission. The advice needs to clearly delineate the problem and importance of change and emphasize that the patient is the one who has the capacity and responsibility to decide to change.
3. Assess the patient's readiness to change. Using the stages of change model developed by Prochaska and DiClemente (12,52,53), the patient is assessed for his or her readiness to change on the spectrum and have a brief intervention that matches the current stage of readiness:

   a) Precontemplation: Patient is not concerned and not considering change. Therefore, the goals of the brief intervention at this stage would focus on exploring the patient's own perception of the state of substance use while clearly identifying and expressing concern about the current problem in a nonjudgmental manner. A trial of abstinence or cutting down to clarify the issue can be recommended for the amenable patient, and follow-up should be encouraged even if the patient is not planning on changing.
   b) Contemplation: Patient is considering change or becoming aware of adverse consequences associated with use. Therefore, the goals of brief intervention at this stage focus on developing discrepancies between values and actions while tipping the decisional balance toward change by eliciting positive and negative aspects of substance use. Summaries of pro and con discussion can be very helpful along with advising a trial of abstinence.
   c) Determination: Patient has decided to reduce or stop use. Therefore, the goals of brief intervention at this stage focus on developing an action plan while addressing residual ambivalence. The clinician should provide a menu of options while assisting the patient in generating and implementing a plan that accounts for the patient's strengths. Additionally, the clinician acknowledges the significance of the decision while educating the patient on the challenges ahead in a supportive and reassuring manner (e.g., relapse would not disrupt the patient-clinician relationship).
   d) Action: Patient is making changes. Therefore, the goals at this stage are supporting and encouraging ongoing change while acknowledging the challenges.
   e) Maintenance: Patient has made changes and is maintaining progress. Therefore, the goals at this stage are validating the patient's resolve and anticipating future challenges as part of relapse prevention.
   f) Relapse: Patient has returned to using. Therefore, the goals at this stage are renewing the process of contemplation and emphasizing the positive aspects of previous success. Discussion of lessons learned is also crucial with a focus on supporting patient's self-efficacy so that recovery seems achievable.

4. Negotiate goals and strategies for change. Using an empathic counseling style with reflective listening such as motivational interviewing (37), the clinician

engages the patient in a discussion of goals and action plan appropriate for the current state of the problem. Interested readers should refer to the seminal work by Miller and Rollnick to learn more about specific skills to elicit and promote change talk (37).

5. Arrange for follow-up treatment. Once the patient and the clinician have negotiated an action plan, the primary care clinician plays an important role in monitoring the patient's progress and compliance. Any medical problem other than substance use (e.g., hypertension) and abnormal physical markers should be monitored and managed by the clinician in collaboration with other involved health care providers. Because resistance and denial (i.e., lack of insight) are common with substance-abusing adolescents and young adults, the patient and/or family might be unwilling to pursue a more extensive evaluation that is clearly warranted (11). If the patient and/or family are declining the clinically indicated further assessment and referral for treatment, then the clinician should consider more frequent follow-up visits with the goal of promoting treatment engagement using motivational interviewing techniques.

13.9 Referral to treatment and the primary care clinician's role in treatment

For the patient who has not responded to brief intervention or has been deemed to need further in-depth assessment or specialized treatment on the primary care clinician's brief psychosocial assessment, the clinician has several key functions to perform in addition to initiating and facilitating access to appropriate referrals for assessment and specialized treatment: (1) participate effectively as a member of the treatment team if required, (2) serve as the gatekeeper to monitor the patient's progress, and (3) carry out needed case management functions as appropriate (12). Determination for the appropriate level of service is usually done at an in-depth assessment by an experienced addiction specialist, but primary clinicians in underserved area or with expertise in substance abuse may choose to assume partial or total responsibility for the assessment function.

The recommended assessment is often based on the patient placement criteria published by the American Society of Addiction Medicine (54) incorporating the following six dimensions: (1) acute intoxication and/or withdrawal; (2) biomedical conditions and complications; (3) emotional/behavioral conditions (e.g., psychiatric conditions, psychological or emotional/behavioral complications of known or unknown origin, poor impulse control, changes in mental status, or transient neuropsychiatric complications); (4) treatment acceptance or resistance; (5) relapse potential or continued use potential; and (6) recovery/living environment (see chapters 5 and 6). For primary care clinicians who will not perform substance abuse assessment, it's still very helpful to be familiar with the six dimensions since primary care clinicians are often the ones managing problems within the first two dimensions and may be counted on to provide medical clearance to facilitate patient entry into specialized substance abuse treatment.

In addition to understanding the clinical basis for specific referrals or treatments, it's imperative for primary care clinicians to establish effective working relationships with addiction and/or mental health treatment professionals and facilities in their communities to ensure that adolescents and young adults have access to treatment appropriate for their developmental, medical, mental health, and psychosocial needs (11). Substance-abusing adolescents and young adults should be managed collaboratively (or comanaged) with addiction or mental health specialist whenever possible and have regular medical home office visits throughout the recovery process. Resources on referrals for primary care clinicians are included elsewhere in the book.

With continuing changes in the health care system in the United States, addiction treatment services are increasingly being provided by primary care clinicians in the context of patient's general medical care (12). Patients often return to their primary care clinicians for follow up care after substance abuse treatment and for continued care of previously diagnosed or emergent medical or psychological conditions, including pharmacotherapy for relapse prevention and/or co-occurring psychiatric conditions. Furthermore, as gatekeepers monitoring the patient's progress, primary care clinicians are often in the best position to encourage recovery support activities such as a structured schedule with prosocial activities (e.g., sports, church, etc.) and mutual self-help support groups (e.g., Alcoholics Anonymous). Discussions of specific treatments and recovery support interventions are covered elsewhere in this book.

With adolescents and young adults who refuse to accept referral to treatment or drop out before completion, the primary care clinicians have several important tasks: (1) continue treating any medical problem including substance-related issues while being mindful of potential complications with certain psychotropic medications; (2) continue to engage the patient in brief interventions focusing on promoting treatment engagement and be prepared to refer the patient for specialized treatment or explore appropriate alternatives that are acceptable to the patient; and (3) encourage family members and friends to participate in appropriate family-based mutual support groups (e.g., Al-Anon) or family-based psychosocial interventions that focus on learning about substance use disorders and minimizing distress and behaviors that perpetuate the patient's substance use pattern.

13.10 Conclusions

Pediatricians and primary care clinicians have important roles to play in identifying, screening, and referring adolescents and young adults with substance use disorders for in-depth assessment or treatment and in delivering brief interventions in patients with milder substance-related problems (12). The recommendations contained in the AAP policy statement are helpful in aiding the pediatrician (11) in performing the full range of tasks involved and may be adapted for primary care clinicians working with young adults:

1. Become knowledgeable about all aspects of SBIRT through training program curricula or continuing medical education that provide current best-practices training.
2. Become knowledgeable about the spectrum and pattern of substance use in adolescents and young adults in their practice area.
3. Ensure appropriate confidentiality in care that complies with state and federal regulations that govern health information privacy and substance abuse treatment.
4. Screen adolescents and young adults for substance use with formal validated screening tools at appropriate primary care visits and respond to screening results with the appropriate brief intervention.
5. Augment interpersonal communication and patient care skills by becoming familiar with motivational interviewing techniques.
6. Develop close working relationships with qualified and licensed professionals and programs that provide comprehensive substance use prevention and treatment services.
7. Facilitate patient referrals to locally available and developmentally appropriate treatments by applying multidimensional assessment criteria.
8. Consider co-occurring psychiatric disorders throughout the SBIRT process
9. Maintain familiarity with the latest SBIRT services including coding regulations and strategies and advocate for availability of quality mental health and substance use services that are integrated into primary care.

Although substance abuse in adolescents and young adults can be a very complex and challenging problem confronting pediatricians and primary care clinicians, implementing a structured and algorithmic approach highlighted in this chapter in the management of substance abuse in adolescents and young adults can enhance the prospect that primary clinicians will be effective at promoting good health outcomes throughout their patient's recovery process.

References

1. Compton WM, Thomas YF, Stinson FS. Prevalence, correlates, disability, and comorbidity of DSM-IV drug abuse and dependence in the United States. Arch Gen Psychiatry 2007;64:566–76.
2. Clark DB, Jones BL, Wood SD, Cornelius JR. Substance use disorder trajectory classes: Diachronic integration of onset age, severity, and course. Addict Behav 2006;31:995–1009.

3. Johnston LD, O'Malley PM, Bachman JG, Schulenberg JE. Monitoring the Future national results on adolescent drug use: Overview of key findings, 2010. Ann Arbor: Institute Social Research, University Michigan, 2011.
4. Substance Abuse and Mental Health Services Administration. Results from the 2010 National Survey on Drug Use and Health: Summary of national findings. NSDUH Series H-41, HHS Publication No. (SMA) 11–4658. Rockville, MD: Substance Abuse Mental Health Services Administration, 2011.
5. Miller NS, Giannini AJ, Gold MS, Philomena JA. Drug testing: Medical, legal, and ethical issues. J Subst Abuse Treat 1990;7(4):239–44.
6. Klein JD, Wilson KM, McNulty M, Kapphahn C, Collins KS. Access to medical care for adolescents: Results from the 1997 common wealth fund survey of the health of adolescent girls. J Adolesc Health 1999;25:120–30.
7. D'Amico EJ, Milse JNV, Stern SA, Meredith LS. Brief motivational interviewing for teens at risk of substance use consequences: A randomized pilot study in a primary care clinic. J Subst Abuse Treat 2008;35:53–61.
8. Knight JR, Harris SK, Sherritt L, Van Hook S, Lawrence N, Brooks T, et al. Prevalence of positive substance abuse screen results among adolescent primary care patients. Arch Pediatr Adolesc Med 2007;161(11):1035–41.
9. Merikangas KR, He JP, Burstein M, Swendsen J, Avenevoli S, Case B, et al. Service utilization for lifetime mental disorders in U.S. adolescents: Results of the National Comorbidity Survey-Adolescent Supplement (NCS-A). J Am Acad Child Adolesc Psychiatry 2011;50(1):32–45.
10. Kulig JW, American Academy of Pediatrics Committee on Substance Abuse. Tobacco, alcohol, and other drugs: The role of the pediatrician in prevention, identification, and management of substance abuse. Pediatrics 2005;115(3):816–21.
11. Committee on Substance Abuse, Levy SJ, Kokotailo PK. Substance use screening, brief intervention, and referral to treatment for pediatricians. Pediatrics 2011;128(5):e1330–40.
12. Center for Substance Abuse Treatment. A guide to substance abuse services for primary care clinicians. Rockville, MD: Substance Abuse Mental Health Services Administration, 1997.
13. Madras BK, Compton WM, Avula D, Stegbauer T, Stein JB, Clark HW. Screening, brief interventions, referral to treatment (SBIRT) for illicit drug and alcohol use at multiple health-care sites: Comparison at intake and 6 months later. Drug Alcohol Depend 2009;99(1–3):280–95.
14. Babor TF, McRee BG, Kassebaum PA, Grimaldi PL, Ahmed K, Bray J. Screening, brief intervention, and referral to treatment (SBIRT): Toward a public health approach to the management of substance abuse. Subst Abuse 2007;28(3):7–30.
15. American Psychiatric Association. Diagnostic and statistical manual of mental disorders, 4th ed., text rev. Washington, DC: American Psychiatric Association, 2000.
16. Whitlock EP, Polen MR, Green CA, Orleans T, Klein J; U.S. Preventive Services Task Force. Behavioral counseling interventions in primary care to reduce risky/harmful alcohol use by adults: A summary of the evidence for the U.S. Preventive Services Task Force. Ann Intern Med 2004;140(7):557–68.
17. U.S. Preventive Services Task Force. Screening for illicit drug use: U.S. Preventive Services Task Force recommendation statement. January 2008. Accessed December 2, 2012 . URL: http://www.uspreventiveservicestaskforce.org/uspstf08/druguse/drugrs.htm
18. Van Hook S, Harris SK, Brooks T, Carey P, Kossack R, Kulig J, et al.; New England Partnership for Substance Abuse Research. The "Six T's": Barriers to screening teens for substance abuse in primary care. J Adolesc Health 2007;40(5):456–61.
19. Britto MT, Tivorsak TL, Slap GB. Adolescents' needs for health care privacy. Pediatrics 2010;126:e1469–76.

20. Lothen-Kline C, Howard DE, Hamburger EK, Worrell KD, Boekeloo BO. Truth and consequences: Ethics, confidentiality, and disclosure in adolescent longitudinal prevention research. J Adolesc Health 2003;33:385–94.
21. Cheng TL, Savageau JA, Sattler AL, DeWitt TG. Confidentiality in health care: A survey of knowledge, perceptions, and attitudes among high school students. JAMA 1993;269:1404–7.
22. Legal Action Center. Confidentiality and communication: A guide to the federal drug & alcohol confidentiality law and HIPAA. New York: Legal Action Center City New York, 2006.
23. Gittler J, Quigley-Rick, Saks MJ. Adolescent health care decision making: The law and public policy. Washington, DC: Carnegie Council Adolescent Development, 1990.
24. Weddle M, Kokotailo P. Adolescent substance abuse: Confidentiality and consent. Pediatr Clin North Am 2002;49:301–15.
25. Appelbaum PS. Clinical practice: Assessment of patients' competence to consent to treatment. N Engl J Med 2007;357:1834–40.
26. Silber TJ. Justified paternalism in adolescent health care. J Adolesc Health 1989;10:449–453.
27. National Institute on Alcohol Abuse and Alcoholism. Helping patients with alcohol problems: A health practitioner's guide. NIH Publication No. 03–3769. Rockville, MD: NIAAA, 2003.
28. Bukstein OG, Bernet W, Arnold V, Beitchman J, Shaw J, Benson RS, et al.; Work Group on Quality Issues. Practice parameter for the assessment and treatment of children and adolescents with substance use disorders. J Am Acad Child Adolesc Psychiatry 2005;44(6):609–21.
29. Thompson MP, Sims L, Kingree JB, Windle M. Longitudinal associations between problem alcohol use and violent victimization in a national sample of adolescents. J Adolesc Health 2008; 42:21–7.
30. Champion HL, Foley KL, DuRant RH, Hensberry R, Altman D, Wolfson M. Adolescent sexual victimization, use of alcohol and other substance, and other health risk behaviors. J Adolesc Health 2004;35:321–8.
31. Goldston DB, Curry JF, Wells KC, Roley M. Assessment and treatment of suicidal behavior. In: Kaminer Y, Winters KC. Clinical manual of adolescent substance abuse treatment. Washington, DC: American Psychiatric Publishing, 2011:349–77.
32. Joiner TE Jr, Conwell Y, Fitzpatrick KK, Witte TK, Schmidt NB, Berlim MT, et al. Four studies on how past and current suicidality relate even when "everything but the kitchen sink" is covaried. J Abnorm Psychol 2005;114(2):291–303.
33. National Institute on Alcohol Abuse and Alcoholism. Alcohol screening and brief intervention for youth: A practitioner's guide. NIH Publication No. 11–7805. Rockville, MD: NIAAA, 2011.
34. Knight JR, Sherritt L, Shrier LA, Harris SK, Chang G. Validity of the CRAFFT substance abuse screening test among adolescent clinic patients. Arch Pediatr Adolesc Med 2002;156:607–14.
35. Subramaniam M, Cheok C, Verma S, Wong J, Chong SA. Validity of a brief screening instrument-CRAFFT in a multiethnic Asian population. Addict Behav 2010;35:1102–4.
36. Dhalla S, Zumbo BD, Poole G. A review of the psychometric properties of the CRAFFT instrument: 1999–2010. Curr Drug Abuse Rev 2011;4:57–64.
37. Miller WR, Rollnick S. Motivational interviewing: Preparing people for change, 2nd ed. New York: Guilford, 2002.
38. Saunders JB, Aasland OG, Babor TF, de la Fuente JR, Grant M. Development of the Alcohol Use Disorders Identification Test (AUDIT): WHO collaborative project on early detection of persons with harmful alcohol consumption-II. Addiction 1993;88(6):791–804.
39. Babor TF, Grant M, Acuda W, Burns FH, Campillo C, Del Boca FK, et al. A randomized clinical trial of brief interventions in primary care: Summary of a WHO project. Addiction 1994;89(6): 657–60.
40. Rubinsky AD, Kivlahan DR, Volk RJ, Maynard C, Bradley KA. Estimating risk of alcohol dependence using alcohol screening scores. Drug Alcohol Depend 2010;108(1–2):29–36.

41. Bush K, Kivlahan DR, McDonell MB, Fihn SD, Bradley KA. The AUDIT alcohol consumption questions (AUDIT-C): An effective brief screening test for problem drinking. Ambulatory Care Quality Improvement Project (ACQUIP). Alcohol Use Disorders Identification Test. Arch Intern Med 1998;158(16):1789–95.
42. Bradley KA, DeBenedetti AF, Volk RJ, Williams EC, Frank D, Kivlahan DR. AUDIT-C as a brief screen for alcohol misuse in primary care. Alcohol Clin Exp Res 2007;31(7):1208–17.
43. Smith PC, Schmidt SM, Allensworth-Davies D, Saitz R. Primary care validation of a single-question alcohol screening test. J Gen Intern Med 2009;24(7):783–8.
44. Ewing JA. Detecting alcoholism: The CAGE questionnaire. JAMA 1984;252(14):1905–7.
45. Maisto SA, Saitz R. Alcohol use disorders: Screening and diagnosis. Am J Addict 2003;12(Suppl 1):S12–25.
46. Humeniuk R, Ali R, Babor TF, Farrell M, Formigoni ML, Jittiwutikarn J, et al. Validation of the Alcohol, Smoking And Substance Involvement Screening Test (ASSIST). Addiction 2008;103(6): 1039–47.
47. Brown RL, Rounds LA. Conjoint screening questionnaires for alcohol and other drug abuse: Criterion validity in a primary care practice. Wis Med J 1995;94(3):135–40.
48. Gavin DR, Ross HE, Skinner HA. Diagnostic validity of the drug abuse screening test in the assessment of DSM-III drug disorders. Br J Addict 1989;84(3):301–7.
49. Smith PC, Schmidt SM, Allensworth-Davies D, Saitz R. A single-question screening test for drug use in primary care. Arch Intern Med 2010;170(13):1155–60.
50. Kaner E, Bland M, Cassidy P, Coulton S, Deluca P, Drummond C, et al. Screening and brief interventions for hazardous and harmful alcohol use in primary care: A cluster randomised controlled trial protocol. BMC Public Health 2009;9:287.
51. Bertholet N, Daeppen JB, Wietlisbach V, Fleming M, Burnand B. Reduction of alcohol consumption by brief alcohol intervention in primary care: Systematic review and meta-analysis. Arch Intern Med 2005;165(9):986–95.
52. Prochaska JO, DiClemente CC, Norcross JC. In search of how people change: Applications to addictive behaviors. Am Psychol 1992;47(9):1102–14.
53. Samet JH, Rollnick S, Barnes H. Beyond CAGE: A brief clinical approach after detection of substance abuse. Arch Intern Med 1996;156(20):2287–93.
54. Fishman M; American Society of Addiction Medicine. ASAM patient placement criteria: Supplement on pharmacotherapies for alcohol use disorders. Philadelphia, PA: Wolters Kluwer Health, Lippincott Williams Wilkins, 2010.

Section III: **Special populations**

14 Substance use disorders in adolescents and young adults: Comorbidity and treatment

Brieana M. Rowles, Aaron Ellington, Andrew R. Tarr,
John L. Hertzer, and Robert L. Findling

Substance use disorders (SUDs) frequently co-occur with other psychiatric disorders in adolescents and young adults. Diagnosing these comorbid conditions can be challenging in young populations. If these conditions are left untreated, the prognosis for youths with comorbid conditions may be particularly poor. This is, in part, owing to the fact that the presence of a comorbid psychiatric disorder in young patients with substance abuse disorders increases the likelihood for problems with family and school, criminal involvement, risky behaviors, and poor treatment adherence and outcomes. Fortunately, evidence-based treatments for these co-occurring conditions have emerged from recent intervention research. This chapter describes the general principles of assessment, diagnosis, and treatment for young patients with co-occurring substance use and psychiatric disorders and outlines recent treatment research for this vulnerable population.

14.1 Introduction

SUDs are fairly common among adolescents and young adults in the United States, with prevalence rates ranging from approximately 8% (1) to approximately 35% (2). Not only are SUDs common, but they also frequently co-occur with other psychiatric disorders. The National Survey on Drug Use and Health reported that in 2010, 22.1% of adolescents aged 12 to 17 (N = 379,000) with substance dependence or abuse in the past year also had a major depressive episode during the same time period (3). Additionally, the most recent practice parameter from the American Academy of Child and Adolescent Psychiatry reported that up to 50% of adolescents with SUDs in clinical populations have a comorbid psychiatric disorder (4).

14.2 Common comorbid psychiatric conditions

Studies of community-based samples of children and adolescents generally report attention-deficit/hyperactivity disorder (ADHD) and disruptive behavior disorders as the most commonly occurring comorbid psychiatric conditions in SUDs, at rates just under 70% (5,6). In addition, ADHD complicated by co-occurring oppositional defiant disorder or conduct disorder (CD) is associated with significant risk for developing SUDs (7). The next most frequently reported comorbid psychiatric conditions at approximately 20%–30% are mood disorders (both depressive disorders and bipolar disorders [BPDs]) (5,8). Anxiety disorders occur at a rate of approximately 20% in children and adolescents with SUDs (5).

14.2.1 Clinical samples

Similar to data from community samples, clinical samples of children and adolescents report rates suggesting that ADHD and disruptive behavior disorders are the most common conditions comorbid with SUDs (9–12). Approximately 40%–50% of young patients diagnosed with an SUD meet diagnostic criteria for comorbid ADHD (9,10,12). It has been suggested that ADHD during childhood/adolescence is a significant risk factor for developing an SUD (13). Further, longitudinal assessments of the relationship of ADHD in adolescence to later SUD have found that not only are co-occurring oppositional defiant disorder or CD significant predictors of SUD (13,14), but also that comorbid CD predicts SUD in pediatric ADHD (15,16). CD has been reported to co-occur in approximately 50% of children and adolescents with an SUD (10–12).

Mood disorders also are commonly comorbid with juvenile SUDs in clinical settings (9,12). Approximately 20% to more than 50% of children and adolescents with SUDs suffer from major depressive disorder (MDD) (4,11,17,18). BPDs occur in 15% to 30% of juvenile SUD cases (19,20). Further, juvenile BPD has been found to be a predictor of later SUD (21), and preliminary data suggest that co-occurring BPD and posttraumatic stress disorder increase the risk of subsequent SUD (22). Posttraumatic stress disorder and other anxiety disorders occur at rates of approximately 10%–40% in juvenile SUD in clinical settings (4,12,18).

While psychotic disorders are not uncommonly comorbid with SUDs, the onset of the psychotic disorder generally occurs in late adolescence to early adulthood (23). Thus, clinical sample data are generally limited to adults. Of note, substance use and SUDs, particularly cannabis use, are associated with earlier age of onset of psychotic symptoms (24–28). Accordingly, adolescents with SUDs may be at increased risk for developing a comorbid psychotic disorder.

14.3 General principles of assessment and diagnosis

Considering the serious risks associated with SUDs and co-occurring psychiatric conditions, and high rates of comorbid individuals, proper assessment is critical. Although validated psychometric instruments are used frequently in scientific investigations, research has shown that only a small number of treatment providers report using formal assessment measures (e.g., self-reports, structured interviews, etc.) when determining proper treatment referrals (29). Lichtenstein et al. (29), for instance, found that the standard practice in mental health settings to generate diagnostic information and determining a basic treatment plan is to conduct an informal or unstructured "clinical interview."

There also has been concern regarding the proper training of clinicians on how to properly diagnose comorbidity in youths with SUDs. Training clinicians to accurately assess comorbid individuals is critical because of the complexities in deciphering various symptoms that overlap in presentation. Clinicians are generally trained to assess and treat one segment: either SUDs or mental health disorders. Additionally, state and federal funding sources for treating comorbid individuals typically pay for one or the other disorder, but generally not both simultaneously (30). Accordingly, patients or clinicians are forced to decide what gets treated first (i.e., sequential treatment) or choose to treat both separately at the same time (i.e., parallel treatment). Research has yielded that both sequential and parallel treatment are less effective and have a higher cost than an integrative approach with properly trained staff (30–33).

Jensen-Doss and Weisz (34) also found that when studying children and adolescents in an outpatient facility, in the absence of "diagnostic agreement" (i.e., the difference between the clinician-given diagnosis and a research-generated diagnosis), there were greater no-shows, cancellations, and dropouts from treatment. When SUD and depression are involved – both high risk factors for suicide in adolescents – diagnostic disagreement can have serious treatment ramifications (29).

According to *Addiction Counseling Competencies: The Knowledge, Skills, and Attitudes of Professional Practice,* Technical Assistance Publication Series 21, published by the Substance Abuse and Mental Health Services Administration (35), appropriate assessment should include a process sensitive to age, gender, racial and ethnic culture, and disabilities that includes but is not limited to: (1) history of alcohol and drug use; (2) physical health, mental health, and addiction treatment histories; (3) family issues; (4) work history and career issues; (5) history of criminality; (6) psychological, emotional, and worldview concerns; (7) current status of physical health, mental health, and substance use; (8) spiritual concerns of the patient; (9) education and basic life skills; (10) socioeconomic characteristics, lifestyle, and current legal status; (11) use of community resources; (12) treatment readiness; and (13) level of cognitive and behavioral functioning. These comprehensive assessment procedures combined with a comprehensive mental health assessment can aid in assessing comorbidity with appropriate precision.

14.4 General principles of treatment

Even when using an integrated treatment approach and a qualified treatment team, treating this population is difficult owing to the multiple issues unique to these patients. Children and adolescents with comorbid disorders are at greater risk for problems with family and school, criminal involvement, and suicidal behaviors than youths with SUDs alone (4). Also, problems related to substance use tend to persist over a longer period of time when the patient has a co-occurring mental health disorder (36). Further, comorbid patients tend to be at increased risk for non-adherence with treatment, poorer treatment outcomes, and greater use of system resources when compared to patients with just a SUD (37).

As noted earlier, psychiatric comorbidity with SUDs is the rule, rather than the exception, and it seems to be essential to treat these co-occurring psychiatric conditions together (4). What follows is an overview of recent treatment research for children and adolescents with SUDs and a co-occurring psychiatric condition (see table 14.1).

14.4.1 ADHD

In general, the rates of substance use are elevated for youths with ADHD, and the presence of oppositional defiant disorder or CD has been shown to further increase the risk and frequency of illicit alcohol and/or drug use (7,38,39). As previously noted, ADHD is one of the most common psychiatric comorbidities in young patients with SUD (9,10,12). Only a few trials have studied the effectiveness of U.S. Food and Drug Administration (FDA)–approved ADHD medications for the treatment of comorbid ADHD and SUD in children and adolescents.

Recently, atomoxetine, a selective norepinephrine reuptake inhibitor, was studied in combination with motivational interviewing (MI)/cognitive behavioral therapy (CBT) for the treatment of co-occurring ADHD and SUD in adolescents. Thurstone et al. (11) randomized 70 adolescents (aged 13–19) meeting diagnostic criteria for ADHD and at least one nontobacco SUD, as well as scoring ≥ 22 on the *Diagnostic and Statistical Manual of Mental Disorders*, fourth edition (*DSM-IV*), ADHD Rating Scale (ARS-IV), to double-blind treatment with atomoxetine + MI/CBT or placebo + MI/CBT for up to 12 weeks. Participants weighing < 70 kg initiated double-blind medication treatment at a dose of 0.5 mg/kg per day to 0.75 mg/kg per day. The dosage was increased 25 mg per week until the total daily dose reached 1.1–1.5 mg/kg per day. Participants weighing ≥ 70 kg initiated atomoxetine versus placebo at 50 mg/day. Dosage for these patients was increased to 75 mg/day during the second week of treatment and to 100 mg/day during the third week.

Adverse events were generally mild; however, participants treated with atomoxetine experienced vomiting more frequently than those treated with placebo, while treatment with placebo was associated with muscle cramps and sadness. Both treatment groups experienced significant reductions in ADHD symptoms during the 12 weeks of treatment, based on total scores on the ARS-IV. Further, based on clinician-administered timeline followback (TLFB) procedures, there was an overall

Table 14.1: Selected treatment studies of substance use disorders and comorbid psychiatric conditions in children and adolescents

Study	*N*	Age range	Inclusion criteria/ psychiatric diagnosis	Design	Medication and mean dose, mg/day*	Outcome**
Attention-deficit/hyperactivity disorder (ADHD)						
Thurstone et al. (11)	70	13–19	ADHD + SUD; *DSM-IV* ADHD checklist score ≥ 22	12-week DB-RPCT; ATX+MI/CBT vs. PCB+ MI/CBT	PT weight < 70 kg = 1.19 mg/kg/day ATX; PT weight ≥ 70 kg = 88.8 mg/day ATX	↓ *DSM-IV* ADHD checklist scores: ATX+MI/CBT = PCB+MI/CBT; ↓ substance use: ATX+MI/CBT = PCB+MI/CBT
Riggs et al. (40)	303	13–18	ADHD + SUD	16-week DB-RPCT; OROS-MPH+CBT vs. PCB+CBT	Maximum dose: 72 mg OROS-MPH	↓ ADHD-RS scores: OROS-MPH+CBT = PCB+CBT; ↓ substance use: OROS-MPH+CBT = PCB+CBT
Depressive disorders						
Findling et al. (42)	34	12–17	Depressive disorder + SUD; CDRS-R score ≥ 40	8-week DB-RPCT	Maximum dose: 20 mg FLX	↓ CDRS-R scores: FLX=PCB; # of positive urine drug screens: FLX = PCB
Hides et al. (43)	60	15–25	MDD + SUD	20-week open trial, 44-week follow-up	N/A	Week 20: 82.7% full or partial remission of MDD; Week 44: 84.0% full or partial remission of MDD

(*Continued*)

Table 14.1: Selected treatment studies of substance use disorders and comorbid psychiatric conditions in children and adolescents (*Continued*)

Study	*N*	Age range	Inclusion criteria/ psychiatric diagnosis	Design	Medication and mean dose, mg/day*	Outcome**
Riggs et al. (44)	126	13–19	MDD + CD + SUD	12-week DB-RPCT; FLX+CBT vs. PCB+ CBT	Maximum dose: 20 mg FLX	↓ CDRS-R scores: FLX+CBT > PCB+CBT; Treatment response (CGI-I ≤ 2): FLX+CBT = PCB+CBT; ↓ substance use: FLX+CBT = PCB+CBT; ↓ CD symptoms: FLX+CBT = PCB+CBT
Cornelius et al. (45)	70	14–25	MDD + CUD	12-week DB-RPCT; FLX+CBT/MET vs. PCB+ CBT/MET	Maximum dose: 20 mg FLX	↓ depressive symptoms: FLX+CBT/MET = PCB+CBT/MET ↓ CUD *DSM-IV* criteria: FLX+CBT/MET = PCB+CBT/MET
Cornelius et al. (46)	50	15–20	MDD + AUD	12-week DB-RPCT; FLX+CBT/MET vs. PCB+ CBT/MET	Maximum dose: 20 mg FLX	↓ depressive symptoms: FLX+CBT/MET = PCB+CBT/SMET ↓ alcohol consumption: FLX+CBT/MET = PCB+CBT/MET
Bipolar disorder (BPD)						
Geller et al. (48)	25	12–18	*DSM-III-R* BPD*** + *DSM-III-R* SDD	6-week DB-RPCT; Li^++IPT vs. PCB+IPT	Mean = 1,769 (401) mg/day Li^+; target serum levels = 0.9–1.3 mEq/L	↓ *DSM-III-R* mood symptoms: Li^++IPT = PCB+IPT; ↓ *DSM-III-R* SDD symptoms: Li^++IPT = PCB+IPT; ↑ CGAS scores: Li^++IPT > PCB+IPT

Psychotic disorders						
Green et al. (49)	262	16–40	First-episode psychosis; lifetime SUD: *n* = 97	12-week DB-RCT; OLZ vs. HPL	Mean modal dose OLZ = 10.2 mg/day; mean modal dose HPL = 4.8 mg/day	Treatment response:**** lifetime SUD: 27%; no SUD: 35%
Sevy et al. (51)	49	16–40	First-episode psychosis + CUD	16-week DB-RCT; OLZ vs. RIS	Mean modal dose OLZ = 15 (6) mg/day; mean modal dose RIS = 4 (2) mg/day	Response rate: OLZ = RIS

*If applicable.

**An "=" sign in the "Outcome" column indicates no significant difference between treatments.

****DSM-III-R* BPD = bipolar I disorder, bipolar II disorder, mania, or major depressive disorder with at least one of the adolescent predictors of future BPD.

****(1) ratings ≤ 3 on the Positive and Negative Syndrome Scale (PANSS) items P1, P2, P3, P5, and P6; (2) ≥ 30% reduction from baseline PANSS score; and (3) a CGI-S score < 4.

↓ = decrease; ADHD-RS = ADHD Rating Scale; ATX = atomoxetine; CBT = cognitive behavioral therapy; CD = conduct disorder; CDRS-R = Children's Depression Rating Scale-Revised; CUD = cannabis use disorder; DB = double-blind; FLX = fluoxetine; HPL = haloperidol; IPT = interpersonal therapy; Li^+ = lithium; MDD = major depressive disorder; MET = motivation enhancement therapy; MI = motivational interviewing; OLZ = olanzapine; OROS-MPH = osmotic-release methylphenidate; PCB = placebo; PT = patient; RCT = randomized controlled trial; RPCT = randomized placebo-controlled trial; RIS = risperidone; SDD = substance dependence disorder; SUD = substance use disorder.

significant decrease in non-nicotine substance use from baseline to week 12 for both treatment groups. Of note, the two groups did not significantly differ from one another in reduction of ADHD symptoms ($p = 0.298$) or in decrease in substance use ($p = 0.110$). Owing to the lack of a significant between-group difference, the authors concluded that the MI/CBT may have contributed to the large treatment response in both the placebo- and atomoxetine-treated groups.

In a similar fashion, Riggs et al. (40) randomized 303 adolescents (aged 13–18) meeting diagnostic criteria for ADHD and at least one nontobacco SUD to double-blind treatment with osmotic-release methylphenidate (OROS-MPH) + CBT or placebo + CBT for up to 16 weeks. Medication treatment was initiated at 18 mg/day of OROS-MPH versus placebo and increased to a maximum daily dose of 72 mg during the first two study weeks. Measures, including the ADHD Rating Scale (ADHD-RS) and the Clinical Global Impression-Improvement (CGI-I) scale, were used to assess for improvements in ADHD symptoms. Substance outcome measures included the TLFB and urine drug screens. In both treatment groups, ADHD symptoms and substance use decreased (all p values < 0.001). However, no significant between-group differences were found. Some secondary outcomes did favor treatment with OROS-MPH, including lower parent ADHD-RS scores and more negative urine drug screens. The authors concluded that CBT for SUD may contribute to ADHD treatment response.

Warden et al. (41) explored potential associations of co-occurring MDD with baseline demographic/clinical characteristics, treatment response, and adherence/retention in a subset of the study participants with ADHD and SUD from the Riggs et al. (40) study. After comparing the 38 patients with comorbid MDD, ADHD, and SUD to the 265 patients without comorbid MDD, the authors found that the adolescents with co-occurring MDD were more likely to have more severe substance use at baseline and during study participation. As a result, the authors concluded that adolescents with ADHD, MDD, and SUD may also require interventions targeting depression.

In summary, considering the large treatment responses in the groups not receiving active medication in the studies described previously, it is possible that psychotherapeutic interventions for substance use that were provided concomitantly with the placebo or active medication may have contributed to the abating of ADHD symptomatology in children and adolescents with ADHD and an SUD in these clinical trials. Further exploration into the effectiveness of psychotherapy in this population appears to be warranted.

14.4.2 Depressive disorders

Both fluoxetine and escitalopram are FDA approved for the treatment of MDD in young patients. However, for some time, fluoxetine was the only approved antidepressant medication for children and adolescents with MDD. Likely for this reason, fluoxetine is the most commonly studied antidepressant medication in young patients with MDD and co-occurring SUD, whether as monotherapy or in combination with psychotherapy.

14.4.2.1 Antidepressant monotherapy

Findling et al. (42) randomized 34 participants (12–17 years) meeting diagnostic criteria for a depressive disorder (MDD, dysthymic disorder, or depressive disorder not otherwise specified) and an SUD to double-blind treatment with either fluoxetine (n = 18) or placebo (n = 16) for up to 8 weeks. It is important to note that the study's final sample size was modest due to that fact that enrollment was terminated following a planned interim futility analysis. In this study, participants were initially given 10 mg of fluoxetine/placebo and could have their dose increased to 20 mg after 4 weeks, based on the discretion of the treating physician. Any participants and their families who were not currently receiving psychotherapy were offered referrals to community-based resources for SUDs during study participation.

The primary efficacy measure was the Children's Depression Rating Scale-Revised (CDRS-R). Although both treatment groups had a reduction in CDRS-R scores, at the end of study participation, placebo-treated patients experienced a greater mean reduction in CDRS-R score than fluoxetine-treated patients. There were no statistically significant between-group differences in treatment-emergent adverse events; one patient in the placebo group and one patient in the fluoxetine group discontinued study participation owing to suicidal ideation. Further, there was not a significant difference in rates of positive urine drug toxicology results between treatment groups.

14.4.2.2 CBT monotherapy

Hides et al. (43) treated 60 participants (15–25 years) with MDD and co-occurring substance misuse or an SUD with individual integrated CBT treatment. Over 20 weeks, study participants received 10 CBT sessions plus case management. Measures used to assess symptoms of depression and anxiety included the Mood and Anxiety Symptom Questionnaire (MASQ), the Hamilton Depression Rating Scale (HAM-D), the Hamilton Anxiety Rating Scale (HAM-A), the Clinical Global Impression (CGI) scale, and the Social and Occupational Functioning Scale (SOFAS). Substance use measures included the TLFB, Alcohol Use Disorders Identification Test (AUDIT), Severity of Dependence Scale (SDS), Readiness to Change Questionnaire (RTCQ), Drug Use Motives Measure (DUMM), and urine drug screens. Study participants were assessed midtrial (10 weeks), post-trial (20 weeks), and at 6-month follow-up (44 weeks). After 20 weeks, 82.7% of the study participants achieved partial or full remission of MDD. Overall, CBT was associated with significant improvements in depression, anxiety, and social and occupational functioning. Additionally, treatment with CBT resulted in significant reductions in the presence and number of SUDs, substance use, severity of dependence on substances, and increased days of abstinence.

14.4.2.3 Combination CBT and antidepressant therapy

Riggs et al. (44) examined the effects of fluoxetine and CBT on adolescents (13–19 years) with MDD, at least one nontobacco SUD, and CD. One hundred twenty-six participants were randomized to double-blind combination treatment with either fluoxetine (20 mg/day) or placebo and CBT for up to 16 weeks. Individual 1-hour CBT sessions were administered at each study visit. For MDD, the main outcome measures were the CDRS-R and the CGI-I, while CD was assessed via self-report of number of symptoms in the past 30 days. Substance use was measured by self-report and urine drug screens. While fluoxetine combined with CBT had greater efficacy than placebo combined with CBT on change from baseline CDRS-R score, no between-group differences were noted on the CGI-I.

Further, both treatment groups reported an overall decrease of self-reported substance use and number of CD symptoms. However, the placebo-CBT group had a significantly higher proportion of substance-free weekly urine screen results than the fluoxetine-CBT group. The authors noted that adverse events in both groups were generally mild and transient. Suicidal ideation (assessed by CDRS-R item #13) decreased overall in both groups; however, five study participants (fluoxetine + CBT, $n = 4$; placebo + CBT, $n = 1$) were evaluated or hospitalized for concerns of worsening suicidality during the study. The authors concluded that treatment with CBT, rather than with fluoxetine, may be associated with both depressive symptom improvement and decreased substance use in children and adolescents with MDD, SUD, and CD, considering the mixed efficacy findings and significant treatment response.

The 12-week efficacy of fluoxetine versus placebo in combination with CBT and motivation enhancement therapy (MET) for the treatment of depressive symptoms and cannabis use was studied by Cornelius et al. (45). Seventy adolescents and young adults (14–25 years) meeting *DSM-IV* criteria for a cannabis use disorder (CUD) and for MDD were randomized to double-blind treatment with either fluoxetine or placebo plus CBT/MET. To maximize participant safety and to minimize the risk of medication side effects, treatment with fluoxetine was initiated at 10 mg/day during the first 2 weeks of study participation and increased to 20 mg/day thereafter. Study participants received nine sessions of CBT/MET.

Both treatment groups showed significant improvements in both self-reported depressive symptoms, based on the Beck Depression Inventory (BDI), and clinician-rated depressive symptoms, based on the HAM-D. However, no between-group differences were found. Further, a significant decrease of approximately 40% was noted across both treatment groups in the number of DSM criteria for cannabis dependence during the study. Cornelius et al. (45) concluded that the lack of between-group differences in both depressive symptoms and cannabis-related symptoms may result from the efficacy of CBT/MET or from limited fluoxetine efficacy.

Similarly, Cornelius et al. (46) explored the acute efficacy of fluoxetine plus CBT/MET versus placebo plus CBT/MET in 50 adolescents and young adults (15–20 years) with MDD and an alcohol use disorder (AUD). Study participants were randomized in a double-blind fashion to either condition for up to 12 weeks of treatment. Treatment with fluoxetine was initiated at 10 mg/day during the first 2 weeks of study participation and increased to 20 mg/day thereafter. Study participants received nine sessions of psychotherapy. Analysis of the BDI and the HAM-D demonstrated significant reductions in depressive symptoms in both treatment groups. Per the Structured Clinical Interview for the *DSM* (SCID) and TLFB, the number of *DSM-IV* AUD symptoms significantly decreased, and the number of days of heavy alcohol use significantly decreased as well in both treatment groups. There were no serious adverse events, and fluoxetine was well tolerated. Of note, the number of days of heavy alcohol use was significantly associated with the lack of remission of BDI depression scores (BDI < 8) at study week 6 and study week 12/end of study.

Similar to Cornelius et al. (45), the authors concluded that the lack of between-group differences in both depressive symptoms and drinking may result from the efficacy of CBT/MET or from limited fluoxetine efficacy. At 2-year follow-up, both treatment groups demonstrated continued improvements in both depressive and alcohol-related symptoms compared to a group of adolescents with MDD and AUD that received naturalistic treatment (47). Again, no significant difference was noted between fluoxetine and placebo, thus suggesting that CBT/MET may be efficacious for the long-term treatment of MDD and AUD in adolescents and young adults.

14.4.2.4 Summary for depressive disorders

In each of the trials outlined previously, both depressive symptoms and substance use decreased during study participation, regardless of treatment intervention. Considering the lack of difference between treatment with fluoxetine and placebo when combined with psychotherapy, it is possible that psychosocial treatments for substance disorders may be beneficial for young patients with MDD and an SUD. Further study of psychotherapeutic interventions in the absence of pharmacotherapy appears to be warranted in this population.

14.4.3 BPD

Treatment research for children and adolescents with co-occurring BPD and an SUD is quite limited. In the only published trial we could identify, under the auspices of a randomized, double-blind, placebo-controlled study in this population, Geller et al. (48) treated 25 study participants (12–18 years) meeting diagnostic criteria for *Diagnostic and statistical manual of mental disorders*, third edition, revised (*DSM-III-R*), criteria for a BPD with either lithium or placebo for up to 6 weeks. Target lithium serum levels during the study were set to 0.9–1.3 mEq/L. Both treatment groups received weekly interpersonal therapy modified for use with families. Based on mood and substance dependence item scores on the Schedule for Affective Disorders and Schizophrenia for School-Age Children (K-SADS), there were no significant differences between the two treatment groups with regard to symptomatic improvement.

However, Children's Global Assessment Scale (CGAS) scores were significantly higher at the end of study participation in participants randomized to lithium. Further, study participants randomized to lithium had significantly fewer positive random urine drug screens when compared to participants randomized to placebo ($p = 0.028$). Treatment with lithium was well tolerated. Despite the administration of interpersonal therapy to all study participants, outcomes for this psychosocial treatment were not measured. Because lithium appears to be efficacious for the treatment of both BPDs and SUD, longer-term and replication studies may be warranted.

14.4.4 Psychotic disorders

There are limited data regarding the treatment of young patients with psychotic disorders and comorbid SUDs, despite the association between substance use and early onset psychotic symptoms (24–28). However, a few studies exploring clinical outcomes of patients with SUDs and psychotic disorders have included participants under the age of 18 years.

Green et al. (49) reported on the rates and effects of co-occurring SUDs in 262 patients (16–40 years) with first-episode psychosis (meeting *DSM-IV* criteria for schizophrenia, schizoaffective disorder, or schizophreniform disorder) receiving double-blind treatment with either olanzapine or haloperidol for up to 12 weeks. Of the 262 study participants, 97 (37%) had a lifetime *DSM-IV* SUD: 74 (28%) with a CUD, 52 (21%) with an AUD, 17 (6%) with a cocaine use disorder, 12 (5%) with a hallucinogen/PCP disorder, and 3 (1%) with a opioid use disorder. Treatment response was defined by the following: (1) ratings ≤ 3 on the Positive and Negative Syndrome Scale (PANSS) items P1, P2, P3, P5, and P6; (2) $\geq 30\%$ reduction from baseline PANSS score; and (3) a CGI-S score < 4.

In both treatment groups, patients with a comorbid SUD were less likely than those without an SUD to meet criteria for response (27% vs. 35%). In the olanzapine group, patients with an AUD were significantly less likely to respond to treatment than patients without an AUD ($p < 0.02$). Patients with an SUD and treated with haloperidol were significantly less likely to complete study participation compared to patients without an SUD and treated with haloperidol ($p < 0.04$). In the olanzapine group, SUD did not affect length of study participation, a finding in contrast to other adverse outcomes associated with the presence of SUD. Green et al. (49) concluded that first-episode psychosis patients are likely to have a co-occurring SUD, and that the presence of these disorders may negatively influence treatment response.

Secondary analysis of data from the acute treatment phase of a prospective, randomized trial of patients (16–40 years) with first-episode psychosis (meeting *DSM-IV* criteria for schizophrenia, schizoaffective disorder, or schizophreniform disorder) (50) compared the efficacy of olanzapine and risperidone in patients with co-occurring CUDs (51). Forty-nine patients with first-episode psychosis and CUD were randomized to treatment with either olanzapine ($n = 28$) or risperidone ($n = 21$) for up to 16 weeks. Sevy et al. (51) found that, in this subset of patients with CUD, neither rates of study completion nor rates of response differed between treatment groups. Additionally, there were no significant differences between treatment groups for the proportion of study participants with CUD using alcohol or cannabis during the trial.

14.4.4.1 Summary for psychotic disorders

In the absence of data, it is difficult to draw definitive conclusions specific to the treatment of young patients with psychotic disorders and comorbid SUDs. Considering a lack of difference between antipsychotic agents with regard to amelioration of psychotic symptoms and effects on substance use, other factors such as side-effect profiles of individual agents may help determine antipsychotic medication selection for young patients with psychotic disorders and comorbid SUDs. However, it appears that the presence of SUDs is associated with worse outcomes, and, accordingly, specific evidence-based treatments for this population are needed.

14.4.5 Anxiety disorders

Despite an association between higher rates of anxiety disorders in those with SUDs (4,12,18), treatment research for children and adolescents suffering from co-occurring anxiety disorders and SUDs is lacking. However, there is evidence to suggest that children and adolescents with anxiety disorders (generalized, separation, and social anxiety disorders) who receive and respond positively to long-term treatment with CBT are less likely to engage in substance misuse in the future compared to patients who do not respond positively to CBT (52).

14.4.6 Treatment recommendations and prognosis

In both community and clinical populations of children and adolescents, SUDs are common and frequently co-occur with other psychiatric conditions. Further, children and adolescents who suffer from both SUDs and psychiatric disorders are more likely to experience negative outcomes when compared to youths with SUDs and no psychiatric comorbidities (4). Fortunately, there are emerging evidence-based treatments for these co-occurring conditions. Recent intervention research suggests that combining psychotherapeutic and pharmacotherapeutic interventions are perhaps the most effective methods of treating this patient population. However, further exploration into effective treatments is warranted, particularly with regard to treatment approaches for patients who do not initially respond to psychotherapy.

In general, prognosis for untreated comorbid patients can be poor. Nevertheless, prognosis can be improved if the following steps are adhered to during the assessment, diagnosis, treatment, and maintenance of these patients: (1) use of validated assessment tools, (2) assessment and treatment by qualified and trained clinicians, (3) making accurate diagnoses of both the SUDs and the mental health disorders, and (4) use of evidence-based and integrated treatment protocols.

Acknowledgments

Dr. Findling receives or has received research support, acted as a consultant, received royalties from, and/or served on a speaker's bureau for Abbott, Addrenex, Alexza, American Psychiatric Press, AstraZeneca, Biovail, Bristol-Myers Squibb, Dainippon Sumitomo Pharma, Forest, GlaxoSmithKline, Guilford Press, Johns Hopkins University Press, Johnson & Johnson, KemPharm Lilly, Lundbeck, Merck, National Institutes of Health, Neuropharm, Novartis, Noven, Organon, Otsuka, Pfizer, Physicians' Post-Graduate Press, Rhodes Pharmaceuticals, Roche, Sage, Sanofi-Aventis, Schering-Plough, Seaside Therapeutics, Sepracore, Shionogi, Shire, Solvay, Stanley Medical Research Institute, Sunovion, Supernus Pharmaceuticals, Transcept Pharmaceuticals, Validus, WebMD, and Wyeth. Drs. Ellington and Hertzer, Ms. Rowles, and Mr. Tarr have no financial ties to disclose. Ms. Rowles completed this project as part of her position as Communications and Analysis Specialist at Case Western Reserve University.

References

1. Kessler RC, Avenevoli S, Costello EJ, Georgiades K, Green JG, Gruber MJ, et al. Prevalence, persistence, and sociodemographic correlates of DSM-IV disorders in the National Comorbidity Survey Replication Adolescent Supplement. Arch Gen Psychiatry 2012;69:372–80.

2. Copeland W, Shanahan L, Costello EJ, Angold A. Cumulative prevalence of psychiatric disorders by young adulthood: A prospective cohort analysis from the Great Smoky Mountains Study. J Am Acad Child Adolesc Psychiatry 2011;50:252–61.
3. Substance Abuse and Mental Health Services Administration. Results from the 2010 National Survey on Drug Use and Health: Mental health findings. NSDUH Series H-42, HHS Publication No. (SMA) 11–4667. Rockville, MD: Substance Abuse and Mental Health Services Administration, 2012.
4. Bukstein OG, Work Group on Quality Issues. Practice parameter for the assessment and treatment of children and adolescents with substance use disorders. J Am Acad Child Adolesc Psychiatry 2005;44:609–21.
5. Kandel DB, Johnson JG, Bird HR, Weissman MM, Goodman SH, Lahey BB, et al. Psychiatric comorbidity among adolescents with substance use disorders: Findings from the MECA study. J Am Acad Child Adolesc Psychiatry 1999;38:693–9.
6. Armstrong TD, Costello EJ. Community studies on adolescent substance use, abuse, or dependence and psychiatric comorbidity. J Consult Clin Psychol 2002;70:1224–39.
7. August GJ, Winters KC, Realmuto GM, Fahnhorst T, Botzet A, Lee S. Prospective study of adolescent drug use among community samples of ADHD and non-ADHD participants. J Am Acad Child Adolesc Psychiatry 2006;45:824–32.
8. Lewinsohn PM, Klein DN, Seeley JR. Bipolar disorder in a community sample of older adolescents: Prevalence, phenomenology, comorbidity, and course. J Am Acad Child Adolesc Psychiatry 1995;34:454–63.
9. Latimer WW, Stone AL, Voight A, Winters KC, August GJ. Gender differences in psychiatric comorbidity among adolescents with substance use disorders. Exp Clin Psychopharmacol 2002;10:310–5.
10. Dennis M, Godley SH, Diamond G, Tims FM, Babor T, Donaldson J, et al. The Cannabis Youth Treatment (CYT) study: Main findings from two randomized trials. J Substance Abuse Treat 2004;27:197–213.
11. Thurstone C, Riggs PD, Salomonsen-Sautel S, Mikulich-Gilbertson SK. Randomized, controlled trial of atomoxetine for ADHD in adolescents with substance use disorder. J Am Acad Child Adolesc Psychiatry 2010;49:573–82.
12. Wu L, Gersing K, Burchett B, Woody GE, Blazer DG. Substance use disorders and comorbid Axis I and II psychiatric disorders among young psychiatric patients: Findings from a large electronic health records database. J Psychiatr Res 2011;45:1453–62.
13. Wilens TE, Martelon MK, Joshi G, Bateman C, Fried R, Petty C, et al. Does ADHD predict substance-use disorders? A 10-year follow-up study of young adults with ADHD. J Am Acad Child Adolesc Psychiatry 2011;50:543–53.
14. Harty SC, Ivanov I, Newcorn JH, Halperin JM. The impact of conduct disorder and stimulant medication on later substance use in an ethnically diverse sample of individuals with attention-deficit/hyperactivity disorder. J Child Adolesc Psychopharmacol 2011;21:331–9.
15. Gau SS, Chong MY, Yang P, Yen CF, Liang KY, Cheng AT. Psychiatric and psychosocial predictors of substance use among adolescents: Longitudinal study. Br J Psychiatry 2007;190:42–8.
16. Brook DW, Brook JS, Zhang C, Koppel J. Association between attention-deficit/hyperactivity in adolescence and substance use disorders in adulthood. Arch Pediatr Adolesc Med 2010;164:930–4.
17. Birmaher B, Ryan ND, Williamson D, Brent DA, Kaufman J, Dahl RE, et al. Child and adolescent depression: A review of the past 10 years. Part I. J Am Acad Child Adolesc Psychiatry 1996;35:1427–39.
18. Lubman DI, Allen NB, Rogers N, Cementon E, Bonomo Y. The impact of co-occurring mood and anxiety disorders among substance-abusing youth. J Affect Disord 2007;103:105–12.

19. Wilens TE, Biederman J, Kwon A, Ditterline J, Forkner P, Moore H, et al. Risk of substance use disorders in adolescents with bipolar disorder. J Am Acad Child Adolesc Psychiatry 2004;43:1380–6.
20. Goldstein BI, Strober MA, Birmaher B, Axelson DA, Esposito-Smythers C, Goldstein TR, et al. Substance use disorders among adolescents with bipolar spectrum disorders. Bipolar Disord 2008;10:469–78.
21. Wilens TE, Biederman J, Adamson JJ, Henin A, Sgambati S, Gignac M, et al. Further evidence of an association between adolescent bipolar disorder with smoking and substance use disorders: A controlled study. Drug Alcohol Depend 2008;95:188–98.
22. Steinbuchel PH, Wilens TE, Adamson JJ, Sgambati S. Posttraumatic stress disorder and substance use disorders in adolescent bipolar disorder. Bipolar Disord 2009;11:198–204.
23. American Academy of Child and Adolescent Psychiatry. Practice parameter for the assessment and treatment of children and adolescents with schizophrenia. J Am Acad Child Adolesc Psychiatry 2001;40:4S–23S.
24. Veen ND, Selten JP, van der Tweel I, Feller WG, Hoek HW, Kahn RS. Cannabis use and age at onset of schizophrenia. Am J Psychiatry 2004;161:501–6.
25. Barnes TR, Mutsatsa SH, Hutton SB, Watt HC, Joyce EM. Comorbid substance use and age at onset of schizophrenia. Br J Psychiatry 2006;188:237–42.
26. Sevy S, Robinson DG, Napolitano B, Patel RC, Gunduz-Bruce H, Miller R, et al. Are cannabis use disorders associated with an earlier age of onset of psychosis? A study in first-episode schizophrenia. Schizophr Res 2010;120:101–7.
27. DeHert M, Wampers M, Jendricko T, Franic T, Vidovic D, De Vriendt N, et al. Effects of cannabis use on age at onset in schizophrenia and bipolar disorder. Schizophr Res 2011;126:270–6.
28. Dragt S, Nieman DH, Schultze-Lutter F, van der Meer F, Becker H, de Haan L, et al. Cannabis use and age of onset of symptoms in subjects at clinical high risk for psychosis. Acta Psychiatr Scand 2012;125:45–53.
29. Lichtenstein DP, Spirito A, Zimmermann RP. Assessing and treating co-occurring disorders in adolescents: Examining typical practice of community-based mental health and substance use treatment providers. Comm Ment Health J 2010;46:252–7.
30. Petersen CL, Zettle RD. Treating inpatients with comorbid depression and alcohol use disorders: A comparison of acceptance and commitment therapy versus treatment as usual. Psychol Rec 2002;59:521–36.
31. Drake RE, Mueser KT, Clark RE, Wallach MA. The course, treatment, and outcome of substance disorder in persons with severe mental illness. Am J Orthopsychiatry 1996;66:42–51.
32. Havassy BE, Shopshire MS, Quigley LA. Effects of substance dependence on outcomes of patients in a randomized trial of two case management models. Psychiatric Serv 2000;51:639–44.
33. Mueser KT, Torrey WC, Lynde D, Singer P, Drake RE. Implementing evidence-based practices for people with severe mental illness. Behav Mod 2003;27:387–411.
34. Jensen-Doss A, Weisz JR. Diagnostic agreement predicts treatment process and outcomes in youth mental health clinics. J Consult Clin Psychol 2008;76:711–22.
35. Substance Abuse and Mental Health Services Administration. Report to congress on the prevention and treatment of co-occurring substance abuse disorders and mental disorders. Washington, DC: U.S. Government Printing Office, 2002.
36. Cosci F, Fava GA. New clinical strategies of assessment of comorbidity associated with substance use disorders. Clin Psychol Rev 2011;31:418–27.
37. Pray ME, Watson LM. Effectiveness of day treatment for dual diagnosis patients with severe chronic mental illness. J Addict Nurs 2008;19:141–9.
38. White HR, Xie M, Thompson W, Loeber R, Stouthamer-Loeber M. Psychopathology as a predictor of adolescent drug use trajectories. Psychol Addict Behav 2001;15:210–8.

39. Molina B, Pelham W. Childhood predictors of adolescent substance use in a longitudinal study of children with ADHD. J Abnorm Psychol 2003;112:497–507.
40. Riggs PD, Winhusen T, Davies RD, Leimberger JD, Mikulich-Gilbertson S, Klein C, et al. Randomized controlled trial of osmotic-release methylphenidate with cognitive-behavioral therapy in adolescents with attention-deficit/hyperactivity disorder and substance use disorders. J Am Acad Child Adolesc Psychiatry 2011;50:903–14.
41. Warden D, Riggs PD, Min SJ, Mikulich-Gilbertson SK, Tamm L, Trello-Rishel K, et al. Major depression and treatment response in adolescents with ADHD and substance use disorder. Drug Alcohol Depend 2012;120:214–9.
42. Findling RL, Pagano ME, McNamara NK, Stansbrey RJ, Faber JE, Lingler J, et al. The short-term safety and efficacy of fluoxetine in depressed adolescents with alcohol and cannabis use disorders: A pilot randomized placebo-controlled trial. Child Adolesc Psychiatry Ment Health 2009; 3:11.
43. Hides L, Carroll S, Catania L, Cotton SM, Baker A, Scaffidi A, et al. Outcomes of an integrated cognitive behaviour therapy (CBT) treatment program for co-occurring depression and substance misuse. J Affect Disord 2010;121:169–74.
44. Riggs PD, Mikulich-Gilbertson SK, Davies RD, Lohman M, Klein C, Stover SK. A randomized controlled trial of fluoxetine and cognitive behavioral therapy in adolescents with major depression, behavior problems, and substance use disorders. Arch Pediatr Adolesc Med 2007;161:1026–34.
45. Cornelius JR, Bukstein OG, Douaihy AB, Clark DB, Chung TA, Daley DC, et al. Double-blind fluoxetine trial in comorbid MDD-CUD youth and young adults. Drug Alcohol Depend 2010;112: 39–45.
46. Cornelius JR, Bukstein OG, Wood DS, Kirişci L, Douaihy A, Clark DB. Double-blind placebo controlled trial of fluoxetine in adolescents with comorbid major depression and an alcohol use disorder. Addict Behav 2009;34:905–9.
47. Cornelius JR, Douaihy A, Bukstein OG, Daley DC, Wood DS, Kelly TM, et al. Evaluation of cognitive behavioral therapy/motivational enhancement therapy (CBT/MET) in a treatment trial of comorbid MDD/AUD adolescents. Addict Behav 2011;36:843–8.
48. Geller B, Cooper TB, Sun K, Zimerman B, Frazier J, Williams M, et al. Double-blind and placebo-controlled study of lithium for adolescent bipolar disorders with secondary substance dependency. J Am Acad Child Adolesc Psychiatry 1998;37:171–8.
49. Green AI, Tohen MF, Hamer RM, Strakowski SM, Lieberman JA, HGDH Research Group, et al. First-episode schizophrenia-related psychosis and substance use disorders: Acute response to olanzapine and haloperidol. Schizophr Res 2004;66:125–35.
50. Robinson DG, Woerner MG, Napolitano B, Patel RC, Sevy SM, Gunduz-Bruce H, et al. Randomized comparison of olanzapine versus risperidone for the treatment of first-episode schizophrenia: 4-month outcomes. Am J Psychiatry 2006;163:2096–102.
51. Sevy S, Robinson DG, Sunday S, Napolitano B, Miller R, McCormack J, et al. Olanzapine vs. risperidone in patients with first-episode schizophrenia and a lifetime history of cannabis use disorders. Psychiatry Res 2011;188:310–4.
52. Kendall PC, Safford S, Flannery-Schroeder E, Webb A. Child anxiety treatment: Outcomes in adolescence and impact on substance use and depression at 7.4-year follow-up. J Consult Clin Psychol 2004;72:276–87.

15 Adolescent girls and substance abuse: Recent trends, risk factors, and consequences

Ruqiya Shama Tareen

Clinicians who treat young adolescents are concerned about the rising rates of initiation of substance abuse in younger adolescents for obvious reasons. Traditionally, we have treated substance abuse as one entity without paying attention to the specific needs based on age, gender, and psychosocial makeup of the particular population. Adolescent and preadolescent girls in their early formative years are abusing alcohol and other substances at a much higher rate than ever before posing a unique challenge for substance abuse providers. This chapter discusses some of the often overlooked complications of substance abuse that are unique to the adolescent female population, including substance abuse associated sexual activity, resultant pregnancies, and associated obstetric/gynecologic psychiatric complications such as perinatal mood disorder.

15.1 Introduction

This chapter considers recent trends, risk factors, and consequences for substance abuse in adolescent females. The rate of substance abuse is on the rise in U.S. youth. According to the Substance Abuse and Mental Health Services Administration (SAMHSA), substance abuse trends are changing dramatically with initiation rates highest in young age and a dramatic shift in gender trends (1,2). The most recent data collected in 2009 showed that 730, 228 patients 12 years and older reported using alcohol and other drugs requiring an admission to an alcohol or drug treatment program. Alcohol remains the most commonly abused substance in adolescents with the highest use among 19-year-olds; in this group, about 15% reported using alcohol. The rate starts declining from there to 12.8% in persons aged 18 to 25 (1,2). Out of these, about 23% were only using alcohol, while 39% reported using other drugs without alcohol, and about 37% reported using both alcohol and at least one other drug at the time of admission (3). Figure 15.1 depicts the recent trends in choice of substances in U.S. adolescents.

15.2 Gender differences in substance abuse

Traditionally, substance abuse is considered to be a more common problem in male adolescents, but in the past decade or so, young girls slowly approached the same level. According to the SAMHSA 2000 report, when looking at the gender

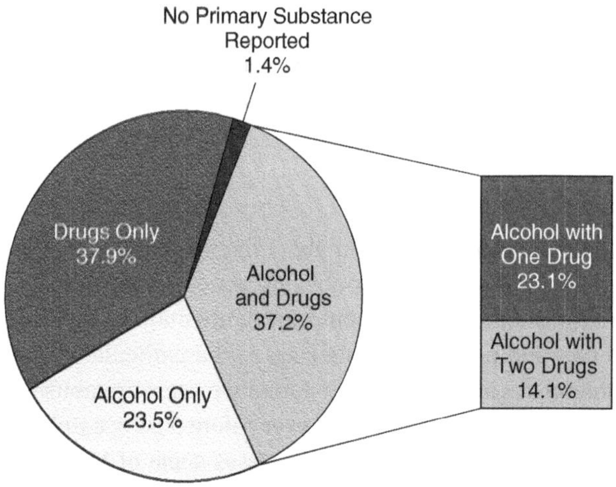

Figure 15.1: Substance Abuse and Mental Health Services Administration treatment data set 2009. Source: Substance Abuse and Mental Health Services Administration (SAMHSA) Treatment Episode Data Set (TEDS), 2009, based on data received through November 3, 2010. (Permission: The Data Spotlight may be copied without permission. Citation of the source is appreciated. Find this report and those on similar topics online at http://www.samhsa.gov/data/.)

distribution in all age groups, males were more than twice as likely (7.7 %) compared to their female counterparts (3.3%) to be abusing or be dependent on alcohol (1). While this may appear to support the general assertion that substance abuse is mainly a disease afflicting men, once one sifts through these data and breaks the data out by age group, the picture changes considerably. For instance, in adolescents 12–17 years of age, the rates of alcohol abuse and dependence were very similar in both genders – 5.2% in boys versus 5.1% in girls (1).

The majority of new substance users, however, were younger, and 56.2% of new initiators were female (1). Moving 5 years forward on this timeline, in 2005, SAMHSA reported that – for the first time – adolescent girls ages 12–17 admitting to current alcohol use surpassed their male peers at the rate of 17.2% females versus 15.9% of males (2). The same pattern was seen in adolescents who started using illicit drugs other than alcohol. More than 55% were younger than age 18 when they first used, and 56.2% were female (2).

15.3 Risk factors for substance abuse in female adolescents

Nongender specific risk and protective factors have been identified that affect substance abuse predisposition in adolescents (see chapter 9). The literature shows, in addition, that young adolescent girls have factors specific to their gender and

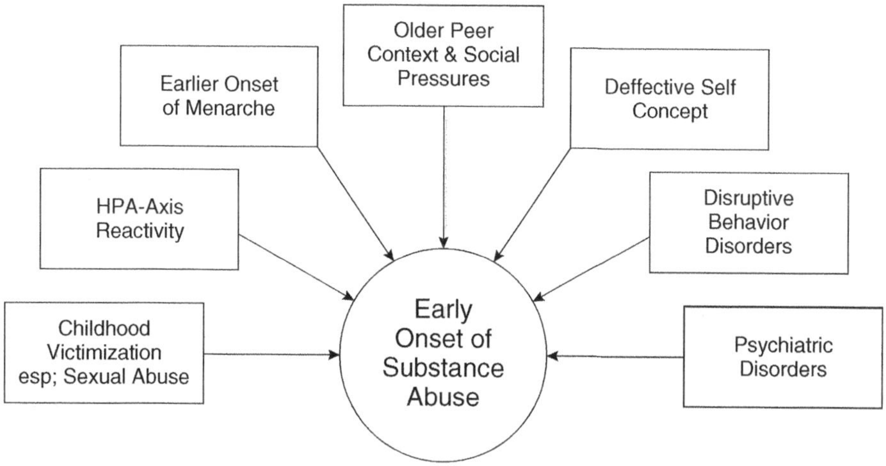

Figure 15.2: Risk factors predisposing to early onset of substance abuse in female adolescents

age (see figure 15.2). Early identification of these risk and protective factors is important because continuation of risks can worsen prognosis and enhancement of protective aspects can improve the course of illness. Figure 15.2 gives a brief overview of some of these risk factors.

15.3.1 Puberty status and timing

Attainment of puberty has been associated with a significant rise in smoking tobacco and cannabis, drinking alcohol, and abusing other substances independent of other variables such as school grade and age (4). Several researchers have suggested a role of pubertal changes and their possible link to this behavior. The age of menarche has been declining at a rate of 1–3 months per decade for more than past 175 years. For instance, in the United States in recent years, puberty has generally been occurring between the ages of 8 and 13 years of age in girls (5). It is well known that adolescents seldom start abusing substances before puberty (4). It has also been established that the earlier the onset of substance abuse, the worse the prognosis (4). The relationship between onset of puberty and initiation of substance abuse has been studied closely (5).

Puberty in this context is examined in two different developmental stages: pubertal status and pubertal timing. Pubertal status refers to morphological changes or development of secondary sexual characteristics, defined in terms of Tanner stages of puberty (5). Puberty timing, on the other hand, is a comparison of one's pubertal standing relative to the same age and same gender peers (5). Girls who mature earlier have a higher risk of starting to abuse substances at an earlier age than their counterparts who are not as sexually matured (4,5). Girls attaining menarche later have shown lesser risk of initiating substance abuse in early teenage years.

There is no definite evidence of how pubertal status and timing are linked to addiction. It has been hypothesized, however, that pubertal timing affects the initiation of substance abuse. For instance, girls who attain puberty earlier than their peers are much more likely to start abusing alcohol or tobacco before age 13 years, which is itself a predictor of developing long-term substance abuse and dependency (6).

Dick et al. followed five consecutive cohorts of Finnish twin girls and surveyed them at 16, 17, and 18 years of age (6). The data revealed that the twin sisters who were discordant for onset of menarche were also discordant in age of onset of substance abuse. The sisters with earlier onset of puberty were about 40% more prone to start abusing substances by age 13 when compared to their twin who achieved menarche later on (6). Attainment of puberty initiates a hormonal cascade that lead to specific changes in cognitive patterns reflective of adolescent behavior. This gives rise to ambivalence and contradictions in an adolescent who might feel out of place among age-matched peers. The initiation of substance abuse earlier in adolescents who mature earlier then age-matched peers may also be due to their identifying and associating with older persons, and their efforts to try to fit within that group by trying to engage in similar types of behavior (7).

15.4 Hormonal changes and emotional reactivity

The hormonal cascade, which is responsible for the hypothalamic-pituitary axis (HPA) that governs the pubertal development, can be divided into two separate processes: the early phase, or adenarche, and the later phase, or goandarche. Adenarche can start as early as 6–9 years of age and is responsible for development of secondary sexual characteristics such as changes in skin and axillary and pubic hairs. This phase is characterized by release of dehydroepiandrosterone from the adrenal cortex without any changes in secretion of cortisol or adrenocorticotropic hormone (8).

Gonadotropin-releasing hormone induces release of luteinizing hormone (LH) and follicle stimulating hormone (FHS) from the pituitary gland. FSH and LH orchestrate the release of estradiol and progesterone from the gonads, which contributes to the development of secondary sexual development. Simultaneously, the linear growth burst is taking place under the influence of growth hormone and insulin-like growth factor-1; cortisol is also involved indirectly in this process. The challenge of physical and sexual development puts the adolescent body and mind under significant stress. Cortisol is critically important in enabling the adolescent to adapt to deal with the challenges of puberty (8).

It has been postulated that HPA reactivity can be compromised in times of puberty, especially in adolescent girls. When adolescent girls during different stages of puberty were challenged with cortisol-releasing hormone (CRH), an increase in cortisol secretion was seen, suggesting a higher stress reactivity and vulnerability to stress (9). These girls not only showed increasing levels of total cortisol secretion following CRH challenge but also had slower reactivity to cortisol, prolonged time to reach peak cortisol levels, and showed slower rate of recovery and return to baseline cortisol levels (9). The baseline cortisol levels continue to increase over the course of different stages of puberty. In comparison, adolescent boys actually showed a decline in baseline level of cortisol over the course of different stages of puberty (9).

This may suggest a gender-specific HPA dysregulation or inefficient response when girls are trying to adapt to the stress of puberty (9). This HPA dysregulation predisposes the adolescent females to dysphoria, irritability, and anxiety during the course of puberty (8,9). This may also explain the significant gender divergence in incidence of psychiatric disorders such as depression and anxiety that emerges around puberty. This increased predisposition to psychiatric disorders at the time when the girls are already under pubertal stress can also predispose to substance abuse (9).

15.5 Childhood sexual abuse

There are several different pathways that may lead to the early initiation of substance abuse in victims of sexual abuse. It has been proposed that psychological trauma suffered by these children alters the normal course of emotional, social, and cognitive development. This, in turn, creates significant hurdles in the already difficult path of mastering age-appropriate normal developmental tasks. These developmental tasks include beginning to define one's own identity, constructing and consolidating self-concept, outlining normal interpersonal boundaries, and figuring out one's place in context of social context. A sexually traumatized young girl, while coping with this added burden, cannot negotiate appropriately with other normal developmental tasks at hands. It is likely that she may succumb to this overpowering psychological liability. Many children and adolescents who are sexually victimized struggle with issues of self-control and behavioral dysregulation and engage in risky behaviors such as early substance abuse initiation (10).

Bailey et al. reported higher potential of initiation of early substance abuse in sexually abused young girls while controlling for all other confounding factors such as age, co-occurring physical abuse, childhood psychopathology (as depression and aggression), family history of alcohol and drug abuse (especially in mothers), and family dysfunction including income level, domestic violence, and parenting practices. The authors concluded that being sexually abused causes these girls to have a depressed self-concept, which leads to behavioral consequences that mediate early onset of substance abuse (10).

15.6 Consequences of substance abuse in female adolescents

Substance abuse is on the rise in all adolescents, but what is more worrisome is that adolescent females are smoking and using other substances much more than previously ever reported. In 2005, among all adolescents aged 12–17, the percentage of females who were currently drinking alcohol was for the first time higher than their male peers of the same age group, at 17.2% versus 15.9% (11). Onset of substance abuse in early age predisposes to lifelong emotional and physical struggles irrespective of gender; also, it poses some very unique challenges for female adolescents as depicted in figure 15.3.

15.7 Substance abuse and sexual activity

According to the U.S. Centers for Disease Control and Prevention (CDC) data collected in 2009, about 9.1% of adolescent female students enrolled in U.S. high schools in 11th grade reported being the victim of physical dating violence (PDV), and about 10.5% of adolescent girls in grades 9–12 reported being forced into a sexual encounter involving intercourse against their wishes (12). This was slightly higher from the PDV rates reported in a similar CDC survey report of 2003, at 8.8% (13). Both surveys reported higher prevalence of PDV and sexual victimization

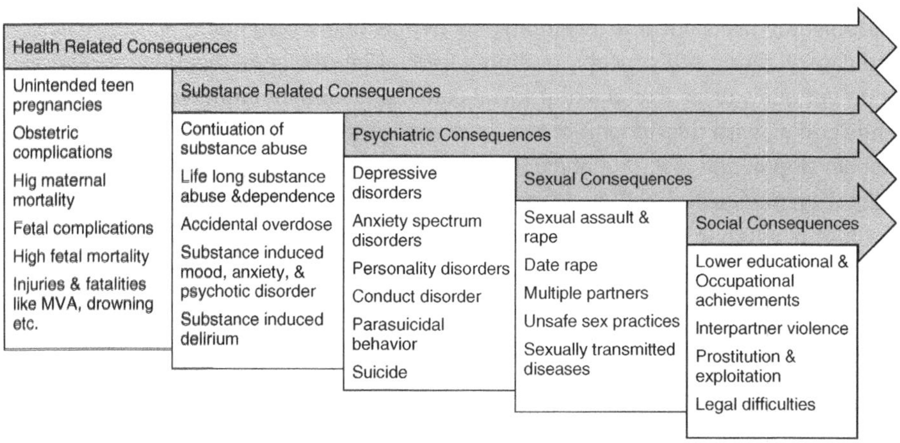

Figure 15.3: Consequences of early onset substance abuse in female adolescents

in African American and Hispanics females versus Caucasian females. From 2002 to 2004, pregnancy-related hospitalizations accounted for 49% of all hospital discharges for adolescent females. During the same period, injury-related visits accounted for one-third of all visits to the emergency department for young girls, and this rate increased by 70% for the groups aged 12–13 and 18–19 (14).

Early initiation of substance abuse of any kind predisposes an adolescent girl to a higher risk of becoming involved in a sexual encounter and a much higher risk of becoming pregnant as a result of it. Cavazos-Rehg et al. studied the connection between the incidence of substance abuse in young high school female students (9th–12th grades) and examined the link between initiation and intensity of substance abuse with engagement in sexual behavior resulting in teen pregnancies (15). They concluded that irrespective of the type of substance being abused (i.e., tobacco smoking, alcohol, or cannabis), initiation of any type of substance abuse was associated with higher risk of sexual activity, which resulted in a higher incidence of teen pregnancies. They also found a dose-dependent relationship in that higher amounts of substances used posed a higher risk of getting pregnant (15). This correlation was true even for tobacco use in girls who started smoking at age 12 or younger and smoked on a daily basis (15).

Some of the risk factors are common and predisposes to both of these high-risk behaviors. In a cross-sectional national survey of high school females that was conducted as part of the National Youth Surveillance System, about 10 % of the 3,000 participants reported having been pregnant at the time this survey was conducted. The rate was higher for Hispanic girls at 13.8% compared to white girls at 7.2%, and there was a significant difference in African American girls at 21.3% (15).

It is believed that the causes of initiating substance abuse early on and engaging in other risky behaviors such as sexual activity are due to loss of an external locus of self-control along with lack of development of an internal inhibitory control that usually is compounded by low parental monitoring and lack of positive role modeling. Also, it is not necessary for one of these behaviors to always precede the other. For instance, the initiation of substance use may be a direct cause of disinhibition resulting from substance use as well as an indirect cause of engaging in sexual behavior because of one sexual partner introducing the other one to substance abuse. Alternatively, substance use may precede sex because of an outside factor or process that includes history of childhood sexual abuse and other forms of victimization, abnormal family dynamics, family history of substance use, and easy availability of drugs (16).

15.8 Substance abuse and unwanted pregnancy

The United States has seen a gradual decline in adolescent pregnancy rates since 1990 that more importantly includes a 34% decline in teen pregnancies in the 15–19 age group over this period of time. However, the 2007 birthrate for adolescent females increased by 4% from 2005 to 2007, or 42.5 births per 1,000 in 15–19 years. The rate was 22.2 births per 1,000 in those 15–17 years of age and 73.9 per 1,000, or 6% higher, in those 18–19 years of age when compared to rates from 2005. For those 10–14 years of age, however, the birthrates were unchanged at 0.6 per 1,000 (17).

One can extrapolate that the increasing trend of initiation of substance abuse earlier in youth may predispose young girls to other risky behaviors including sexual activity leading to an increase in birthrate and pregnancy, as well as birth-related health risks. In the United States, adolescent girls aged 15–19 years who became pregnant reported that for 81% of them, pregnancy was unintended (18). About 40% of these pregnancies end in termination (18).

15.9 Substance abuse and psychiatric disorders

The relationship between psychiatric disorders and substance abuse is bidirectional. On the one end of this spectrum, psychiatric disorders are a risk factor for developing and continuing substance abuse; on the other hand, adolescents may present with psychiatric disorders as a short or long-term sequelae of the substance abuse itself (see chapter 14). Research has demonstrated that pubertal development may have a different impact on the psychological development of girls versus boys. The ratio between testosterone and estradiol changes during the pubertal stage, and while this happens in all adolescents in same way irrespective of gender, somehow it affects the emotional tone differently according to gender. In pubertal girls, the impact on emotional tone is more negative predisposing them to mood disorders, while in boys it has a more protective effect (19).

Puberty is the key age where divergence in the prevalence of depressive disorders between the two genders will start and eventually reach a 2:1 ratio. This ratio remains steady throughout the rest of the female reproductive span until it declines and becomes equal to men around menopause. Girls score higher on a standardized depression scale between ages 12 and 16, while in prepuberty years, the scores stayed steady from ages 8 to 11 (20). Likelihood of co-occurrence of psychiatric and addictive disorders in adulthood increases significantly if both disorders start early on in life (20).

The prevalence of depressive disorders in adulthood increases from 10% in the general population to 30%–50% in the presence of a co-occurring substance abuse disorder; also, this rate may be much higher in adolescents (21). In efforts to elucidate links between depression and addictive processes in the adolescent population, Rao et al. discussed three different ways in which both psychiatric and addictive disorders appear to have a common origin (21). Genetic studies have shown a strong predilection for both psychiatric and substance abuse disorders in probands if there is a history of either type of disorder in the family of origin (see chapter 3). Family history of substance abuse or psychiatric disorders also predispose to an earlier onset of either depressive or addictive disorder (21). Both types of disorders also appear to have involvement of reward and motivation pathways located in the meso-corticolimbic dopamine (MCD) system of brain (see chapter 2) (21).

Depression presents as a downregulation of this pathway when a person develops anhedonia, low energy, withdrawal from activities, and amotivation. On the other hand, a drug-addicted individual may desperately be trying to activate these pathways by repeatedly and increasingly using higher amounts of substances to avoid a dysphoric state (21). Many depressive symptoms are encountered in withdrawal states from many substances of abuse including but not limited to nicotine, alcohol, and other psychostimulants (see chapters 7, 9, 11, and 16). The MCD system reinforces many of the euphoric or stimulating effects of drugs of abuse so that withdrawal from these substances is associated with lower levels of dopamine in this system and associated structures such as the nucleus accumbens and amygdala (21). Functional neuroimaging of brains of depressed people have shown loss of volume and decreased activity in these areas, suggesting a role of the MCD system.

There is also an increase in dopamine level in the striatum following treatment with antidepressants, indicating a role of dopamine in both types of disorders. Serotonergic deficiency, which is a major neurotransmitter in the pathophysiology of depression, is also shown to be deficient in alcohol withdrawal states, whereas resuming alcohol intake is associated with increase in serotonin level (21). There are also findings that support a common role of cholinergic and GABA-ergic systems in depressive and addictive disorders (21). The fact that many co-occurring disorders respond to treatment with psychotropic medication supports this common underlying origin of both disorders (21).

15.10 Perinatal mood disorders

In adolescent girls, substance abuse may pose unique challenges that include the added burden of unwanted pregnancy and its psychiatric sequelae. Girls who become pregnant are at a major risk to develop depressive disorders while pregnant and major psychiatric problems after delivery. They usually also have many other psychosocial risk factors that further make them more vulnerable for developing perinatal mood disorders (see table 15.1 and figure 15.4).

Adolescent mothers are at much higher risk of becoming depressed or have a relapse of preexisting mood disorders whether unipolar or bipolar disorder. However, sometimes perinatal mood disorders in this age group may not present as a full-blown major depressive or bipolar disorder, and symptoms may be ill defined making the diagnosis difficult. Perinatal depression predisposes these adolescents

Table 15.1: Common risk factors predisposing to pregnancy and perinatal mood disorders

- Previous history of depression or anxiety spectrum disorders
- Substance abuse
- Family history of substance abuse
- Major life stressors
- Family history of depression
- Childhood sexual abuse and history of other forms of trauma
- Interpartner violence
- Poor social support

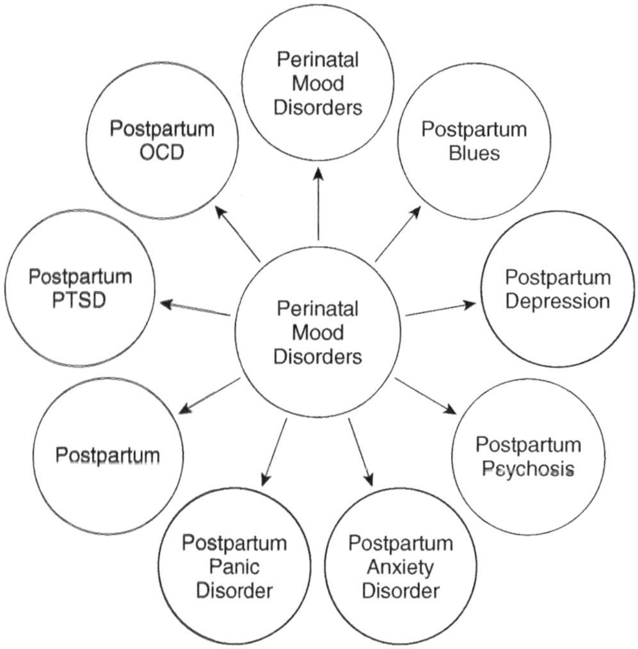

Figure 15.4: Spectrum of perinatal psychiatric disorders

to increased risk of obstetric complications including preeclampsia, low fetal weight gain, premature delivery, and a higher risk of cesarean section.

The perinatal period is also known as a period when adolescents with a history of other psychiatric disorders including various anxiety spectrum disorders (especially obsessive compulsive disorder [OCD] and posttraumatic stress disorder [PTSD]), may show worsening of symptoms or resurgence of a dormant problem. Perinatal depression is highly comorbid with symptoms of generalized anxiety, OCD, and panic disorder.

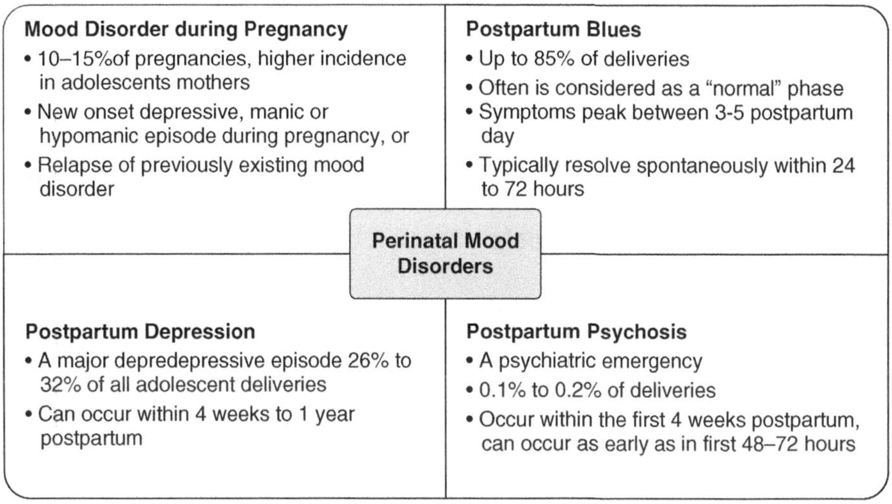

Figure 15.5: Types of perinatal mood disorders

Adolescent mothers who were subjected to sexual abuse as children may have a sudden relapse of PTSD symptoms such as nightmares and flashbacks along with a tendency for avoidance and hypervigilance. Adolescent mothers with history of eating disorder may have a very difficult time during pregnancy. Pregnancy-related weight changes may lead to serious issues with their body image, causing them to starve, binge, purge, or restrict particular foods in order to preserve their ideal body image, characteristic of eating disorders.

Depression may worsen during the third trimester, and the severity of depressive symptoms may be directly proportional to younger age as well as drug abuse (including nicotine and alcohol) along with other psychosocial stressors. Young mothers with depression are at an increased risk for giving birth prematurely and having instrument-assisted vaginal deliveries and cesarean sections. Adolescent mothers have much lower resilience ability than older women impacting their ability to develop a positive adaption to pregnancy and to be able to cope with the responsibilities of motherhood (22). Figure 15.5 outlines various psychiatric disorders that may complicate the perinatal period.

15.11 Spectrum of perinatal mood disorders

15.11.1 Postpartum blues

Clinicians often consider this as a normal phase of the postpartum period, as it occurs in about 85% of deliveries irrespective of the age of mom. The symptoms peek between 3 and 5 days postpartum. The new mothers feel fatigued and complain of having no energy or appetite. They are irritable, acutely hypersensitive to any emotional stimuli, excessively worried about the baby, and easily overwhelmed. At times, they feel they have no feelings for the baby. No treatment is necessary as the blues' phase is usually over within a week (23).

15.11.2 Postpartum psychosis

This is a very rare but serious disorder complicating about only 0.1%–0.2% of deliveries. Women with a history of bipolar disorder have a 50% chance of developing a postpartum psychotic episode. The risk is much higher in the first pregnancy, but if they had a postpartum psychotic episode, this increases the risk of having another psychotic episode in subsequent pregnancies by 57% (24). The symptoms start within the first 4 weeks postpartum but may occur as early as in the first 48–72 hours (24). Most cases of postpartum psychosis are a severe manic or depressive episode of bipolar disorder with psychotic features. Symptoms can be of varied nature, including auditory and visual hallucinations and delusions of religious nature or involving a good-versus-evil struggle. Delusions with a focus on the infant can be quite dangerous because these mothers can harm their infants. In essence this is a true psychiatric emergency requiring immediate psychiatric admission and management (24).

15.11.3 Postpartum depression (PPD)

PPD complicates about 4.8%–15% of deliveries, and this wide range depends on the different diagnostic criteria used. These adolescent mothers are at a much higher risk of developing PPD, as high as 47% of the adolescent deliveries (24). Diagnosis of PPD may not occur in a timely manner for some of them – predisposing these young mothers and their babies to various complications. Even when diagnosed, up to 15% of these women continue to have active symptoms lasting for as long as 24 weeks after the onset of the index episode (24). The *Diagnostic and Statistical Manual of Mental Disorders*, fourth edition, text revision (*DSM-IV-TR*), defines PPD as occurring within 4 weeks postpartum; however, recent research suggest that a PPD episode can occur within 1 year postpartum with a peak incidence at 12 weeks postpartum (25). PPD symptoms include sleep disturbances, low energy, lack of appetite, anhedonia (especially lack of interest in the baby and impaired responses to the infant's cues), persistent depressed mood with frequent crying spells, suicidal ideation, and at times infanticide ideation (24,25).

15.12 Substance abuse and suicide risk in young girls

The link of substance abuse to suicidality is complex due to the multiple compounding psychosocial factors involved in most of these cases and also the fact that at times, it is very difficult to discern which came first. Is it the suicidality that leads to daredevil behavior including substance abuse or it is substance abuse that leads to depressive symptoms and suicidality? Behnken et al. looked at alcohol abuse as a mediator between forced sexual activity and suicidality in young girls (26). About 28% of girls reported binge drinking, and this behavior was found to be highly associated with suicidal behavior in this sample. About 11% of these girls also reported being a victim of forced sexual intercourse. The study indicated a link between binge drinking to both forced sexual intercourse and suicidality (26). The association between alcohol and suicidal ideation remained strong even when one controls for sexual assault.

The pathway of mediation from forced sexual activity to suicidality was weakened when alcohol was taken out of the equation. These associations remained constant when examined across races in Caucasian, Hispanic, and African American girls. The risk of going from suicidal ideation to attempting and even completing suicide in this group of girls was much higher in the adolescent group (26). Substance abuse predisposed them to impulsivity, disinhibition, aggression, and above all poor decision making – a perfect combination for suicidal behavior. It has also been reported that when substance abuse is not involved in a sexual assault, the victim is more likely to have better coping skills and better ability to deal with stress related to trauma (26).

15.13 Impact of substance abuse on adolescent mother and offspring

Many psychoactive drugs are known to produce deleterious maternal and fetal effects in young pregnant women. The most notable one is alcohol in the well-documented fetal alcohol syndrome (FAS) (see chapter 18). FAS is composed of a constellation of phenotypic features of various degrees along with developmental delays and cognitive difficulties (27). Expression of FAS occurs on a wide spectrum ranging from fetal alcohol effects to an alcohol-related neurodevelopmental disorder and fetal alcohol syndrome. The physical features vary significantly among affected children, ranging from mild deformities to about 8% of the infants having microcephaly; furthermore, 28% show growth retardation, and 16% have typical facial features (27).

The features of FAS include midfacial hypoplasia, short upturned nose, and other facial features; limb and joints anomalies; sensorineural hearing loss; and cardiovascular defects. Behavioral and cognitive effects include hyperactivity, attention problems, sensory integration difficulties, frequent temper tantrums, and fine motor difficulties. Approximately 75% of these children fall in the mild-to-moderate range of mental retardation (27).

Smoking tobacco increases the risk of spontaneous miscarriage in a dose-dependent fashion, with risk increasing when five or more cigarettes a day are being smoked (28). Other maternal fetal risks observed in pregnant women smoking cigarettes are appetite suppression, low birth weight, higher plasma levels of carbon monoxide in mothers and fetus, decreased placental blood circulation, higher heart rate and decreased heart rate variability in the fetus, and a much higher level of nicotine and its by-products in amniotic fluid. The role of hundreds of carcinogens and other toxic substances found in cigarettes is not very well defined at this time. A survey of 173,687 children with congenital malformation showed that smoking was associated with higher risks of developing cardiovascular, musculoskeletal, and gastrointestinal malformations, as well as many other types of congenital malformations involving almost all systems.

Neurodevelopmental delays associated with nicotine exposures include language delays, lower global cognitive scores, and externalizing behaviors such as agitations, aggression, conduct disorder, and future risk of developing antisocial behavior (29). Temperamental difficulties and internalizing behaviors have also been documented. Increased risks of developing childhood cancer and infertility in the children exposed to smoking in utero as well as secondhand smoke have been reported (29).

Other drug abuse has been on the rise in adolescent girls including cocaine abuse (see chapter 11). Cocaine-abusing pregnant girls are at high risk for spontaneous abortion, abruptio placenta, and preterm delivery. Fetal exposure to cocaine results in decreased birth weight and head circumference. Neurodevelopmental effects of cocaine are not very well understood; however, children exposed in utero to cocaine achieve lower scores on standardized tests (30).

15.14 Substance abuse and unintentional injuries

Alcohol is found to be responsible for about 36% of accidental deaths in adolescents from 15 to 20 years of age, while 20% of these were in children under age 15 (see chapter 9). Alcohol is also associated with 51% of traumatic brain injuries suffered in the adolescent age group (31). Alcohol-related fatal and nonfatal injuries are a major problem in the adolescent age group. In 2005, about 13% of adolescents 12 years or older reported driving under the influence of alcohol at least once in the preceding year, this corresponds to 31.7 million adolescents (31).

15.15 Prevention and treatment strategies specific for adolescent girls

The first step in devising any long-term treatment plan is to identify risk and protective factors and to devise a prevention strategy. The United States has seen a relative decline in substance abuse since the 1970s, but this decline has not been seen in the female population; in fact, in some age groups, it has been on rise, especially rates of earlier initiation of substance use in preteen girls (32). Studies have shown that even in age-matched controls when boys and girls are managed with the same protocols, the response rate in girls is more likely to be dependent on the risk factors predisposing them to substance abuse in first place (32).

Some of the risk factors are not gender specific such as poor psychosocial support, low socioeconomic conditions, lack of self-control, low academic achievement, and current home environment. Girls are more likely to report gender-specific risk factors such as negative self-image, low self-worth, anxiety, depression, tendency to internalize stress, negative body image and dieting, and eating disorders (32). Physical and sexual abuse was also twice as commonly reported in girls than boys. These gender differences in risk factors were most prominent in the 12- to 13-year-old age group, but the difference dissipates slowly as age progresses (32).

Traditionally substance abuse programs have not focused on gender, racial, and ethnic differences in the population served. There is growing evidence that in order to be effective, existing substance abuse programs need to identify the specific risk and protective factors in the population they are serving especially in adolescent and female patients. Some of the previously used models can be modulated to address more gender-related issues such as gender-specific issues in cognitive or social-ecological theory. In addition, recent gender-specific theories are emerging that can be implemented to improve the outcomes and prognosis in adolescent females (32). Some of these theories are briefly described subsequently.

15.15.1 Self-in-relation theory of women development

It has been proposed that good attachment is central to developing a girl's self-development in the context of the world around them. This is in contrast to the traditional model that all individuals strive for developing their own identity by separation and individuation, which was considered a critical milestone of this age group (32). Adolescent girls are more likely to become self-sufficient adults with a better worldview if they are interdependent on strong positive relationships. These strong healthy interpersonal connections give rise to greater knowledge of self and others, understanding of self-worth, confidence in self, zest, and motivation. It is important to develop programs specifically for preadolescent and adolescent girls that foster stronger, healthier connections within the family, teachers, or counselor, or through programs where such relationships can be fostered with peers and older women (32).

15.15.2 Social-structural model

There are several theories under this model that identify that men and women have different societal roles; also, socialization experiences are perceived and experienced vastly differently by preadolescent girls and boys (32). Any deviant social behavior such as substance abuse that is learned during this stage of development is the product of learned social behavior. In our society, peers, parents, teachers, and culture expect young girls to conform to societal gender specification. Girls are assigned this gender role very early on in life, limiting their abilities of self-actualization. They may feel suffocated in this traditional mold, and this may lead to internalization behaviors including but not limiting to substance abuse.

15.15.3 Theory of gender and power

This theory focuses on the gender-based differential in heterosexual relationships and how they impact on the social and cultural context of women's health practices. The theory identifies three important areas of struggle for women in such dyadic relationship: division of labor, division of power, and structure of social norms as well as affective responses (32). This is a very important framework for understanding the high risk of substance abuse in adolescent girls who are physically and sexually abused and emotionally controlled.

A substance abuse program that constructs the rehabilitation and recovery framework around this model is going to help these adolescent girls to move forward from a passive to a more assertive role. When we empower young girls in this way, they learn better coping skills and will not have to rely on substance abuse to overcome such learned helplessness because of the abuse they have endured (32).

Gender-informed or gender-specific substance abuse treatment programs should provide treatment plans that focus on the following several important areas (32) (see figure 15.6):

1. Improving self-efficacy: This involves employing strategies to develop and enhance self-esteem as well as improve self and body image in these young girls.
2. Developing competencies: Coach preadolescent and adolescent girls on how to change existing self-destructive behaviors and engage them in learning better coping strategies, which they can use in problem solving in different areas of their lives, including interpersonal communications.

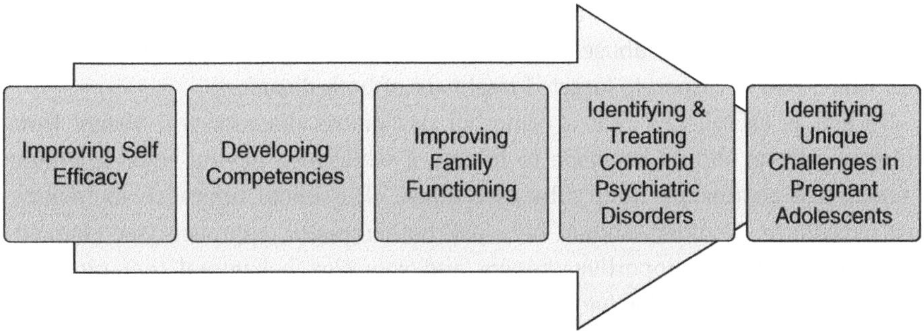

Figure 15.6: Substance abuse prevention and treatment strategies specific for adolescent girls

3. Promoting healthy lifestyle: Educating about how the risk-taking behaviors (such as substance abuse, unsafe sex, etc.) impact the emotional and physical well-being and how to overcome this with healthy lifestyle choices.
4. Improving family functioning: Family therapy is part of most of traditional substance abuse programs, but this needs to be more tailored toward female adolescent issues by facilitating better interpersonal communications and strengthening the family bonds by identifying power imbalances.
5. Treatment of comorbid psychiatric illness: Given that a large number of female adolescents suffer from dual diagnosis, it is imperative to incorporate psychiatric care while they are in substance abuse rehabilitation programs to enhance compliance with the program and to improve outcomes.
6. Identifying unique challenges in treating pregnant adolescents: This is often neglected, and many programs have difficulties with providing care aimed at improving pregnancy outcomes and teaching parenting skills.

In essence, several gender-informed psychosocial models are now available and need to be incorporated in our traditional system of providing substance abuse treatment. If we choose to ignore gender differences, long-term outcomes and prognosis could worsen. Gender-specific programs are important to alter the course and prognosis of substance abuse disease in young women. Also, if they become pregnant while abusing substances and continue to do so during pregnancy, their children are also at high risk for negative outcomes (32).

15.16 Treatment of comorbid psychiatric illness

The bidirectional relationships of psychiatric comorbidities make it difficult to ascertain what level of treatment is necessary at a given time. It is very challenging to make a clinical distinction between primary psychiatric disorders with comorbid substance abuse and substance-induced psychiatric disorders. Taking time to obtain a careful history and to construct a chronological account of emergence of psychiatric disorders with substance abuse may help a clinician to devise an individualized plan, which may incorporate targeted treatment of both disorders.

Once it is established that a comorbid psychiatric disorder will benefit from treatment, efforts should be made to initiate it while also paying equal attention to encourage abstinence from substance abuse. The initial approach to treating most psychiatric disorders should be a psychotherapeutic approach (see chapters 5 and 6). Individual supportive therapy and cognitive behavioral therapy (CBT) have been shown to be effective in treating mild uncomplicated cases of depression as well as personality and anxiety spectrum disorders. CBT focuses on eliciting negative schemas that patients may have developed about themselves, their relationships with family and friends, and their general worldview. CBT attempts to challenge these negative schemata and help patients change them in a positive direction. This helps these adolescents to develop a better understanding of their illness, improve compliance with their substance abuse treatment, and improve overall prognosis as well as long-term abstinence.

Use of psychotropic medication will be necessary in patients with severe anxiety spectrum or depressive disorders who have failed to respond to psychotherapeutic interventions (see chapter 6). The decision to treat a comorbid psychiatric illness depends on the nature and severity of illness, and its impact on co-occurring substance abuse disorders. More likely than not, a comorbid psychiatric illness decreases compliance with the goals of substance abuse treatment programs and leads to a relapse and recovery revolving door. Selective serotonin reuptake inhibitors (SSRIs) are now considered the first-line medications for the management of anxiety and depression in these patients. All SSRIs are considered equal in efficacy, but only a few are officially approved for use in the pediatric population (32). At present, fluoxetine is approved for use in children ≥8 years of age for depression and in those ≥7 years for OCD. Fluvoxamine is approved in patients ≥8 years, sertraline in patients ≥6 years, and escitalopram for adolescents ≥12 years of age for OCD (33) (see chapters 6 and 14).

Once a decision is made to treat, the choice of an SSRI depends on various factors such as the specific side-effect profile, whether this medication has produced good results in this patient previously or even has shown a good response in a family member, contraindications, the availability of acceptable formulations (i.e., solution or suspension), and its cost (33). Cost is an important factor as some of the newer SSRIs are not covered by major formularies or insurance plans. One should also take into account every measure possible to improve compliance with these medications. For instance, prescribing a medication with single daily dosing is usually preferable to two or three times a day dosing (33).

The U.S. Food and Drug Administration has issued an advisory and black-box warning about emergence of suicidal ideation during the initial phase of SSRI treatment; this development has changed the prescribing behaviors of many primary care physicians and pediatricians in recent years leading to a reluctance in some to prescribe SSRIs. It is, however, recommended that the use of SSRIs in children and adolescents be taken in consideration in situations where it is indicated, and these pediatric patients should be followed closely, especially in the earlier phase of treatment, to monitor for any suicide risk (33).

15.17 Treatment of substance abuse in pregnant adolescents

The cocaine epidemic of the 1980s in the United States was the first time that pregnant substance-abusing women became a focus of medical attention. Most of that attention, however, revolved around the obstetric emergencies and complications in these women, and little attention was paid to the unique challenges these females posed for the existing traditional rehabilitation and recovery programs (34) (see chapter 18). Most substance abuse programs still continued to focus on traditional male-focused models when treating pregnant adolescents and failed to take into account that these young women are "not alone" in their struggle for recovery. They have to deal with the added psychological and physical burden of pregnancy while working on their recovery. While going through the rigors of abstinence, they have to take care of their children and deal with a multitude of related psychosocial stressors and often scarce resources that are available to them (34).

Most researchers in the area of substance abuse management agree that screening for substance abuse should be done early on for all pregnant women irrespective of age, socioeconomic background, and their presentation (see chapter 4). Brief screenings tools such as the 4P-Plus questionnaire have been shown to be very effective and can be easily administered in a busy primary care or obstetrics practice (34). Engaging pregnant substance abusers in a substance abuse program is challenging. These young girls are usually facing many other psychosocial stressors and may lack the supportive and empathetic network needed to enhance their chances of long-term recovery.

Most young women do not divulge their substance abuse to their obstetric providers fearing the consequence of losing their children. Creating a safe and trusting environment for these women is important to build a therapeutic relationship. Developing a comprehensive program where these mothers can keep their children with them while engaging in recovery with the involvement of local child protective services has demonstrated a better retention rate (35). Pregnant women who successfully complete a comprehensive residential rehabilitation program of sufficient duration were shown to be more likely to remain abstinent, have fewer psychiatric comorbidities, be gainfully employed, and have better parenting skills and attitudes. More recently, motivational interviewing and computer-based motivational intervention have revealed good results in this high-risk group (35).

Table 15.2: Core competencies for delivery of gender-specific substance abuse treatment

Competencies	Description
Gender difference	Differences in physiology, cognition, emotions, social development, communication patterns, roles, socialization, risks, and resiliency affect the prevention, treatment, and recovery needs.
Biopsychosocial and spiritual	It is critical that staff delivering substance abuse care understand how sociocultural identities differ among women and girls and may lead to different health outcomes.
Violence and trauma	Vulnerability to violence and trauma must be addressed in prevention efforts as well as other mental health and substance abuse services.
Physical and medical problems	Higher risk of physical and medical problems in women and girls and identifying the risk factors like intimate partner violence, rape/ sexual abuse, and childhood abuse and neglect.
Societal expectations and sexuality	Acceptance and inclusion of women with lived experiences of mental health problems, substance abuse, and trauma in the delivery of comprehensive, gender-responsive services and recovery-oriented care.
Boundaries	Acceptance and inclusion of women in the delivery of comprehensive, gender-responsive services where staff delivers care with self-awareness and appropriate boundaries.
Physiological demands	Demands of puberty, pregnancy, perimenopause, and menopause and the accompanying physiological, psychological, and developmental changes, with changing risks, opportunities, and support needs.
Parenting and family context	Consideration of culturally sensitive, family-centered work with a woman's family is critical to her wellness and recovery, including working with children, intimate partners, and other family members.
Socioeconomic considerations	Navigation, access, use, and coordination among community resources and systems may be necessary for women's success in prevention and treatment programs.
Stigma	Address the impact of stigma and stereotypes on recovery for women and girls, as well as the skills and attitudes required to address these challenges.

Adapted from: Substance Abuse and Mental Health Services Administration. Addressing the needs of women and girls: Developing core competencies for mental health and substance abuse service professionals. HHS Pub. No. (SMA) 11–4657. Rockville, MD: SAMHSA, 2011.

Most pharmacological interventions used for substance abuse disorders are not well studied in the pregnant population for obvious reasons. Two notable exceptions are the use of methadone and buprenorphine (see chapters 6 and 10). A recently published prospective multicenter study compared 90 women taking buprenorphine

versus 45 women who were managed on methadone, considered a gold standard in treating pregnant women with opioid dependence (36). The study reported no significant differences between these two strategies; both drugs showed equal efficacy, and there were no differences in outcome measures such as pregnancy outcomes, birth outcomes, or severity of neonatal abstinent syndromes (36). This is of special significance in the adolescent population because opioid abuse and dependence is on the rise in this age group, mostly in the form of prescription opioid abuse (see chapter 10).

15.18 Future of substance abuse treatment

In past few years, there has been growing awareness of the lack of focus on the female population in the existing system of substance abuse management programs. SAMHSA has recognized this concept, and in March of 2009, a panel started developing the competencies for substance abuse health care providers, specifically for adolescent girls and women. The task was to identify some overarching core concepts as a foundation to develop the competencies to address the specific needs of this population group (37) (see table 15.2).

15.19 Conclusions

Rapidly rising rates of substance abuse in young girls pose unique challenges that are not commonly understood by health care providers. Substance abuse rehabilitation and recovery programs usually provide a male-oriented approach, which fails to recognize the specific needs of the female population. There is a growing need to focus on understanding the protective and risk factors of preteen and teenage age girls early on to provide prevention, timely intervention, and abstinence efforts within a gender-specific treatment approach. Investment in developing comprehensive substance abuse and recovery programs will not only result in positive outcomes in these adolescent girls but will also decrease the likelihood of negative outcomes in their offspring.

References

1. SAMHSA, Office of Applied Studies, National Household Survey on Drug Abuse, 2000. Accessed December 2, 2013. URL: http://www.icpsr.umich.edu/icpsrweb/SAMHDA/studies/3262?q=national+house+hold+survey+2Date
2. Substance Abuse and Mental Health Services Administration. Results from the 2005 National Survey on Drug Use and Health: National findings. NSDUH Series H-30, DHHS Publication No. SMA 06–4194. Rockville, MD: Office of Applied Studies, 2006.

3. Substance Abuse and Mental Health Services Administration (SAMHSA) Treatment Episode Data Set (TEDS), 2009, based on data received through November 3, 2010. Accessed Dec 2, 2013. URL: http://www. store.samhsa.gov/list/series?name=Treatment-Episode-Data-Set-TEDS
4. Patton GC, McMorris BJ, Toumbourou JW, Hemphill SA, Donath S, Catalano RF. Puberty and the onset of substance use and abuse. Pediatrics 2004;114:300–6.
5. Ganong WF. Physiology of reproduction in women. In: DeCherney AH, Nathan L. Current diagnosis & treatment obstetrics and gynecology, 10th ed. New York: McGraw-Hill, 2007.
6. Dick DM, Rose RJ, Viken RJ, Kaprio J. Pubertal timing and substance use: Associations between and within families across late adolescence. Dev Psychol 2000;36:180–9.
7. Al-Sahab B, Ardem CI, Hamadeh MJ. Age at menarche and current substance use among Canadian adolescent girls: Results of a cross-sectional study. BMC Public Health 2012;12:195–202.
8. Blumenthal H. Relations among pubertal maturation, cortisol reactivity, pubertal timing, and social anxiety symptoms among female adolescents. ProQuest Dissertations and Theses, Univ of Arkansas, 2009.
9. Stroud LR, Papandonatos GD, Williamson DE. Sex differences in cortisol response to corticotropin releasing hormone challenge over puberty: Pittsburgh Pediatric Neurobehavioral Studies. Psychoneuroendocrinol 2011;36(8):1226–38.
10. Bailey JA. McCloskey LA. Pathways to adolescent substance use among sexually abused girls. J Abnorm Child Psychol 2005;33(1):39–53.
11. Substance Abuse and Mental Health Services Administration. Results from the 2005 National Survey on Drug Use and Health: National findings. NSDUH Series H-30, DHHS Publication No. SMA 06–4194. Rockville, MD: Office of Applied Studies, 2006.
12. Shaw FE, Casey CG. Centers for Disease Control and Prevention. Surveillance summaries. MMWR 2010;59:SS-5.
13. Black MC, Noonan R, Legg M, Eaton D, Breiding MJ. Physical dating violence among high school students-United States. MMWR 2006;55:532–5.
14. MacKay, Duran C, Andrea AP. Adolescent health in the United States. Hyattsville, MD: National Center Health Statistics, 2008–1034, 2008.
15. Cavazos-Rehg PA, Bierut LJ, Cottler LB. Substance use and the risk for sexual intercourse with and without a history of teenage pregnancy among adolescent females. J Stud Alcohol Drugs. 2011;72(2):194–8.
16. Palen LA, Smith EA, Cladwell LL, Mathews C, Vergnani T. Transitions to substance use and sexual intercourse among South African high school students. Subst Use Misuse 2009;44 (13):1872–87.
17. Hamilton BA, Martin JA, Ventura SJ. Births: Preliminary data for 2007. Natl Vital Stat Rep 2009;57:12.
18. Finer LB, Henshaw SK. Special tabulations, commissioned by the National Campaign to Prevent Teen and Disparities in Rates of Unintended Pregnancy in the United States, 1994 and 2001, Perspect Sex Repro H 2006;38(2):90–6.
19. Angold A, Costello EJ, Worthman CM. Puberty and depression: The roles of age, pubertal status and pubertal timing. Psychol Med 1998;28(1):51–61.
20. Twenge J, Nolen-Hoeksema S. Age, gender, race, socioeconomic status, and birth cohort differences on the Children's Depression Inventory: A meta-analysis. J Abnorm Psychol 2002;111 (4):578–88.
21. Rao U. Links between depression and substance abuse in adolescent's neurobiological mechanisms. Am J Prev Med 2006;31(6):S161–74.
22. Salazar-Pousada D, Arroyo D, Hidalgo L, Pérez-López FR, Chedraui P. Depressive symptoms and resilience among pregnant adolescents: A case-control study. Obstet Gynecol Int 2010:1–7.

23. O'Keane V, Lightman S, Patrick K, Marsh M, Papadopoulos AS, Pawlby S. Changes in the maternal hypothalamic-pituitary-adrenal axis during the early puerperium may be related to the postpartum 'blues'. J Neuroendocrinol 2011;23(11):1149–55.
24. Doucet S, Dennis C, Letourneau N. Differentiation and clinical implications of postpartum depression and postpartum psychosis. J Obstet Gynecol Neonatal Nurs 2009;38(3):269–79.
25. American Psychiatric Association. Diagnostic and statistical manual of mental disorders, 4th ed., text rev. Washington, DC: APA, 2000.
26. Behnken MP, Le YCL, Temple JR. Forced sexual intercourse, suicidality, and binge drinking among adolescent girls. Addict Behav 2010;35:507–9.
27. Jones MW, Bass WT. Fetal alcohol syndrome. Neonatal Netw 2003;22(3):63–70.
28. Economides D, Braithwaite J. Smoking, pregnancy and the fetus. J R Soc Health 1994;114 (4):198–201.
29. Melo M, Bellver J, Soares SR. The impact of cigarette smoking on the health of descendants. Expert Rev Obstet Gynecol 2012;7(2):167.
30. Loebstein R, Koren G. Pregnancy outcome and neurodevelopment of children exposed in utero to psychoactive drugs: The motherisk experience. J Psychiatry Neurosci 1997;22(3):192–6.
31. Sleet DA, Ballesteros MF, Borse NN. A review of unintentional injuries in adolescents. Annu Rev Public Health 2010;31:195–212.
32. Amaro H, Blake SM, Schwartz PM. Developing theory-based substance abuse prevention programs for young adolescent girls. J. Early Adolescence 2001;21(3):256–93.
33. Kamboj MK, Tareen RS. Management of nonpsychiatric medical conditions presenting with psychiatric manifestations. Pediatr Clin North Am 2011;58:219–41.
34. Chasnoff IJ, McGourty RF, Bailey GW. The 4P's Plus screen for substance use in pregnancy: Clinical application and outcomes. J. Perinatol 2005;25(6):368–74.
35. Lester BM, Twomey JE. Treatment of substance abuse during pregnancy. Women's Health 2008;4:67–77.
36. Lacroix I, Alain Berrebi A, GaripuyD. Buprenorphine versus methadone in pregnant opioid-dependent women: A prospective multicenter study. Eur J Clin Pharmacol 2011;67(10):1053–9.
37. Substance Abuse and Mental Health Services Administration. Addressing the needs of women and girls: Developing core competencies for mental health and substance abuse service professionals. HHS Pub No. (SMA) 11–4657. Rockville, MD: Substance Abuse Mental Health Services Administration, 2011.

16 Prescription stimulant and other substance abuse in college students

Brandon Johnson and Jeffrey Newcorn

Substance abuse among college students has been the focus of considerable recent attention, given the high prevalence of use/abuse in this population, the nature of the drugs that are abused, the specific contextual issues that fuel abuse in this population, and the potentially dire outcomes of substance use in this population. It is hoped that better understanding the types of substance abuse that most often occur in the college age population, the specific contextual factors that support substance abuse in this population, and the various available methods of prevention and treatment of substance abuse that have been developed for college students will contribute to more informed approaches to managing this problem.

16.1 Introduction

Substance abuse among college students requires specific attention because of the unique circumstances and characteristics of drug-taking behavior in this population. In 2011, the rate of illicit substance use among full-time college students was 22% (1). In addition to clear-cut substance abuse, there are significantly higher rates of binge alcohol use among full-time college students as opposed to others aged 18–22. The risk of substance use in the college population is potentiated by decreased parental supervision, a new and complex social structure that often includes communal living, and a view of substance intoxication as being relatively normative.

Consequences of substance use can have a profound impact on young adults and are a major public health concern in the United States. Alcohol-related deaths alone in college students reached 1,825 in 2005. In 2001, 10.5% of college students reported being injured because of drinking, 12% were hit or assaulted by another college student, and 2% reported sexual assault related to alcohol. Furthermore, 28.9% of college students reported driving while under the influence of alcohol, contributing to a significant risk of alcohol-related motor vehicle accidents (2). Another significant aspect of substance abuse in college students is its relation to comorbid mental health disorders and suicide. One study found that suicidal ideation was higher in students with nicotine dependence, alcohol-related problems, and illicit drug use (3). Prevention and treatment of substance use disorders in college students may help to diminish these adverse outcomes and reduce the public health burden from this population.

Certain trends highlight the environmental influences of college life and their role in substance use. For example, college-bound 12th graders were found to have a lower than average use of all illicit substances while they were in high school compared to those who did not attend college. However, the eventual use of illicit substances by this group when they reached college was found to equal or in some cases exceed the use of their noncollege peers. This "catching up" effect may in part be related to important contextual issues; the fact that college students often leave the parental home for the first time and tend to defer marriage leaves them more independent than they were in high school, but also not grounded in either their family of origin or a new family (4).

Increased academic demand and pressure to succeed may drive some college students to use substances as a coping mechanism, or even to misuse substances in an attempt to enhance academic performance. Of note, a national health survey found that college students reported the highest use in the past year of Adderall (i.e., mixed amphetamine salts, a stimulant medication prescribed for attention-deficit/hyperactivity disorder [ADHD]; see section 16.6) compared to several other demographic groups. This increased use among college students may be attributable to the desire to stay awake and focused during study time, as well as completion of course work (4). Issues related to abuse of prescription stimulants will be covered in detail subsequently.

The goals of this chapter are to discuss the use of various licit and illicit substances of abuse by the college student population, including demographics and recent trends of use, relationship to use of other substances, co-occurrence of psychiatric disorders, consequences of using specific substances, and implications for prevention and treatment.

16.2 Alcohol

In addition to the types of alcohol abuse seen in other populations (see chapter 9), binge drinking is particularly common in the college age population. Binge drinking is usually defined as having five or more drinks in a row on a single occasion for men, or four or more drinks for women (5). As this type of drinking is one of the main forms of alcohol use during the college years, it should be specifically queried in clinical assessment.

16.2.1 Prevalence and demographic features

Drinking increases rapidly during the young adult years, and alcohol use peaks during these years (i.e., ages 18–24). The prevalence of alcohol abuse and dependence also peaks during this age range. Roughly 38% of college students meet criteria for an alcohol use disorder – 31.6% meet criteria for alcohol abuse, and 6.3% meet criteria for alcohol dependence (6). In one survey of college students (5), the prevalence of binge drinking in the 2 weeks prior to the survey was 50% in men and 39% in women. In the same study, more than one-fifth of college students binged three or more times in the 2-week period queried. Risk factors for higher rates of binge drinking in this population include male gender, Caucasian race, residing in a fraternity, being involved in athletics, binge drinking as a high school senior, and viewing parties as very important (5). In support of the previous findings, results of another study indicate that high school drinkers are three times more likely to meet criteria for alcohol dependence during the first year of college than nondrinkers (7).

There is not a consensus about whether college students drink more than their noncollege peers. Carter et al. found that college students drink more and with increased frequency compared to their noncollege peers; however, these differences were thought to be due to factors other than college attendance itself (8). One such factor is the nature of the living situation; alcohol dependence was highest in men and women living in dormitories, while the highest levels of alcohol abuse were by men living off campus. Age was also determined to be an important factor in drinking habits. Increased frequency of drinking was found in younger college students and tended to decrease later in college. The latter finding is in contrast to drinking patterns of noncollege drinkers, whose drinking continues to increase throughout young adulthood.

16.2.2 Consequences

The frequent occurrence and potentially dire consequences of alcohol use disorders in college students illustrate that this problem is a major public health concern. Compiling data from multiple national public health resources, Hingson et al. reported that in 2005 college drinking accounted for 1,825 student deaths, 599,000 injuries, and 97,000 instances of sexual assault or date rape (2). Factors associated with adverse consequences from drinking include participation in athletics, living in dormitories, being a member of a fraternity/sorority, and spring break trips (9,10).

16.2.3 New methods of ingestion

Alcohol is consumed and abused by college students in several nontraditional ways. One new method of consumption involves combining alcohol with energy drinks. Energy drinks are highly marketed to the young adult population, and it is estimated that 51% of college students consume them. Studies attempting to elucidate the reasons for mixing energy drinks with alcohol have concluded that college students mix the two in order to quicken the onset of intoxication and reduce fatigue after drinking, and because they don't like the taste of alcohol (11).

Dangers associated with the combination include misjudgment of level of intoxication, the drinker's erroneous belief that he/she is are able to perform tasks that require fine motor control, and increased intent of drinkers to drive home (12). Also of concern are findings that college students who consume alcohol mixed with energy drinks are significantly more likely to report marijuana, cocaine, and Ecstasy use. Increased rates of high-risk sexual behaviors were also found in this population (12).

Another alarming recent development involves ingestion via the so-called "alcohol enema." This method involves placing a tube in the consumer's rectum and pouring beer through the tube, directly into the rectum. This practice is extremely dangerous as it avoids first-pass metabolism by the liver and increases the blood alcohol concentration very rapidly. A handful of cases of dangerous intoxication or death by this method have made national headlines in the United States. No studies have yet been conducted to determine the prevalence of this method of ingestion.

16.2.4 Prevention and treatment

Nelson et al. examine the rate of college binge drinking and the rate of adult binge drinking by state and found the two to be highly correlated (13). This study also showed an inverse relationship between the rates of college binge drinking and the number of laws in a state that restrict the promotion and sale of high quantities of alcohol. The rate of adult binge drinking and number of regulatory laws were determined to be independent predictors of college binge drinking. It is therefore reasonable to conclude that stricter regulation of alcohol sales may result in decreased binge drinking among college students.

Parental involvement is another important factor mediating alcohol use disorders in college. Kaynak et al. found that higher levels of parental monitoring during high school correlated with a decreased risk for alcohol dependence in the first year of college (7). Several parent-based interventions attempt to educate parents of incoming freshmen about the risks of college drinking, with the goal of increasing discussion between parents and students about alcohol use and abuse, and decreasing parental permissiveness regarding drinking. Measures of program effectiveness document a decrease in the frequency of alcohol use as well as the occurrence of high-risk drinking in participants (7).

The specific circumstances and culture of college campuses may contribute to the high rates of alcohol use disorders in college students in important ways, and these can be targeted in prevention and treatment programs. Of note, amendments to the Higher Education Act of 1965, which specify policies to prevent the use of illicit drugs and abuse of alcohol, are often not stringently enforced on college campuses. These regulations mandate that colleges share information with students and employees about the dangers of drug and alcohol consumption as well as available treatment options.

In 2012, the U.S. Department of Education's Office of the Inspector General published a report indicating that enforcement of the substance use policies in the Higher Education Act has been almost nonexistent (14). Better enforcement of, and compliance with, these policies may help change the culture of college campuses, where many students report that drinking is an expected aspect of college life.

Treatment of alcohol use disorders in college students requires the same steps as treating alcohol use disorders in other age groups. Prochaska and DiClemente's stages of change (15) are especially pertinent to this population, and motivational interviewing (16) is accepted as the gold standard for therapeutic intervention. Particular problems in implementing these interventions in the college population include the inconsistent availability of resources and ongoing uncertainty as to how best to deliver the treatments.

Early intervention, via brief structured interventions administered before or shortly after the onset of negative consequences of alcohol consumption, has been found to be particularly effective in reducing the frequency and consequences of alcohol use disorders. One example of such a program is the Brief Alcohol Screening Intervention for College Students. This intervention involves two face-to-face interviews. The first encounter is a motivational interview, and the second gives personalized feedback based on student drinking behavior. Students undergoing this intervention were found to have a significant reduction in alcohol consumption as well as alcohol-related problems (17). The method of delivering alcohol education services may also influence the success of the outcome. Fachini found that face-to-face interventions as opposed to computerized interventions may be better received by the student and may create a stronger commitment to change (17).

16.3 Nicotine

Despite extensive public health initiatives and costly government taxes on cigarettes, 18.1% of the U.S. population continues to smoke (18). Among college students, rates are at least as high or even higher; one recent study found that 35.3% of college students smoke cigarettes to varying degrees. Factors found to correlate with higher smoking level include having more friends that smoke, drinking, binge drinking, and more "other" tobacco use (19). Of note, many students in the latter study were nondaily smokers, who represent a growing subgroup of the smoking population. Despite the previous belief that nondaily smoking is a pathway to daily smoking, or conversely to quitting, evidence suggests that nondaily smoking behavior can be sustained for long periods of time and poses serious health risks (20).

One important subset of nondaily smokers in college is the group of "social smokers." These individuals tend to smoke almost exclusively in the presence of peers – usually at parties, bars, or nightclubs. Schane et al. found that social smokers tend not to label themselves as smokers, do not consider themselves addicted, and often do not understand the negative consequences of their smoking (20). Consequently, this type of smoker shows little interest in quitting and believes he/she can quit at any time.

In addition to cigarettes, other means of smoking have become popular among college students (e.g., smoking tobacco through a hookah). As many as 50% of students who smoke tobacco with a hookah do not smoke cigarettes, and they tend to view hookah smoking as safer than cigarette smoking (21). However, smoking tobacco via a hookah one time delivers 20 times the number of carcinogens as one cigarette (22). Cigar use is also on the rise among college students, and there are a significant number of students who smoke cigars who do not smoke cigarettes (21). Consequently, smoking prevention efforts need to highlight the risks tobacco products other than cigarettes.

Important relationships exist between nicotine addiction and mental illness. Nearly every known psychiatric disorder has been shown to be associated with increased smoking rates, including affective disorders such as major depressive disorder and bipolar disorder, and psychotic disorders such as schizophrenia. In particular, nicotine use and depression are highly comorbid and can each potentiate the other (23). Multiple anxiety disorders including posttraumatic stress disorder, panic disorder, generalized anxiety disorder, social anxiety disorder, and specific phobia have also been associated with increased risk of smoking (24). The link between smoking and psychiatric disorder is even clearer with regard to ADHD. A review by McClernon et al. highlighted that patients with ADHD have a higher rate of smoking, initiate smoking earlier, smoke larger quantities of cigarettes, and are less likely to quit compared to their non-ADHD counterparts (25). This strong association may be related to overlap in neurobiological and/or genetic substrates that underlie ADHD and smoking. In particular, both dopaminergic and nicotinic systems are implicated in the two disorders (25).

16.3.1 Treatment

Smoking cessation continues to be a major U.S. public health priority. Traditional methods of smoking cessation include the use of nicotine patches and gums, behavior modification therapies, or the combination (see chapter 7). Pharmacological agents influencing reward circuits in the brain, such as bupropion and varenicline, have shown efficacy in clinical trials; both of the previously discussed medications are approved by the U.S. Food and Drug Administration (FDA) for smoking cessation. More recent data suggest that a combination of varenicline, bupropion, and a serotonin reuptake inhibitor may be more effective than varenicline alone in enhancing smoking cessation (26).

Due to the fact that nondaily smoking and binge drinking are highly comorbid behaviors in college students, concomitant treatment of alcohol use disorders may be an important strategy for smoking cessation in this population (27). Targeting comorbid non–substance abuse psychiatric disorders can also play an important role. As an example, a variety of psychopharmacological therapies have been studied as possible adjunctive treatments for smoking cessation in patients with ADHD. In one study, osmotic-release methylphenidate (OROS-MPH; a long-acting, sustained-delivery form of the stimulant methylphenidate) was found to decrease ADHD symptoms but did not impact smoking cessation (28).

However, another study (29) found that non-Caucasian patients had a statistically significant increase in smoking cessation when treated with adjunctive OROS-MPH compared to Caucasian patients. Further study is necessary to better understand the apparent discrepancies across the latter two studies. Treatment of nicotine dependence can also overlap with treatment for mood and anxiety disorders. As discussed previously, bupropion, a medication that can be used for smoking cessation, is also a commonly used treatment for depression and anxiety.

16.4 Marijuana

Marijuana is second only to alcohol in frequency of use among college students. A survey of college students across the United States found that 37.6% had tried marijuana at least once, and 15.9% had used in the prior month (30) (see chapter 8). Another study found that among past-year college users, 25% met the criteria of the *Diagnostic and Statistical Manual of Mental Disorders*, fourth edition (*DSM-IV*), for a cannabis abuse disorder (31).

One factor that seems to influence marijuana use among college students is the perception of how much their peers use the substance. The American College Health Association (ACHA) survey cited previously found that college students perceived that 81.8% of their peers had used marijuana in the last month (30). There is concern that the perception by abstainers that a vast majority of their peers are using may compromise their ability to maintain abstinence (31).

One tool for correcting misconceptions regarding peer use is the eCHECKUP TO GO (e-TOKE), a web-based marijuana intervention for college students currently abstaining from marijuana. In a pilot study using this instrument, e-TOKE was found to aid in decreasing the misperception of exaggerated use among peers. While there was no significant difference in initiation of marijuana use between the e-TOKE group and the control group, students who used this tool did report less perceived disapproval from their peers regarding their abstention (32).

16.4.1 Consequences

Marijuana use can be associated with a variety of adverse outcomes, both acutely and as a function of chronic use (see chapter 8). Difficulties with psychomotor function, attention, memory, and learning have been associated with acute cannabis intoxication, and these may persist after a short period of abstinence (33). In a study of at-risk marijuana users in college (more than five times in the past year), the most common marijuana-related impairments were concentration problems, driving while high, missing class, and putting oneself at risk for physical injury (31). Many of the at-risk users in this study did not meet the criteria for a cannabis use disorder according to *DSM-IV* criteria. This finding underscores the importance of recognizing and targeting students for treatment even if they do not have a formal cannabis use disorder diagnosis (31).

16.4.2 Association with other conditions and implications for prevention and treatment

While marijuana use can have negative health consequences on its own, it is also important to consider the potential for comorbidity of marijuana, tobacco, and alcohol use. Among college students who smoked marijuana in the past 30 days, 38% also smoked cigarettes, and 69% binge drank (34). Due to the high level of comorbid use of these substances, treatment and prevention measures that target multiple substance use may prove to be more effective than targeting any single drug of abuse.

In addition to established behavioral treatments for cannabis dependence (e.g., motivational enhancement, 12-step programs, and cognitive behavioral therapy), there is new research on pharmacological agents that may be effective in promoting cannabis cessation (35). Gray et al. studied the over-the-counter agent N-acetylcysteine (NAC) as a possible treatment for cannabis use in adolescents between the ages of 15 and 21, based on the ability of this agent to upregulate the cystine-glutamate exchanger in the nucleus accumbens (36). The cystine-glutamate exchanger has been shown in animal models to be downregulated during chronic administration, and administration of NAC has been shown to reduce drug-seeking behavior (37). Results of the Gray study were encouraging; there was a significant reduction in positive urine toxicology in the NAC-treated group versus the placebo group (36).

16.5 Cocaine

According to statistics collected by the Substance Abuse and Mental Health Services Administration (2008), cocaine abuse is most prevalent among young adults in the United States and has been on the rise in recent years (38); 2.6% of college students reported last-year use in 1996 compared with 5.1% in 2007 (39) (see chapter 11). A high rate of exposure to opportunities for cocaine use has been shown to correlate with increased rate of use. By the end of the fourth year of college, as many as 36% of students have had the opportunity to use cocaine at least once, and 13% have used cocaine at least once. Of those students who reported having the opportunity, 37% used cocaine at some point during 4 years of college (40). Cocaine users are more likely to be male, Caucasian, and meet criteria for a comorbid alcohol or cannabis use disorder.

Possible gender differences should be considered; in the Kasperski study, there was a nonsignificant trend for female college students who use cocaine to be more likely than their male peers to meet criteria for cocaine abuse (8.4% vs. 5.4%) and cocaine dependence (9.3% vs. 2.5%) (40). Although alcohol use and related consequences receive the most attention from college administrators, cocaine use also poses a serious health risk for college students because cocaine use is relatively common and often concurrent with other substance use.

16.6 Prescribed stimulants

A growing and particularly pernicious problem in the college age population is the misuse, diversion, and abuse of prescription stimulants, which are prescribed for ADHD (see chapters 10 and 11). ADHD is a neuropsychiatric disorder that affects between 2% and 8% of the U.S. college student population (41). Stimulant medications are considered the gold-standard treatment for ADHD, though a variety of nonstimulant medications and psychosocial treatment options are also available.

Recent emphasis on the frequent continuation of this disorder into adulthood has contributed to increasing use of prescription stimulant medications in the college population. However, accompanying the appropriate and justified increase in use of prescription stimulants in this population are important concerns about nonmedical use, diversion, and abuse potential (42). In one study, specific risk factors for the nonmedical use of prescription stimulants among college students included being male, Caucasian, Jewish, affiliated with a fraternity or sorority, and having a lower grade-point average (42).

College students may misuse prescription stimulants to improve concentration, increase alertness and energy, as a study aid, and to attain euphoria (43). The communal nature of college living and the relatively visible nature of daily living habits in this setting likely represent additional important risk factors for diversion of stimulants in this population.

Of note, not all stimulant medications carry the same risk of misuse. College students are more likely to misuse short- or intermediate-acting formulations than long-acting formulations. This is particularly true for students who report using the medication to get high (43,44). One possible reason for this difference in abuse potential is that the short-acting stimulants produce a more immediate upsurge in stimulant blood level and resultant dopamine release and thereby induce more of a euphoric effect than their longer-acting counterparts. Also of interest is the route of administration of stimulants when they are misused. One study found that nearly all misusers used an oral route of administration (95.3%), but 38.1% did report snorting the medication (44). Several studies have shown that mixed amphetamine salts (MAS; i.e., Adderall) and MAS-XR are the most commonly diverted stimulants in the college population (43,44).

ADHD is the most frequent FDA-approved indication for stimulant medication use. The increasing number of prescriptions written, however, has led many to question the appropriateness of the ADHD diagnosis in an as yet undefined subgroup of individuals who are prescribed stimulants. Musso et al. noted that the base rate of malingering in the face of external incentives is 10.2% (45). Possible incentives for feigning ADHD and thereby receiving prescriptions for stimulant medications include the potential for improved performance, recreational use, and selling the medication illicitly. In addition, feigning a diagnosis of ADHD can result in receiving academic accommodations that may further improve performance. How to more carefully determine which students should be legitimately prescribed stimulants and academic accommodations for ADHD and weeding out those with malingering behavior remains the subject of much discussion.

Examples of misuse of prescription stimulants include using more of the drug than has been prescribed, mixing the drug with alcohol or other drugs, or using the drug to intentionally get high. In one study among college students using prescribed stimulants for ADHD, 40% reported misuse of some kind in the last year; 36% reported using too much of their stimulant, 19% reported general misuse, and 19% reported intentionally using their stimulant with other drugs (43). Another study found that 25% of college students who were prescribed stimulants for ADHD used the medication to get high (46). In the Sepulveda study, college students who initiated use of prescribed stimulants for ADHD during college were more likely to misuse their medications than those who initiated treatment at an earlier age (43).

A similar but somewhat different problem is the diversion of prescription stimulants (i.e., providing access to those who do not have a prescription). Data from one study showed that more college students report illicit use of prescription stimulants than medical use, and that the leading source of obtaining the medication was through friends or peers. In the same study, 54% of college students who were legitimately prescribed stimulants for the treatment of ADHD were approached to sell, trade, or give away their medication each year (42). Diversion of medication occurred in 36% of students who had received a prescription for stimulants. Among those who reported personal misuse of their stimulants, the rate of diversion was even higher (57%) (43). Similarly, Upadhyaya found that 29% of students prescribed stimulants reporting that they had given or sold their medication to someone else at some point in time (46).

16.6.1 Associations/risk factors for misuse and diversion

Multiple studies have linked the misuse of prescription stimulants with increased use of other substances, including cigarette smoking, binge drinking, marijuana use, and other drug use (43,46). Students with ADHD who had active ADHD symptoms were more likely to use tobacco or drugs other than alcohol or marijuana (46). While the relationships among ADHD symptoms, stimulant treatment, and use of other substances is intriguing, it is unclear what the nature of the associations are; does misuse of ADHD medications lead to other substance abuse, or vice versa? One theory posits that nicotine use among students with active ADHD symptoms represents self-medicating because nicotine is known to enhance dopaminergic neurotransmission and has been shown to improve attention in individuals with ADHD (47). Due to the increased level of other substance use in students who misuse prescription stimulants, one must consider these individuals to be at increased risk for the negative outcomes associated with those other substances as well.

16.6.2 Prevention and treatment

Prevention and treatment strategies include the following: (1) better control of ADHD symptoms, which will likely decrease risk for subsequent drug abuse; (2) considering the full range of therapeutic options (i.e., not just stimulant medications) for treating youth with ADHD; (3) counseling college students about the potential personal and legal risks of misuse and diversion; and (4) impressing on college students that safety of prescribed stimulants can only be assured within the designated therapeutic range and in patients who have been adequately screened for risk of adverse effects (including potentially lethal cardiovascular adverse effects). Following from the previous discussion, counseling college students should include specific discussion about the likelihood of being asked to share their prescription stimulants with friends, methods of properly storing their medication, and potential safety issues that can occur if individuals who have not been screened medically use their drugs.

Educating physicians who treat ADHD in college students is an important strategy for several reasons. As previously noted, short-acting stimulant formulations are more likely to be misused than long-acting formulations; therefore, use of long-acting stimulants as a first choice option when stimulants are prescribed is likely to decrease the amount of stimulant misuse. In addition to altering the pharmacokinetic distribution curve (i.e., generally slower onset of effect and distribution of drug over a longer period of time), some of the long-acting formulations offer additional protection in that the medication can't be crushed and delivered in an alternative form.

Another option for restricting the use of immediate release stimulants is to consider the use of approved nonstimulant medications where appropriate – that is, atomoxetine for ADHD (FDA approved for this indication in this age group) (48); bupropion for depression with ADHD symptoms (approved for depression in this age group and documented off-label efficacy in ADHD) (49,50); and long-acting alpha-2 agonists (FDA approved in children under 18 years but no doubt useful in older patients) (51). In addition, it is important to consider evidence-based psychosocial approaches, which teach and support improved organizational skills (52,53).

As noted previously, several studies have shown that MAS (i.e., Adderall) and MAS-XR are the most commonly diverted stimulants in the college population (43,44). While further study is required to determine whether this is due to higher rates of prescription and availability of these formulations, or other factors related to the formulations themselves, use of methylphenidate compounds (i.e., a different class of stimulants) preferentially might be potentially useful. When using amphetamine compounds, preferentially prescribing the long-acting amphetamine formulation lisdexamfetamine (i.e., dextro-amphetamine, which is covalently bound to the naturally occurring amino acid, l-lysine, which renders it inert until metabolized gradually in the blood stream) would also seem to minimize risk of diversion.

Finally, as it has been shown that college students can easily feign ADHD symptoms, it is important to educate physicians to use structured rating scales and validated interviews in making the diagnosis, and to consider the possibility that at least some individuals inappropriately seeking prescription stimulants know the diagnostic criteria and feign positive responses (54). Consequently, it is important to collect information regarding other contextual and developmental characteristics of the disorder and also consider whether there is sufficient impairment to warrant treatment.

16.7 Conclusions

Substance abuse among college students has been the focus of considerable recent attention, given the high prevalence of use/abuse in this population, the nature of the drugs that are abused, the specific contextual issues that fuel abuse in this population, and the potentially dire outcomes of substance use in this population. It is hoped that better understanding the types of substance abuse that most often occur in the college age population, the specific contextual factors that support substance abuse in this population, and the various available methods of prevention and treatment of substance abuse that have been developed for college students will contribute to more informed approaches to managing this problem.

References

1. Substance Abuse and Mental Health Service Administration. Results from the National Survey on Drug Use and Health: Summary of national findings. NSDUH Series H-44, HHS Publication No. (SMA) 12–4713. Rockville, MD: Substance Abuse and Mental Health Service Administration, 2012.

2. Hingson RW, Zha W, Weitzman ER. Magnitude of and trends in alcohol-related mortality and morbidity among U.S. college students ages 18–24, 1998–2005. J Stud Alcohol Drugs 2009;16 (Suppl):12–20.
3. Skala K, Kapusta ND, Schlaff G, Unseld M, Erfurth A, Lesch OM, et al. Suicidal ideation and temperament: An investigation among college students. J Affect Disord 2012;141(2–3):399–405.
4. Johnston LD, O'Malley PM, Bachman JG, Schulenberg JE. Monitoring the future national survey results on drug use, 1975–2011. Vol. 2, College students and adults ages 19–50 years. Ann Arbor: Institute Social Research, University Michigan, 2012.
5. Wechsler H, Dowdall G, Davenport A, Castillo S. Correlates of college student binge drinking. Am J Public Health 1995;85:921–6.
6. Knight JR, Wechlser H, Kuo M, Seibring M, Weitzman ER, Schuckit MA. Alcohol abuse and dependence among US college students. J Stud Alcohol 2002;63:263–70.
7. Kaynak O, Meyers K, Caldeira KM, Vincent KB, Winters KC, Arria AM. Relationships among parental monitoring and sensation seeking on the development of substance use disorder among college students. Addict Behav 2012;38:1457–63.
8. Carter AC, Brandon KO, Goldman MS. The college and noncollege experience: A review of the factors that influence drinking behavior in young adulthood. J Stud Alcohol Drugs 2010; 71:742–50.
9. Lee CM, Maggs JL, Rankin LA. Spring break trips as a risk factor for heavy alcohol use among first-year college students. J Stud Alcohol 2006;67:911–6.
10. Presley CA, Meilman PW, Leichliter JS. College factors that influence drinking. J Stud Alcohol 2002;14(Suppl):82–90.
11. Marczinski CA. Alcohol mixed with energy drinks: Consumption patterns and motivations for use in U.S. college students. Int J Environ Res Public Health 2011;8(8):3232–45.
12. Snipes DJ, Benotsch EG. High-risk cocktails and high-risk sex: Examining the relation between alcohol mixed with energy drink consumption, sexual behavior, and drug use in college students. Addict Behav 2012;38:1418–23.
13. Nelson TF, Naimi TS, Brewer RD, Wechsler H. The state sets the rate: The relationship among state-specific college binge drinking, state binge drinking rates, and selected state alcohol control policies. Am J Public Health 2005;3:441–6.
14. Kelly TA, McGuinness TM. Treatment of alcohol-dependent college students. J Psychosoc Nurs Ment Health Serv 2012;50(10):15–8.
15. Prochaska JO, DiClemente CC. Stages of change in the modification of problem behaviors. Prog Behav Modif 1992;28:183–218.
16. Miller WR. Motivational interviewing. In: Hersen M, Rosqvist J, eds. Encyclopedia of behavior modification and cognitive behavior therapy. Vol. 1, Adult clinical applications. Thousand Oaks, CA: Sage, 2005:383–9.
17. Fachini A, Aliane PP, Martinez EZ, Furtado EF. Efficacy of brief alcohol screening intervention for college students (BASICS): A meta-analysis of randomized controlled trials. Subst Abuse Treat Prev Policy 2012;7:40.
18. Centers for Disease Control and Prevention. Behavioral risk factor surveillance system survey data. Atlanta, GA: U.S. Department Health Human Services CfDCaP, 2008.
19. Berg CJ, Ling PM, Hayes RB, Berg EN, Nehl E, Choi WS, et al. Smoking frequency among current college student smokers: Distinguishing characteristics and factors related to readiness to quit smoking. Health Educ Res 2012;27(1):141–50.
20. Schane RE, Glantz SA, Ling PM. Nondaily and social smoking: An increasingly prevalent pattern. Arch Intern Med 2009;169:1742–44.

21. Primack BA, Sidani JE, Agarwal AA, Donny EC, Shadel WG, Eissenberg TE. Prevalence of and associations with water-pipe smoking among US university students. Ann Behav Med 2008;36:81–6.
22. Sepetdjian E, Shihadeh A, Saliba NA. Measurement of 16 polycyclic aromatic hydrocarbons in narghile waterpipe tobacco smoke. Food Chem Toxicol 2008;46:1582–90.
23. Tsuang MT, Francis T, Minor K, Thomas A, Stone WS. Genetics of smoking and depression. Hum Genet 2012;131:905–15.
24. Lasser K, Boyd JW, Woolhandler S, Himmelstein DU, McCormick D, Bor DH. Smoking and mental illness: A population-based prevalence study. JAMA 2000;284:2606–10.
25. McClernon FJ, Kollins SH. ADHD and smoking: From genes to brain to behavior. Ann NY Acad Sci 2008;1141:131–47.
26. Issa JS, Abe TO, Moura S, Santos PCJL, Pereira AC. Effectiveness of coadministration of varenicline, bupropion, and serotonin reuptake inhibitors in a smoking cessation program in the real-life setting. Nicotine Tob Res 2013;15(6):1146–50.
27. Harrison ELR, Desai RA, McKee SA. Nondaily smoking and alcohol use, hazardous drinking, and alcohol diagnoses among young adults: Findings from the NESARC. Alcohol Clin Exp Res 2008;32(12):2081–7.
28. Winhusen T, Somoza E, Brigham GS, Liu, D, Green CA, Covey LS, et al. Does treatment of attention deficit hyperactivity disorder (ADHD) enhance response to smoking cessation intervention in ADHD smokers? A randomized trial. J Clin Psychiatry 2010;71(12):1680–8.
29. Covey LS, Hu MC, Winhusen T, Weissman J, Berlin I, Nunes EV. OROS-methylphenidate or placebo for adult smokers with attention deficit hyperactivity disorder: Racial/ethnic differences. Drug Alcohol Depend 2010;110:156–9.
30. American College Health Association. American College Health Association-National College Health Assessment II: Reference group executive summary spring 2012. Hanover, MD: American College Health Association, 2012.
31. Caldeira KM, Arria AM, O'Grady KE, Vincent KB, Wish ED. The occurrence of cannabis use disorders and other cannabis-related problems among first-year college students. Addict Behav 2008;33:397–411.
32. Elliot JC, Carey KB. Correcting exaggerated marijuana use norms among college abstainers: A preliminary test of a preventive intervention. J Stud Alcohol Drugs 2012;73:976–80.
33. Kalant H. Adverse effects of cannabis on health: An update of the literature since 1996. Progr Neuro-psychopharmacol Biol Psychiatr 2004;28(5):849–63.
34. Primack BA, Kim KH, Shensa A, Sidani JE, Barnett TE, Switzer GE. Tobacco, marijuana, and alcohol use in university students: A cluster analysis. J Am Coll Health 2012;60:5:374–86.
35. Danovitch I, Gorelick DA. State of the art treatments for cannabis dependence. Psychiatr Clin North Am 2012;35(2):309–26.
36. Gray KM, Carpenter MJ, Baker NL, DeSantis SM, Kryway E, Hartwell KJ, et al. A double-blind randomized controlled trial of N-Acetylcysteine in cannabis-dependent adolescents. Am J Psychiatry 2012;169(8):805–12.
37. Moussawi K, Pacchioni A, Moran M, Olive MF, Gass JT, Lavin A, et al. N-Acetylcysteine reverses cocaine-induced metaplasticity. Nat Neurosci 2009;12:182–9.
38. Substance Abuse and Mental Health Services Administration. Results from the 2007 National Survey on Drug Use and Health: National findings. DHHS Publication No. SMA 08–4343. Rockville, MD: Office of Applied Studies, 2008.
39. Johnston LD, O'Malley PM, Bachman JG, Schulenberg JE. Monitoring the future national survey results on drug use, 1975–2006. Vol. 2, College students and adults ages 19–45 years. NIH Publication No 07–6206. Bethesda, MD: National Institute Drug Abuse, 2007.

40. Kasperski SJ, Vincent KB, Caldeira KM, Garnier-Dykstra LM, O'Grady KE, Arria AM. College students' use of cocaine: Results from a longitudinal study. Addict Behav 2011;36: 408–11.
41. Weyandt LL, DuPaul G. ADHD in college students. J Attent Disord 2006;10(1):9–19.
42. McCabe SE, Knight JR, Teter CJ, Wechsler H. Non-medical use of prescription stimulants among US college students: Prevalence and correlates from a national survey. Addiction 2005;99: 96–106.
43. Sepulveda DR, Thomas LM, McCabe SE, Cranford JA, Boyd CJ, Teter CJ. Misuse of prescribed stimulant medication for ADHD and associated patterns of substance use: Preliminary analysis among college students. J Pharm Pract 2011;24(6):551–60.
44. Teter CJ, McCabe SE, LaGrange K, Cranford JA, Boyd CJ. Illicit use of specific prescription stimulants among college students: Prevalence, motives, and routes of administration. Pharmacotherapy 2006;26(10):1501–10.
45. Musso MW, Gouvier WD. "Why is this so hard?" A review of detection of malingered ADHD in college students. J Attention Disord 2012;5:1–16.
46. Upadhyaya HP, Rose K, Wang W, O'Rourke K, Sullivan B, Deas D, et al. Attention-deficit/hyperactivity disorder, medication treatment, and substance use patterns among adolescents and young adults. J Child Adolesc Psychopharmacol 2005;15(5):799–809.
47. Kollins SH, McClernon J, Fuemmeler BF. Association between smoking and attention-deficit/ hyperactivity disorder symptoms in a population-based sample of young adults. Arch Gen Psychiatry 2005;62:1142–7.
48. Alder LA, Wilens T, Zhang S, Dittmann RW, D'Souza DN, Schuh L, et al. Atomoxetine treatment outcomes in adolescents and young adults with attention-deficit/hyperactivity disorder: Results from a post hoc, pooled analysis. Clin Ther 2012;34(2):363–73.
49. Solhkhah R, Wilens TE, Daly J, Prince JB, Van Patten SL, Biederman J. Bupropion SR for the treatment of substance-abusing outpatient adolescents with attention-deficit/hyperactivity disorder and mood disorders. J Child Adolesc Psychopharmacol 2005;15(5):777–86.
50. Wilens TE, Prince JB, Waxmonsky J, Doyle R, Spencer T, Martelon M, et al. An open trial of sustained release bupropion for attention-deficit/hyperactivity disorder in adults with ADHD plus substance use disorders. J ADHD Relat Disord 2010;1(3):25–35.
51. Sallee FR, McGough J, Wigal T, Donahue J, Lyne A, Biederman J. Guanfacine extended release in children and adolescents with attention-deficit/hyperactivity disorder: A placebo controlled trial. J Am Acad Child Adolesc Psychiatry 2009;48(2):155–65.
52. Solanto MV, Marks DJ, Wasserstein J, Mitchell K, Abikoff H, Alvir JM, et al. Efficacy of metacognitive therapy for adult ADHD. Am J Psychiatry 2010;167(8):958–68.
53. Safren SA. Cognitive-behavioral approaches to ADHD treatment in adulthood. J Clin Psychiatry 2006;67(8):46–50.
54. Conners CK, Erhardt D, Epstein JN, Parker JDA, Sitarenios G, Sparrow E. Self-ratings of ADHD symptoms in adults I: Factor structure and normative data. J Attention Disord 1999;3(3):141–51.

17 Sports doping by adolescent athletes

Dilip R. Patel and Donald E. Greydanus

Use of drugs and nutritional supplements is widespread in collegiate-, professional-, and elite-level sports. Although, less is known about the use of drugs and supplements to enhance sports performance in high school age athletes, such use does occur and is a reason for grave concern.

Research on these products remains limited, and athletes rely on word of mouth from fellow sports enthusiasts, coaches, nutrition store personnel, advertisements, and other unscientific sources for information on what drugs, herbs, or other available agents will help them improve their athletic performance or their lives in general. This chapter reviews the use by athletes of anabolic agents, human growth hormone, clenbuterol, creatine, stimulants, and erythropoietin.

17.1 Introduction

For thousands of years, humans have sought the use of medicines, herbs, and other chemicals to improve their lives in various ways. Some scholars have interpreted the story of Adam and Eve in Genesis as a story of the original humans seeking to be strong (wise) like God (1). Extensive pharmacopoeias have been developed in China and India over the past eons (2). The first classifier of medicinal herbs is noted by historians as the Chinese emperor Shen-Nung 2737 BC, and there is a classic recorded painting of him holding *Ephedra* (ma huang) leaves (3). An early historical record of medical treatments is the Ebers Papyrus (1500 BC), which lists more than 700 medicines of various origins (mineral, vegetable, and animal) (2,4).

In recorded history, competitive athletes have used various mixtures of animal and plant origins, taken from known and unknown products, in attempts to improve their athletic performance and gain the perceived benefits of victory (5). For example, athletes during the Greek and Roman games used wines, mushrooms, and opioids; stimulants (i.e., strychnine) were popular at the beginning of the 20th century. Galen, the famous Greek who became the physician to the gladiators of ancient Rome, observed the belief of athletes of his time (AD 180) that consuming mushrooms and herbal teas was beneficial to their overall performance (3). In 1886, a cyclist died during a race in France because of a stimulant overdose (3). Such sports-doping practices have continued in advocates of sport and others to the present age, even though such practices have been banned by sports officials. For example, the death of a British athlete at the Tour de France in 1967 was attributed to the use of amphetamines complicated by a state of dehydration, and nine riders were ruled ineligible for the Tour de France in 2006 because of suspected sports doping (6).

Athletes of the past and of today have been willing to take various chemicals even without any proof of their benefit, in the hope of improving their general health or their sports performance (7). Over thousands of years, athletes have consulted experts from the ancient days of sorcery and alchemy to modern-day biochemistry and pharmacology to find effective yet safe performance-enhancing drugs (5). The milieu of "victory at any cost" that existed millennia ago continues to the present. In 1982, Goldman and colleagues asked 198 world-class athletes if they would take a chemical that would guarantee them success but would lead to their death in 5 years; in this survey, 52% reported they would take this chemical, and this report remained at this level in repeat surveys between 1982 and 1995 (8,9). Connor and Mazanov posed this Faustian bargain to members of the general public in Australia; they noted that only 2 of the 250 individuals surveyed agreed to take such a chemical. These sagacious members of the general public were not obsessed with victory at any cost (9).

As we enter a new millennium and century, it is sobering to realize that only a handful of the thousands of available herbal remedies of old or of modern chemistry have been shown to actually work as prescribed to better one's health (2,4,10). Proof of improving sports performance with various chemicals (including herbs) is even more limited. Yet, today's athletes are taking various products (see table 17.1) in ever-increasing numbers because they are driven to succeed to obtain the perceived glories of winning in contemporary society (11–21). The teenage athlete should be carefully counseled that there are few substances (if any) that consistently and safely improve the performance of a well-trained individual. Also, the use of these agents has considerable potential to cause physical and psychological

Table 17.1: Partial list of drugs and supplements misused by athletes as ergogenic products

- Alpha-lipoic acid
- Anabolic steroids
- Androstenedione
- Antioxidants (vitamin C, vitamin E, beta-carotene)
- Amphetamines
- Bee pollen
- Beta-blockers (i.e., propranolol)
- Beta-hydroxy-beta-methylbutyrate
- Blood
- Boron
- Caffeine
- Calcium
- Carnitine
- Choline
- Chrysin
- Chromium
- Clenbuterol
- Coenzyme Q10
- Creatine
- Diuretics (furosemide, spironolactone, hydrochlorothiazide)
- Dihydroepiandrostenedione
- Engineered dietary supplements
- Ephedrine
- Erythropoietin
- Folic acid
- Ginkgo biloba
- Ginseng
- Glycerol
- Human-growth hormone
- Inosine
- Insulin-like growth factor-I
- Iron
- Niacin
- Nicotine
- Nonsteroidal anti-inflammatory drugs (ibuprofen, mefenamic acid, naproxen, etc.)
- Omega-3 fatty acids
- Oxygen
- Pantothenic acid
- Phosphorus
- Pyridoxine (vitamin B6)
- Selenium
- Vanadium
- Zinc

damage. Misuse of drugs in this manner should be discouraged. Our sports youth live in a modern-day Faustian dilemma often with the encouragement of coaches, trainers, parents, the media, and other members of society obsessed with success at any price.

17.2 Protection for consumers

Some progress was made in the 20th century to help consumers understand whether or not the medications or chemical agents they take are beneficial and safe. In 1906, the Pure Food and Drug Act required foods and drugs, which were sent between various states, to be provided with accurate labels. It was not required that medications be tested for safety until the 1938 Federal Food, Drug and Cosmetic Act (FFDCA). It was also not required that these drugs be proven effective for their intended use until the 1962 Harris-Kefauver Amendment of the FFDCA. However, the 1994 Dietary Supplement Health and Education Act (DSHEA) reversed some of these gains acquired over the previous 88 years. DSHEA allowed products classified as dietary supplements to avoid the scrutiny applied to drugs or medications. Thus, manufacturers of dietary supplements (defined as a vitamin, mineral, herb, other botanic, amino acid, metabolites of these products, related metabolites, related concentrations, or extracts or combinations) do not need to prove safety or efficacy of their products. All that is needed is to note that their products "maintain health or normal structure and function" (10).

This opened up the commercial floodgates to various agents used by athletes in the hope that the products they use are ergogenic (see table 17.2) (22–24). It is important for physicians and medical educators to be aware of these various products and to be willing to provide education to society and their patients about what is known and not known about these products (18,25,26).

Research on these products remains limited and athletes rely on word of mouth from fellow sports enthusiasts, coaches, nutrition store personnel, advertisements, and other unscientific sources for information on what drugs, herbs, or other

Table 17.2: Manufacturers' claims of ergogenic agents

- Serve as an energy source
- Decrease fatigue in sports events
- Increase lean body mass and strength
- Decrease adipose tissue
- Alter weight in desirable directions
- Improve aerobic capacity
- Enhance motor capacity
- Improve appearance
- Enhance overall sports performance

available agents will help them improve their athletic performance or their lives in general (24). Most research has been done on adult men, who are involved in competitive athletics and not on teenage athletes. The potency and purity of nutritional agents are not known and the long-term effects of these various substances are also unknown at present. However, the use of ergogenic agents remains popular, and more than 30,000 individual commercial products are available throughout the world (20,27,28). Unproven claims (see table 17.1) remain while the hope of victory burns strong in athletes of all ages whether competing at the high school level (or below) or at the Olympic level of competition (29,30).

17.3 Definitions

The term *doping* is derived from the Dutch word *dop* in reference to the practice of providing race horses with an opium mixture to act as a stimulant and enhance victory of the competing animal (17). Sports doping refers to the attempt of improvement or stimulation of sports performance in *Homo sapiens* in the eternal quest for victory at any cost. The promise of having a drug that is a true sports-doping chemical often belies an eternal quest for the product having an ergogenic quality, and this term is derived from the Greek words *ergon* (to work) and *gennan* (to produce). The International Olympic Committee defines doping as "... use of an expedient (substance or method) which is potentially harmful to athletes' health and/or capable of enhancing their performance, or the presence in athletes' body of a prohibited substance or evidence of the use thereof or evidence of the use of prohibited method" (26).

The American Academy of Pediatrics defines performance-enhancing agents as "... any substance when taken in nonpharmacological doses specifically for the purposes of improving sports performance. A substance should be considered performance enhancing if it benefits sports performance by increasing strength, power, speed or endurance (ergogenic) or by altering body weight or body composition" (22).

17.4 Anabolic agents

Anabolic steroids or anabolic-androgenic steroids (AASs) are a class of chemicals that are synthetic derivatives of testosterone and represent a drug class often abused by adolescent and adult athletes (31). The roots of their use can be traced to more than 6 millennia ago when ancient farmers noted the quieting or passive effects that castration had on animals (32). Testosterone was isolated in 1935 and developed to improve metabolism; it was used by athletes to gain strength as early as the 1940s. Concern over the use of anabolic steroids by athletes led to an inaugural definition of

Table 17.3: Examples of anabolic steroids

Oral	Injectable	Topical
Oxandronolone	Testosterone cypionate	Testosterone gel
Oxymetholone	Testosterone enanthate	Testosterone transdermal
Stanozolol	Nandrolone phenpropionate	
	Nandrolone decanoate	

sports doping by the International Olympic Committee (IOC) in 1964, the banning of these drugs by the IOC, the start of antidoping programs by the IOC in 1967, and the first official testing for these chemicals at the 1976 Montreal Olympic Games (5).

The term *anabolic* refers to the stimulation of protein synthesis, whereas *androgenic* implies the stimulation of male secondary sex characteristics. The terms *steroids* and *steroid hormones* refer to chemicals that are derived from cholesterol and include corticosteroids and sex hormones (i.e., testosterone, estrogen, and progesterone). Anabolic steroids stimulate several receptors: androgen, estrogen, progestin, and glucocorticoid. Some examples of oral and injectable anabolic steroids are listed in table 17.3. The U.S. Food and Drug Administration (FDA) has classified these chemicals as Schedule II drugs since 1990. Adequate training and protein intake are necessary for maximal effect on protein synthesis in muscle tissue and the individual response is variable. Anabolic steroids have become the sine qua non of the Faustian bargain awaiting our youth.

17.4.1 Epidemiology

According to the Monitoring the Future study, AASs are used predominantly by males. In 2011, annual prevalence rates were1.0%, 1.4%, and 1.8% for boys in grades 8, 10, and 12, respectively, compared with 0.4%, 0.4%, and 0.5% for girls. It is clear that many youth try anabolic steroids including one-third who are not athletes (31–35). Various studies over the past few decades confirm that 5%–11% of high school boys and 0.5%–2.5% of high school girls in the United States have tried anabolic steroids; of these, 50% used these chemicals before 16 years of age, and 33% of these youth were not athletes (31,33,36–50).

These youth have limited knowledge of the dangers of these drugs (41,51–53). Abuse of these chemicals may be increased in the nonathletic population versus the athletic adolescent population (52). Adolescents who take anabolic steroids may also be involved in other high-risk behaviors, including illicit drug use such as cocaine, alcohol, cigarettes, marijuana, smokeless tobacco, and various injectable drugs (43,47–55). Adolescents obtain these drugs from many sources, even from veterinary suppliers. Although abuse of anabolic steroids by American professional athletes has decreased somewhat in recent years, the use of these and other drugs by famous athletes has long encouraged teenagers to try these substances (56–58). Youth often believe that these chemicals are natural hormones and are endorsed by their sports heroes (54). Many teenagers are convinced that these drugs are valuable and worth any risk, even in very high doses.

Oral anabolic steroids are 17-alpha-alkylation chemicals that slow liver inactivation and cause much of the liver side effects of these drugs. The injectable forms are from 19-beta-esterification processes and pose infectious disease risks, including hepatitis (B and C) and HIV/AIDS. The therapeutic doses of such drugs as used for treatment of various medical disorders are 8–30 mg depending on the particular drug being used. Because teenage athletes are often not afraid (nor informed) of risks, they may use prolonged and heavy (supraphysiological) doses. They may use these drugs in various combinations in a method called stacking, that is, cycles of 6–12 weeks on and then off (47,53,59). Increasing a drug dose in a cycle is called pyramiding, and doses may be 10 to more than 40 times the usual therapeutic doses (59). While taking several drugs together (i.e., stacking), some athletes use up to 200 mg per day. These athletes may not have any fear of side effects in their quest for ergogenic qualities or even in attempts to simply improve appearance.

17.4.2 Effects

Numerous studies have established that AAS use results in increased muscle mass, muscle size, and maximal voluntary strength, especially when used in combination with proper training and adequate protein intake (60). Because the gains from AAS use in aerobic capacity are minimal at best, their popularity among endurance athletes is difficult to understand.

Athletes use anabolic steroids in the hope of increasing lean body mass, strength, and/or aggressiveness; as noted, some only wish to improve appearance (33,61). Athletes at particular risk for the use of anabolic steroids include those engaged in sports such as weight lifting, shot putting, discus throwing, bodybuilding, sprinting, football, and wrestling. Whether or not athletes get a significant increase in athletic performance remains controversial, and individualized results are the norm.

17.4.3 Adverse effects

Side effects of anabolic steroids are legion and are reviewed in table 17.4 (33,45,46,62–74).

Table 17.4: Side effects of anabolic steroids

Behavioral	Aggressiveness, irritability, depression, addiction
Cardiovascular	Lower high-density lipoprotein, increased low-density lipoprotein, cardiac hypertrophy, sudden cardiac death
Endocrine and metabolic	Suppression of hypothalamic-pituitary-testicular axis, hyperglycemia, decreased follicle stimulating hormone, decreased luteinizing hormone, hepatic dysfunction, liver tumors, peliosis hepatis, gynecomastia, acne
Unique to female	Hirsutism, cliteromegaly, menstrual irregularity, amenorrhea, deep voice, coarsening of skin
Unique to male	Decreased spermatozoa, decreased testosterone levels, reduced testicular size, prostatic enlargement
Unique to children	Acceleration of maturation, premature fusion of growth plates, virilization in boys, masculinization in girls
Related to injections	Systemic infections, local infections
Musculotendinous	Increased risk for tendon ruptures

17.4.4 Use of additional or concomitant doping agents with AAS

Users of AAS may use other drugs as well (48). For example, they may use human growth hormone (hGH), methamphetamine, or clenbuterol (see later discussion) to augment the anabolic effects of AAS. Human chorionic gonadotropin (HCG) may be added to raise testosterone synthesis and counter the anabolic steroid–induced effect of testicular atrophy. Diuretics (e.g., furosemide, spironolactone, and hydrochlorothiazide) may be used to reduce fluid retention, produce the desired rippled look, or dilute urine to subvert a drug-screening regimen. The use of diuretics to lose weight quickly is not an unusual plan of wrestlers. The use of such medications can result in increased weakness such that a wrestler can be injured by competing against a stronger opponent. Electrolyte dysfunction and other side effects of diuretics may complicate the picture. Pulmonary embolism has been reported in a high school wrestler using such a regimen (74).

Stimulants may be taken along with AAS to increase the drive for exercise and competition, whereas antiacne medications are used to deal with the anabolic steroid–induced acne. Antiestrogens (such as tamoxifen or clomiphene) may be used to prevent the male feminization effects (i.e., gynecomastia) of anabolic steroids. These athletes may use other drugs as well in the course of their training, such as antibiotics, corticosteroids (i.e., prednisone), and analgesics (e.g., morphine, propoxyphene, meperidine, oxycodone, and others). Narcotics and other illicit drugs are abused for their pleasure-granting effects as well. Corticotrophin (ACTH) is used to raise levels of internally produced corticosteroids and to produce a sense of euphoria.

17.4.5 Prevention

Anabolics have been banned by the IOC, the National Collegiate Athletic Association (NCAA), the National Football League (NFL), and many other sporting associations. However, it is often difficult for the adolescent user to stop because many young people have difficulty understanding the consequences of their actions (concrete thinking) and have difficulty avoiding the win-at-all-cost attitude prevalent in the global sports milieu (29,30,41,56,57,75–78). It is important to educate youth about these sports-doping agents (59). Parents and coaches must be taught about these chemicals, and they should not encourage the use of such potentially dangerous chemicals under the guise of "Winning is everything!"

Although there may be some medical indications for these drugs (i.e., treatment of HIV-associated wasting or chronic renal failure), seeking to improve sports performance should not be one of the medical indications to use these drugs (11,44,79). The effort to ban anabolic steroids has now been complicated with the appearance of designer steroids, the first of which was norbolethone that was initially detected by a laboratory in Los Angeles in 2002 (5). Other identified designer steroids include madol (desoxy-methyl testosterone) and tetrahydrogestrinone. Unfortunately, experts and amateurs in the biochemistry industry continue to produce such drugs, and the cat-and-mouse game between sports dopers and sports officials will continue in perpetuity.

17.5 Dihydroepiandrostenedione (DHEA)

DHEA is a mildly androgenic hormone naturally produced in the adrenal glands and testes. It is the precursor to testosterone (as well as dihydrotestosterone) and estrogen. Although DHEA is banned by the FDA and has no proven ergogenic effects, it is used by athletic teens and adults as an alternative to anabolic steroids (31,48,80). The ergogenic attempt is based on a hope and hype that DHEA will increase testosterone and an anabolic insulin-like growth factor (IGF-I). Despite animal studies having shown some DHEA-induced liver toxicity, it is marketed to adults (middle-aged and older) as an over-the-counter alternative to anabolic steroids with additional unproven claims of promoting euphoria, enhancing libido, delaying cardiovascular disease, preventing cancer, and boosting one's immunity (17). Research is limited on DHEA (65). One study evaluated men (average age 24 years) who used 1,600 mg per day for 4 weeks; serum testosterone levels were not altered (81). Another study called the Andro Project also noted no ergogenic qualities of DHEA (82).

DHEA is given at a dose of 50–100 mg per day for 6–12 months in oral or injectable forms, up to 1,600 mg. Side effects may occur as with ingestion of sex hormones. At doses of more than 100 mg/day, gynecomastia (irreversible) in men and hirsutism in women can occur; cancer (prostate or endometrial) may be worsened (83). DHEA should be considered an anabolic steroid, and teenagers should be advised not to use it. The FDA has ruled that it has no medical usage, and it has been banned from the National Hockey League, the IOC, and the NFL, among others.

17.6 Androstenedione

Androstenedione is another androgen produced by the adrenal gland and testes; it is a precursor of estrogen and testosterone (as well as dihydrotestosterone) and is found in Scotch pine tree pollen (84–86). It is used as a T-booster in hope of increasing testosterone; serum testosterone/estrogen ratios are normalized within 1 day of stopping this drug. High doses (such as 100–300 mg per day and 60 minutes before an event) may increase lean muscle mass and strength. Studies note that 300 mg of androstenedione increases testosterone, estrone, and estradiol levels by more than 100 mg (26). It is often used in combination with different anabolic steroids in various cycling methods (80).

Androstenedione is a banned chemical with unknown long-term safety. Side effects are the same as noted with anabolic steroids; the potency and safety of available products are unknown. It should be avoided with growing athletes and for those at risk for prostate or breast cancer. Androstenedione and other steroidal supplements may be packaged with various other chemicals, such as ephedrine, caffeine, saw palmetto, and others (65).

17.7 hGH

hGH has been used especially by power and speed athletes in attempts to increase lean muscle mass and strength, often in combination with anabolic steroids (11,31). However, ergogenic effects have not been proven, even when using supraphysiological doses (87). Although tests are available, it is difficult to detect all users, and the user runs the risk of having an impure product obtained illegally (88,89). Recombinant DNA technology has provided recombinant hGH to those able to pay the high cost of this agent (more than US$3,000 per month) (89). A survey of more than 200 high school male athletes noted that 5% were on hGH (48). The question of hGH purity as a natural product was previously raised with the development of Creutzfeldt-Jakob disease. Side effects of hGH supplementation may include jaw enlargement, gigantism, hypertension, hyperglycemia, fluid retention, carpal tunnel syndrome, slipped capital femoral epiphysis, and pseudotumor cerebri (18,89). Although several amino acids (arginine, ornithine, lysine, and tryptophan) are used to induce release of hGH, doses usually used do not significantly raise hGH in the body.

17.8 Gamma hydroxybutyrate (GHB)

GHB ("Liquid Ecstasy," "G," "Georgia home boy") is a central nervous system depressant that leads to euphoria and lowering of inhibition (90,91). GHB is popular with bodybuilders with the hype and hope of increasing growth hormone release during sleep and enhancing muscle growth. GHB can be made at home with recipes found on the Internet and with ingredients easily purchased. It is made as a clear liquid or white powder; tablets or capsules are available. It is also used as a date rape pill to enhance sexual assault; as a colorless, odorless, and tasteless liquid, it is easily slipped into party drinks to produce sedation and amnesia; effects are noted in 10–20 minutes and last for 4 hours. It is quickly cleared from the body and is hard to detect. Thus, it has become a popular date rape drug. An overdose can lead to profound respiratory depression, coma, and death.

Because the U.S. government is cracking down on GHB use, some are taking GHB metabolites or precursors, such as gamma butyrolactone and even the industrial solvent, 1,4-butanediol (BD). After ingestion of GBH, it becomes GHB. Some companies are substituting BD for GHB, even though BD has been declared a potentially life-threatening drug by the FDA. It is marketed as a dietary supplement in various sleep aid and muscle builder products. Although it is promoted to enhance sexual performance, BD slows breathing and can lead to unconsciousness, emesis, seizures, and death.

17.9 Clenbuterol

Clenbuterol is a beta-2 agonist bronchodilator (substituted phenylethanolamine) that is used with anabolic steroids in attempts to improve lean body mass and decrease adipose tissue (11,44,54,92–94). It is available in Europe, Central America, and South America. Clenbuterol can be given orally with full absorption, whereas aerosol and injection forms are also available. If used therapeutically for asthma, the dose is 0.02–0.04 mg per day; if used ergogenically, a dose of 0.02–0.16 mg per day is tried. Clenbuterol can be used in a 2-day on and 2-day off cycle for several weeks and then stopped before the athletic event, because it can be detected for 2–4 days after the last dose.

However, it is not proven that it increases muscle mass and reduces adipose tissue, certainly not to the extent attributed to anabolic steroids. Several side effects are observed, including tachycardia, headaches, anxiety, dizziness, nausea, tremor, and insomnia. Concern is raised that it may lead to arrhythmias, myocardial

Table 17.5: Substances and methods prohibited by -governing bodies

Main categories of prohibited substances	• Anabolic agents • Peptide hormones, growth hormones, and related substances • Beta-2 agonists • Hormone agonists and metabolic modulators • Diuretics and other masking agents
Main categories of prohibited methods	• Enhancement of oxygen transfer • Chemical and physical manipulation • Gene doping
Main categories of prohibited substances	• Stimulants • Narcotics • Cannabinoids • Glucocorticoids

Source: U.S. Antidoping Agency. Accessed December 20, 2012. URL: http://www.usada.org/prohibited-list

infarction, cardiac muscle hypertrophy, and cerebrovascular accidents. It is banned by many sport agencies, including the IOC, U.S. Olympic Committee, NCAA, and others.

To avoid sanctions for using a medication (even with a prescription) at Olympic competition levels, rules of the World Anti-Doping Code must be followed in which the International Standard for Therapeutic Use Exemptions are used (95). Sports doping has been viewed by authorities as being an unfair and unethical advantage in sports competition. The IOC developed a medical commission in 1967, and they have produced a list of substances that are prohibited (table 17.5) for athletes to use as well as various antidoping regulations (96). Specific screening for prohibited drugs was initiated at the 1972 Munich Olympic Games. In 1999, the World Anti-Doping Agency was developed, and this agency organized a worldwide effort to standardize and enforce antidoping regulations (31). Athletes must be careful even with prescription drugs that are prescribed for them or misuse of medications that are being prescribed for someone else (97).

17.10 Creatine

Creatine is an essential amino acid synthesized from arginine, glycine, and methionine, mainly in the kidneys, and to a lesser extent in the liver and pancreas. It is available in milk, meat, fish, and other foods, although meat and fish are the main food sources and supply more than half of the daily requirement (27,28,31,80, 90,98). The usual diet provides 1–2 g of creatine per day. It is a tasteless crystalline powder that is readily dissolved in liquids and is usually marketed as creatine monohydrate or with phosphorus (99). At all levels of competition (from high school to professional), creatine is the most popular nutritional supplement sold today as an ergogenic agent (27,28,31,90,98,100–104).

All but 5% of creatine is stored in skeletal muscle (especially the fast twitch, type II muscle), two-thirds as a phosphorylated form, and one-third as free creatine. This substance serves as an energy substrate for the contraction of skeletal muscle in the body. Cells with high-energy requirements use creatine in the form of phosphocreatine, which functions as a donor of phosphate to produce adenosine triphosphate (ATP) from adenosine diphosphate. Cells in the skeletal muscles store enough phosphocreatine and ATP for about 10 seconds of high-intensity action (80,100). The purpose of creatine supplementation is to increase resting phosphocreatine levels in muscles and free creatine to briefly postpone fatigue, with potential ergogenic results (99,100). Phosphocreatine maintains high energy ATP levels, acts as a proton buffer, and can lead to reduced glycolysis. When the phosphocreatine levels decrease, glycolysis increases. Maximal exercise eventually stops because of muscle fatigue, probably because of accumulation of lactate and hydrogen ions in addition to a decrease in ATP.

Studies in adult athletes suggest that with creatine supplementation there may be a 5%–15% improvement in short-term (less than 30 seconds), repetitive/intermittent, high-intensity exercise (18,27,28,102,105–107). Creatine is beneficial for those in power sports (i.e., football and sprinters), but not for those in endurance sports (e.g., swimming). Some athletes may have a low intracellular concentration of creatine and thus may respond to it, whereas those with a higher level do not respond. Most in vivo studies show no improvement in sports performance (80). Also, no studies report any improvement with long-term endurance activities.

Athletes use different dosage regimens for creatine supplementation (108–115). The work of Harris and colleagues has led to the current practice of many athletes using a loading dose of 20 g per day (5 g four times a day) for 5–7 days followed by 2–5 g per day for maintenance (113,114). Other loading and maintenance doses are also used. For example, research suggests an equally beneficial effect may be seen with 3 g per day versus a loading dose of 20 g per day (115). The loading routine may maximize the amount of phosphocreatine in muscles, whereas a maintenance dose may keep muscles filled. Positive results are best with an active exercise program, although there is no need to take creatine specifically before or during exercise. Increased weight may result because of fluid (water) retention and not increased protein synthesis (114). An increase of 0.7–3 kg in 1 month has been reported; weight gain can be maintained on 5 g per day of creatine during a 10-week period of detraining and maintained 4 weeks after its use is stopped.

Although creatine is generally regarded as safe, there may be side effects and risks, especially when consuming more than 20 g per day. The best-known effect is weight gain because of fluid (water) retention. Other adverse effects that are often cited but not proven include anecdotal reports of muscle cramps, strains,

Table 17.6: Recommendations of the international society of sports nutrition for use of creatine

- The athlete is past puberty.
- The athlete is involved in competitive training in which creatine supplementation may be beneficial.
- The athlete is consuming a well-balanced, performance-enhancing diet.
- The athlete and the athlete's parents understand the effects of creatine supplementation.
- The athlete's parents approve of creatine supplementation.
- The athlete takes supplementation under proper professional supervision.
- Quality creatine supplements are used.
- That athlete does not exceed recommended dosages.

Source: International Society of Sports Nutrition. Accessed December 18, 2012. URL: http://www.jissn.com/content/4/1/6

dehydration in hot/humid weather, renal function deterioration, suppression of endogenous synthesis, and possible cardiac muscle hypertrophy. Other anecdotal concerns include abdominal pain, dyspnea, nausea, emesis, diarrhea, anxiety, fatigue, migraine headaches, seizures, myopathy, and atrial fibrillation (17,80). Supplementation does reduce endogenous creatine production, with unknown results on the body. Although it is not banned by any major sports groups, the American College of Sports Medicine recommends that those less than 18 years of age should not use creatine (115). Recommendations of the International Society of Sports Nutrition for use of creatine use in children are listed in table 17.6.

17.11 Stimulants

17.11.1 Ephedrine

Ephedrine is a medication that can have beneficial effects in disease states (e.g., asthma), but which is not acceptable to various sports medicine committees because of potential harmful effects (18,20,116,117). It is an example of using a stimulant drug to seek improvement in one's performance in training or competition. Although not proven to be ergogenic, it has been used by various athletes in this regard. Other stimulants include amphetamine and caffeine. They are used to reduce the sense of being tired, lessen the feeling of pain, and heighten aggressiveness (45). As noted earlier, stimulants have been used by athletes over the eons as performance-enhancing chemicals. The Incas in South America chewed coca leaves to help them run long distances (1).

In the case of ephedrine, many believe its sympathomimetic action gives the user an unfair advantage and is thus banned. However, such beta-2 agonists such as terbutaline and salbuterol are accepted in the Olympics if the athlete has documented asthma and informs the Olympic Committee of their use. The purpose is to allow the athlete proper treatment of a verified disorder (i.e., asthma), but not to allow him or her to gain an unfair advantage over the competitors (i.e., using stimulants).

Ephedrine alkaloids are derived from ephedra herbs (also called ma huang). Athletes use dietary supplement products that contain ma huang to improve muscle tone and energy levels, although there is no proof of these claims (10,17). Numerous adverse event reports have been investigated by the FDA. These incidents involved otherwise healthy young to middle-aged adults who developed various complications while on these products; these included hypertension, arrhythmias, anxiety, tremors, insomnia, seizures, paranoid psychoses, cerebrovascular accidents, myocardial infarctions, and death (118). In 2004, the FDA banned sale of all dietary supplements containing ephedra.

17.11.2 Caffeine

Caffeine is a xanthine derivative that is used by many athletes (31,119). In a study of 520 British athletes, 36.1% reported use of creatine, while caffeine use as a sports-doping agent was reported by 23.8% (104). It may improve performance in steady-state endurance activities that rely on fat for fuel because this chemical increases lipid metabolism. It increases the release of free fatty acids from adipocytes and stimulates catecholamine activity (44,120). Studies have noted that ingestion of two to three cups of coffee (100–150 mg of caffeine per cup) increases the endurance of individuals cycling to exhaustion on bicycle ergometers. Coffee seems to reduce the perception of fatigue and allow further performance. However, an excessive amount increases sympathomimetic stimulation, which can interfere with overall athletic performance. Its diuretic effect can also interfere with such performance. Excessive amounts are banned from competition and is defined by NCAA as more than 15 mg/mL in the urine; this usually results from ingestion of six to eight cups of coffee. Other sources of caffeine include tea, over-the-counter pills for sleepiness, and some analgesic pills that contain caffeine.

17.12 Blood doping and erythropoietin (EPO)

Blood doping (blood boosting or blood packing), in which athletes receive transfusions of their own blood, is an attempt to increase aerobic performance (31,121,122). Hemoglobin levels may reach 19–20 g/dL, especially during intense competition (e.g., cycling competition at high altitudes), which leads to dehydration (44).

EPO is a renal glycoprotein that stimulates red cell production (31,121,122). Recombinant EPO (rEPO) is used to increase aerobic capacity and thus has become popular with endurance athletes (e.g., runners and cyclists) (44). rEPO is difficult to detect and has a half-life of 20 hours. As noted with blood doping, several side effects are reported, including increased blood viscosity, hypertension, coronary artery occlusion, cerebrovascular accidents, seizures, and sudden death. Dehydration from intense sports activity may trigger some of these complications. It is as effective in increasing aerobic capacity as blood doping and its use is banned (121,122).

17.13 Miscellaneous sports-doping agents

Beta-blockers (i.e., propranolol, clinetrol, and metoprolol) have been used to reduce anxiety, lessen hand tremor, control tachycardia, and reduce hypertension. Hand control is important in sports such as archery and riflery; these athletes may also use benzodiazepines and barbiturates for relief of anxiety and insomnia (44). Potential side effects of beta-blockers include various well-known cardiovascular, hematologic, central nervous system, and gastrointestinal symptomatology (5).

Ergolytic illicit drugs include alcohol (also used in small amounts for hand control), marijuana, nicotine, cocaine, amphetamines, and others (55). Nicotine may improve central nervous system attention span in some but may also worsen hand steadiness. Insulin has been misused in sports by some because of its anabolic and anticatabolic effects. Drug testing has been developed to detect this practice (123). Selective androgen receptor moderators (SARMs) are a class of drugs with the potential for use and abuse as sports-doping agents, and drug-testing technology is being developed to detect SARMs (124). A selective progesterone receptor modulator is an agent that works on the progesterone receptor with an agonist action on some tissues and an antagonist action in others. Sodium bicarbonate is an alkaline salt that has been used to delay fatigue during bouts of exercise that are limited by acidosis; this may be helpful in cases where the blood flow can increase to accommodate an increase in the by-products of increased muscles at work (17,44). Nonsteroidal anti-inflammatory agents have been used to relieve pain and allow athletes to increase their performance despite painful injuries; this can lead to greater, more permanent injuries (44). Such medications have erroneously been used to quicken healing of muscle soreness after exercise. Side effects of such medications include gastrointestinal bleeding, reduced platelet aggregation, reduced renal perfusion, increased salt/water retention, and thermal regulation dysfunction with resultant heat illness. Another agent falsely used as an anti-inflammatory agent by athletes is dimethyl sulfoxide. This chemical has been available in over-the-counter preparations and is rubbed onto sore or injured areas. Its effectiveness as an anti-inflammatory agent has never been proved by research, and its production does not occur under standards acceptable for human use.

There are many other substances sold as ergogenic agents, such as ginkgo biloba, ginseng, yohimbine (yohimbe), coenzyme Q10, and others as listed in table 17.1 (17,125). The purity and safety of these products are not guaranteed, but this does not prevent youth and other athletes from using them in high amounts. Clinicians providing sports medicine care to youth, whether through anticipatory guidance or direct sports medicine management, should educate their young patients about the never-ending hype and hyperbole of these ergogenic products (11,17,25,126).

17.14 Conclusions

The ancient Olympic Games took place from 776 BC to AD 393, and sports doping was quite common among athletes of ancient societies (5). The modern Olympic Games began in 1886 in Athens, Greece, under the influence of Baron Pierre de Coubertin who emphasized the need for sports to honor competition over winning (3). Unfortunately, the milieu of "winning is everything" persists, and athletes will accept the Goldman challenge in their pursuit of performance-enhancing drugs. Most consumed agents do not improve performance, and risks of severe adverse effects continue to complicate the Faustian dilemma that athletes at all levels face in the early 21st century. Sports doping is also a part of the greater issue of illicit drug use that is so prevalent in youth and adults of the world (52,56,57). Our children and youth must be educated about proper exercise and nutrition. They are curious about using potential sports-doping chemicals of all types (127). We must teach our children and adolescents that sports doping is neither a safe nor effective way to succeed in the game of life on or off the field (128). We need to reinstate Baron Pierre de Coubertin's view of competition over victory as the raison d'être for sports participation among our children and youth. Sports doping is an important cause of hors de combat in contemporary 21st century sports society.

Acknowledgment

Adapted with permission from: Greydanus DE, Patel DR. Sports doping in the adolescent: The Faustian conundrum of Hors de combat. Pediatr Clin North Am 2010;57:729–50.

References

1. Csaky TZ. Doping. J Sports Med Phys Fitness 1972;12(2):117–23.
2. Grollman AP. Alternative medicine: The importance of evidence in medicine and medical evidence. Foreword: Is there wheat among the chaff? Acad Med 2001;76:221–3.
3. De Rose EH. Doping in athletes: An update. Clin Sports Med 2008;27:107–30.
4. Porter R. The greatest benefit to mankind: A medical history of humanity. New York: WW Norton, 1998.
5. Botrè F, Pavan A. Enhancement drugs and the athlete. Neurol Clin 2008;26:149–67.

6. Lippi G, Franchini M, Guidi GC. Switch off the light on cycling, switch off the light on doping. Br J Sports Med 2007. Accessed January 2, 2013. URL: http://dopingjournal.org/noteworthy/achive/2007_11_01<archive.html
7. Gregory AJ, Fitch RW. Sports medicine: Performance-enhancing drugs. Pediatr Clin North Am 2007;54(4):797–806.
8. Goldman B, Bush PJ, Klatz R. Death in the locker room. London: Century, 1984:32.
9. Connor JM, Mazanov J. Would you dope? A general population test of the Goldman dilemma. Br J Sports Med 2009;43:871–2.
10. Talalay P, Talalay P. The importance of using scientific principles in the development of medicinal agents from plants. Acad Med 2001;76:175–84.
11. Greydanus DE. Use and abuse of drugs and supplements. In: Bhave S, Patel DR, Greydanus DE, eds. Sports medicine. New Delhi: Jaypee Brothers Medical Publishers, 2008:122–33.
12. Greydanus DE, Patel DR. Sports doping in the adolescent athlete. Asian J Paediatr Prac 2000; 4(1):9–14.
13. Fragakis S, Thompson C. Popular dietary supplements, 3rd ed. Chicago: American Dietetic Association, 2007.
14. Catlin DH, Fitch KD, Ljungqvist A. Medicine and science in the fight against doping in sport. J Intern Med 2008;264(2):99–114.
15. Rogol AD. Sports, hormones and doping in children and adolescents. In: Ghigo E, Lanfranco F, Strasburger CH, eds. Hormone use and abuse by athletes. New York: Springer, 2011;51–62.
16. Castillo EM, Comstock RD. Prevalence of use of performance-enhancing substances among United States adolescents. Pediatr Clin North Am 2007;54(4):663–75.
17. Greydanus DE. Performance enhancing drugs and supplements. In: Patel DR, Greydanus DE, Baker R, eds. Pediatric practice: Sports medicine. New York: McGraw-Hill Medical Publishers, 2009:63–77.
18. Wang D. Understanding performance-enhancing drug use. Conn Med 2012;76(8):487–91.
19. Fitch K. Proscribed drugs at the Olympic Games: Permitted use and misuse (doping) by athletes. Clin Med 2012;12(3):257–60.
20. Petroczi A, Naughton DP. Supplement use in sport. J Occup Med Toxicol 2007;2:4.
21. Petroczi A, Naughton DP. The age-gender-status profile of high performing athletes taking nutritional supplements: Lessons for the future. J Int Soc Sports Nutr 2008;5:2.
22. American Academy of Pediatrics policy statement: Use of performance enhancing substances. Pediatrics 2005;116:1103–6.
23. Catlin DH, Murray TH. Performance enhancing drugs, fair competition and Olympic sport. JAMA 1996;276:231.
24. Clarkson PM, Thompson HS. Drugs and sport: Research findings and limitations. Sports Med 1997;24:366.
25. Sampson W. The need for educational reform in teaching about alternative therapies. Acad Med 2001;76:248–50.
26. International Olympic Committee. Accessed January 2, 2013. URL: http://www.ioc.org
27. Volek JS, Kraemer WJ. Creatine supplementation: Its effect on human muscular performance and body composition. J Strength Cond Res 1996;10:200–10.
28. Williams MH, Branch JD. Creatine supplementation and exercise performance: An update. J Am Coll Nutr 1998;17:216–34.
29. Patel DR, Greydanus DE, Pratt HD. Youth sports: More than sprains and strains. Contemp Pediatr 2001;18:45.
30. Pratt HD, Patel DR, Greydanus DE. Sports and the neurodevelopment of the child and adolescent. In: DeLee JC, Drez DD, Miller MD, eds. Orthopaedics sports medicine. Philadelphia, PA: WB Saunders, 2003:624–42.

31. Greydanus DE, Patel DR. Sports doping: Use of drugs and supplements to enhance performance. Int Public Health J 2009;1(4):1–7.
32. Dotson JL, Brown RT. The history of the development of anabolic-androgenic steroids. Pediatr Clin North Am 2007;54(4):761–9.
33. Kerr JM, Congeni A. Anabolic-androgenic steroids: Use and abuse in pediatric patients. Pediatr Clin North Am 2007;54(4):771–85.
34. Graham MR, Davies B, Grace FM, et al. Anabolic steroid use: Patterns of use and detection of doping. Sports Med 2008;38(6):505–25.
35. Sjöqvist F, Garle M, Rane A. Use of doping agents, particularly anabolic steroids, in sports and society. Lancet 2008;371(9627):1872–82.
36. Buckley WE, Yesalis CE III, Friedl KE, Anderson WA, Streit AL, Wright JE. Estimated prevalence of anabolic steroid use among male high school seniors. JAMA 1988;260:3441–6.
37. Faigenbaum AD, Zaichkowsky LD, Gardner DE, et al. Anabolic steroid use by male and female middle school students. Pediatrics 1998;101:E6.
38. Foley JD, Schydlower M. Anabolic steroid and ergogenic drugs use by adolescents. Adolesc Med State Art Rev 1993;4(2):341–52.
39. Johnson MD, Jay MS, Shoup B, et al. Anabolic steroid use by male adolescents. Pediatrics 1989;83:921–4.
40. Kindlundh AM, Isacson DG, Berglund L, et al. Doping among high school students in Uppsala, Sweden: A presentation of the attitudes distribution, side effects, and extent of use. Scand J Soc Med 1998;26:71.
41. Komoroski EM, Rickert VI. Adolescent body image and attitudes to anabolic steroid use. Am J Dis Child 1992;146:823–8.
42. Massad SJ, Shier NW, Koceja DM, et al. High school athletes and nutritional supplements: A study of knowledge and use. Int J Sport Nutr 1995;5:232.
43. Middleman AB, Faulkner AH, Woods ER, et al. High-risk behaviors among high school students in Massachusetts who use anabolic steroids. Pediatrics 1995;96:268–72.
44. Patel DR, Greydanus DE. The adolescent athlete. In: Hofmann AD, Greydanus DE, eds. Adolescent medicine, 3rd ed. Stamford, CT: Appleton Lange, 1997:607–38.
45. Pope HC Jr, Katz DL. Psychiatric and medical effects of anabolic-androgenic steroid use. Arch Gen Psychiatry 1994;51:375–82.
46. Tanner SM, Miller DW, Aongi C. Anabolic steroid use by adolescents: Prevalence, motives, and knowledge of risks. Clin J Sport Med 1995;5:109–15.
47. Rogal AD, Yesalis CE III. Anabolic-androgenic steroids and the adolescent. Pediatr Ann 1992;21:175–88.
48. Sturmi JE, Diorio DJ. Anabolic agents. Clin Sports Med 1998;17:261–82.
49. Yesalis CE, Kennedy NJ, Kopstein AN, et al. Anabolic-androgenic steroid use in the United States. JAMA 1993;270:1217–21.
50. DuRant RH, Rickert VI, Ashworth CS, et al. Use of multiple drugs among adolescents who use anabolic steroids. N Engl J Med 1993;328:922–6.
51. Monitoring the future. Accessed January 2, 2013. URL: http://www.Monitoringthefuture.org
52. Harmer PA. Anabolic-androgenic steroid use among young male and female athletes: Is the game to blame? Br J Sports Med 2010;44:26–31.
53. DuRant RH, Escobodo LG, Heath GW. Anabolic steroid use, strength training and multiple drug use among adolescents in the United States. Pediatrics 1995;96:23–6.
54. Heischober BS, Hofmann AD. Substance abuse. In: Hofmann AD, Greydanus DE, eds. Adolescent medicine, 3rd ed. Stamford, CT: Appleton Lange; 1997:703–39.
55. Schydlower M, Rogers PD. Adolescent substance abuse and addictions. Adolesc Med State Art Rev 1993;4:227–477.

56. Greydanus DE, Patel DR. Substance abuse in adolescents: Current concepts. Curr Probl Pediatr Adolesc Health Care 2005;35(3):78–98.
57. Greydanus DE, Patel DR. Substance abuse in adolescents: Current concepts. Disease-a-Month 2005;51(7):392–431.
58. Josefson D. Concern raised about performance enhancing drugs in the United States. BMJ 1998;317:702.
59. American Academy of Pediatrics. Adolescents and anabolic steroids: A subject review. Committee on sports medicine and fitness. Pediatrics 1997;99:1–7.
60. Brower KJ. Anabolic steroids. Psychiatr Clin North Am 1993;16:97–102.
61. Casavant MJ, Blake K, Griffith J, et al. Consequences of use of anabolic androgenic steroids. Pediatr Clin North Am 2007;54(4):677–90.
62. Bhasin S, Storer TW, Berman N, et al. The effects of supraphysiologic doses of testosterone on muscle size and strength in normal men. N Engl J Med 1996;335:1–7.
63. Kanayama G, Hudson JI, Pope HG Jr. Long-term psychiatric and medical consequences of anabolic-androgenic steroid abuse: A looming public health concern? Drug Alcohol Depend 2008; 98(1–2):1–12.
64. Blue JG, Lombardo JA. Steroids and steroid-like compounds. Clin Sports Med 1999;18:667–89.
65. Kashkin KB, Kleber HD. Hooked on hormones? An anabolic steroid addiction hypothesis. JAMA 1989;262:3166–70.
66. Yesalis CE III, Streit AL, Vicary JR, et al. Anabolic steroid use: Indications of habituation among adolescents. J Drug Educ 1989;19:103–16.
67. Duclos M. Use, abuse, and biomedical detection of anabolic steroids and glucocorticoids in sports. Ann Endocrinol (Paris) 2007;68(4):308–14.
68. Malone DA, Dimeff RJ, Lombardo JA, et al. Psychiatric effects and psychoactive substance use in anabolic-androgenic steroid users. Clin J Sport Med 1995;5:25–31.
69. Cohen JC. Hypercholesterolemia in male power lifters using anabolic-androgenic steroids. Phys Sportsmed 1988;16:49–59.
70. Dickerman RD, Schaller F, Prather I, et al. Sudden cardiac death in a 20-year old bodybuilder using anabolic steroids. Cardiology 1995;86:172–3.
71. Ferenchick GS. Are androgenic steroids thrombogenic? N Engl J Med 1990;322:476.
72. Fisher M, Applyby M, Rittoo D, et al. Myocardial infarction with extensive intracoronary thrombus induced by anabolic steroids. Br J Clin Pract 1996;50:222–3.
73. Kennedy MC, Lawrence C. Anabolic steroid abuse and cardiac death. Med J Aust 1993;158:346–8.
74. Luckstead EF, Greydanus DE. Use and abuse of drugs. In: Medical care of the athlete. Los Angeles: Practice Management Information, 1993:195–205.
75. Greydanus DE, Pratt HD. Psychosocial considerations for the adolescent athlete: Lessons learned from the United States experience. Asian J Paediatr Prac 2000;3:19–29.
76. Patel DR, Pratt HD, Greydanus DE. Adolescent growth, development and psychosocial aspects of sports participation: An overview. Adolesc Med State Art Rev 1998;9:425–40.
77. Mulcahey MK, Schiller JR, Hulstyn MJ. Anabolic steroid use in adolescents: Identification of those at risk and strategies for prevention. Phys Sportsmed 2010;38(3):105–13.
78. Wood RI, Stanton SJ. Testosterone and sport: Current perspectives. Horm Behav 2012;61(1): 147–55.
79. Dobs AS. Is there a role for androgenic anabolic steroids in medical practice? JAMA 1999; 281:1326–7.
80. Creatine and androstenedione – Two "dietary supplements". Med Lett Drugs Ther 1998;40:105–6.
81. Nestler JE, Barlascini CO, Clore JN, et al. Dehydroepiandrosterone reduces serum low density lipoprotein levels and body fat, but does not alter insulin sensitivity in normal men. J Clin Endocrinol Metab 1988;66:57–61.

82. Broeder CE, Quindry J, Brittingham K, et al. The Andro Project. Arch Intern Med 2000;160:3093–104.
83. Shelby MK, Crouch DJ, Black DL, Robert TA, Heltsley R. Screening indicators of dehydroepiandrosterone, androstenedione, and dihydrotestosterone use: A literature review. J Anal Toxicol 2011;35(9):635–55.
84. Di Luigi L. Supplements and the endocrine system in athletes. Clin Sports Med 2008;27:131–51.
85. Smurawa TM, Congeni JA. Testosterone precursors: Use and abuse in pediatric athletes. Pediatr Clin North Am 2007;54(4):787–96.
86. Johnson M. Anabolic steroid use in adolescent athletes. Pediatr Clin North Am 1990;37:111.
87. Buzzini S. Abuse of growth hormone among young athletes. Pediatr Clin North Am 2007;54:823–43.
88. Erotokritou-Mulligan I, Bassett EE, Kniess A, et al. Validation of the growth hormone (GH)-dependent marker method of detecting GH abuse in sport through the use of independent data sets. Growth Horm IGF Res 2007;17(5):416–23.
89. Kamboj M, Patel DR. Abuse of growth hormone by athletes. Int Public Health J 2009;3:10–8.
90. Lattavo A, Kopperud A, Rogers PD. Creatine and other supplements. Pediatr Clin North Am 2007;54(4):735–60.
91. Denham BE. Association between narcotic use and anabolic-androgenic steroid use among American adolescents. Subst Use Misuse 2009;44(14):2043–61.
92. Parr MK, Koehler K, Geyer H, et al. Clenbuterol marketed as dietary supplement. Biomed Chromatogr 2008;22(3):298–300.
93. Beckett AH. Clenbuterol and sport. Lancet 1992;340:1165.
94. Roberts CA. The impact of long-term clenbuterol on athletic performance in horses. Vet J 2009;182(3):377.
95. Hilderbrand RL. The world anti-doping program and the primary care physician. Pediatr Clin North Am 2007;54(4):701–11.
96. Barroso O, Mazzoni I, Rabin O. Hormone abuse in sports: The antidoping perspective. Asian J Androl 2008;10(3):391–402.
97. Alaranta A, Alaranta H, Helenius I. Use of prescription drugs in athletes. Sports Med 2008;38(6):449–63.
98. Rogol AD. Drugs of abuse and adolescent athlete. Ital J Pediatr 2010;36:19.
99. Stricker PR. Other ergogenic agents. Clin Sports Med 1998;17:283–97.
100. Clark JF. Creatine and phosphocreatine: A review of their use in exercise and sport. J Athletic Train 1997;32:45–51.
101. Engelhardt M, Neumann G, Berbalk A, et al. Creatine supplementation in endurance sports. Med Sci Sports Exerc 1998;30:1123–9.
102. Greenhaff P. Creatine and its application as an ergogenic aid. Int J Sport Nutr 1995;5:S100–10.
103. Grindstaff PD. Effects of creatine supplementation on repetitive sprint performance and body composition in competitive swimmers. Int J Sport Nutr 1997;7:330–46.
104. Petroczi A, Naughton DP, Mazanov J, et al. Performance enhancement with supplements: Incongruence between rationale and practice. J Int Soc Sports Nutr 2007;4(1):19.
105. Brannon TA, Adams GR, Conniff C, et al. Effects of creatine loading and training on running performance and biochemical properties of rat skeletal muscle. Med Sci Sports Exerc 1997;29:489–95.
106. Greenhaff PL, Casey A, Short AH, et al. Influence of oral creatine supplementation on muscle torque during repeated bouts of maximal voluntary exercise for men. Clin Sci 1993;84:565–71.
107. Williams M. Nutritional ergogenics and sports performance. President's Council Phys Fitness Sports Res Digest 1998;3:1–8.

108. Burke LM, Pyne DB, Telford RD. Effect of oral creatine supplementation on single effort sprint performance in elite runners. Int J Sport Nutr 1996;6:222–33.
109. Cooke WH, Grandjean PW, Barnes WS. Effect of oral creatine supplementation on power output and fatigue during bicycle ergometry. J Appl Physiol 1995;78:670–3.
110. Mujika I, Chatard JC, Lacoste L, et al. Creatine supplementation does not improve sprint performance in competitive swimmers. Med Sci Sports Exerc 1996;28:1435–41.
111. Buford TW, Kreider RB, Stout JR, Greenwood M, Campbell B, Spano M, et al. International Society of Sports Nutrition position stand: Creatine supplementation and exercise. J Int Soc Sports Nutr 2007;4:2–8.
112. Cristani A, Romagnoli E, Boldrini E. Sport's medicalization. Recenti Prog Med 2007;98(9):433–6.
113. Harris R, Sderlund K, Hultman E. Elevation of creatine in resting and exercise muscles of normal subjects by creatine supplementation. Clin Sci 1992;83:367–74.
114. Hultman E, Sderlund K, Timmons JA, et al. Muscle creatine loading in men. J Appl Physiol 1996;81:232–7.
115. Terjung RL, Clarkson P, Eichner ER, et al. American College of Sports Medicine roundtable: Physiological and health effects of oral creatine supplementation. Med Sci Sports Exerc 2000;32:706–17.
116. Keisler B, Hosey R. Ergogenic aids: An update on ephedra. Curr Sports Med Rep 2005;4:231–5.
117. Bent S, Tiedt TN, Odden MC, et al. The relative safety of ephedra compared to other herbal products. Ann Intern Med 2003;138:468–71.
118. U.S. Food and Drug Administration website. Accessed December 20, 2010. URL: http://www.fda.org
119. Burke LM. Caffeine and sports performance. Appl Physiol Nutr Metabol 2008;33(6):1319–34.
120. Duchan E, Patel ND, Feucht C. Energy drinks: A review of use and safety for athletes. Physician Sportsmedicine 2010;38:1–9.
121. Pommering TL. Erythropoietin and other blood-boosting methods. Pediatr Clin North Am 2007;54(4):691–9.
122. Jelkmann W, Lundby C. Blood doping and its detection. Blood 2011;118(9):2395–404.
123. Thevis M, Thomas A, Schanzer W. Mass spectrometric determination of insulins and their degradation products in sports drug testing. Mass SpectromRev 2007. Accessed January 2, 2013. URL: http://dopingjournal.org/noteworthy/achive/2007_11_01<archive.html
124. Thevis M, Kohler M, Maurer J, et al. Screening for 2-quinolinone-derived selective androgen receptor agonists in doping control analysis. Rapid Commun Mass Spectrom 2007;21(21):3477–86.
125. Powers SK, Hamilton K. Antioxidants and exercise. Clin Sports Med 1999;18:525–36.
126. Patel DR, Luckstead EF. Sport participation, risk taking and health risk behaviors. Adolesc Med State Art Rev 2000;11:78.
127. Petroczi A, Naughton DP. Popular drugs in sports: Descriptive analysis of the enquiries made via the Drug Information Database (DID). Br J Sports Med 2009;43:811–7.
128. Martinsen M, Bratland-Sanda S, Eriksson AK, et al. Dieting to win to be thin? A study of dieting and disordered eating among adolescent elite athletes and non-athlete controls. Br J Sports Med 2010;44:70–6.

18 Prenatal drug exposure: Maternal and fetal issues

Colleen Dodich, Shalin Patel, and Amanda Williams

Although teenage pregnancy has been on the decline, substance abuse in the pregnant adolescent population is still a problem that needs to be addressed. The rate of illicit drug use in pregnant teenagers was 20.9% for ages 15–17 and 8.2% for ages 18–25 for the combined 2010–2011 time frame. It is important to screen all women, particularly teenagers, for substance abuse during their initial obstetric visit because substance abuse can encompass all ages and socioeconomic groups. This chapter reviews the recommended screening tools that are available to the practitioner along with parameters used to determine the need for laboratory testing. Substance use, abuse, tolerance, and dependence are all defined as well. Also discussed are the main substances that are abused by this population of adolescents and the management and follow-up that are needed for each substance. The maternal, fetal, and neonatal complications caused from these substances are also addressed. The substances described in this chapter include alcohol, nicotine, marijuana, opioids, cocaine, amphetamines/methamphetamines, benzodiazepines, and inhalants.

18.1 Introduction

Teenage pregnancy has been on the decline for many years with a record low in 2010, yet the teen birthrate in the United States is still higher than most of its industrialized counterparts. The birthrate in 2010 for adolescents aged 15–19 was 34%. This is a nearly 10% drop from 2009 and the lowest number of teenage births reported in more than 60 years (1,2). Unfortunately, although teenage pregnancy is on the decline, teenage drug use during pregnancy is still a problem (see chapter 15). The rate of illicit drug use in pregnant teenagers was 20.9% for ages 15–17 and 8.2% for ages 18–25 for the combined 2010–2011 time frame. For the younger teenagers, the rate of illicit drug use is similar between those who are pregnant and those who are not (1).

It is important to screen all women, particularly teenagers, for substance abuse during their initial obstetric visit because substance abuse can encompass all ages and socioeconomic groups. This screening should then be repeated throughout the pregnancy, such as every trimester. The youngest women report the greatest substance abuse while pregnant. The American College of Obstetricians and Gynecologists promotes screening for substance abuse as a part of complete obstetric care and recommends asking all pregnant women about their use of alcohol, tobacco, and illicit drugs. Early screening and diagnosis of substance abuse or dependence can lead to earlier intervention and management, which can thus lead to improved maternal and neonatal outcomes (3).

There can be barriers to this screening process, though. First, substance abusers, particularly teenagers, may not present for prenatal care for a host of different reasons. They may not know they are pregnant, or be in denial, and they may also have a sense of guilt, shame, and/or fear surrounding the pregnancy. If substance abuse is also part of the picture, that shame, guilt, and fear can be increased. When the adolescent does present for obstetric care, they may not initially be upfront in regard to substance abuse, because they may feel that they will be reprimanded, subjected to legal consequences, have their child taken away from them, or further ostracized. They may also be in denial that their substance use is a big deal or that it will harm themselves or their unborn child. It is important for the provider to cultivate a trusting environment with the patient so that a truthful history can be obtained.

Although all illicit substance abuse is potentially harmful to both the mother and the fetus, it is important to determine the pattern of drug use for correct diagnosis, management, and monitoring of adverse effects to both the mother and baby. Substance use is considered to be sporadic consumption of a drug with no adverse effects from that usage. In some countries, sporadic alcohol use during pregnancy is not considered harmful. Per defined criteria based on the *Diagnostic and Statistical Manual of Mental Disorders*, fourth edition (*DSM-IV*), substance abuse is consumption of a drug that causes adverse effects leading to clinically significant impairment or distress to the user. It is further defined as a manifestation of one of the following criteria within a 12-month period: recurrent use resulting in failure in work, school, or home obligations; recurrent use in hazardous situations; recurrent substance-related legal problems; or recurrent social or interpersonal problems due to the substance. The frequency of use may vary depending on the substance being abused and the individual abuser's needs and wants.

Substance dependence, as defined by the *DSM-IV* criteria, includes a pattern of use that leads to impairment or distress with the manifestation of at least three of the following criteria in the past 12 months: tolerance, withdrawal symptoms, increase or more frequent usage than intended, inability to cut down when desiring to do so, exorbitant amounts of time spent in substance-related activities, decrease or cessation of important social or work-related activities due to substance use, or continued use of the substance despite knowledge of harm (both to the mother and to the fetus). Substance tolerance is defined as the need to increase the amount of drug taken to achieve the same effect (3,4).

There are numerous risk factors that should alert providers to an increased risk of substance abuse. A young age at conception is a risk factor on its own; thus all pregnant teenagers should be screened. In addition to age, a late start to prenatal care, inconsistent prenatal care, an unstable home environment, concomitant sexually transmitted infections (STIs), relational problems, and problems with school or work may signal a substance abuse problem. Also, changes in behavior during appointments, depression symptoms, weight loss, or other health concerns may point to substance abuse. If the pregnant adolescent has had other children who are no longer under her care, a partner with an abuse problem, a family history of substance abuse, a personal history of drug abuse, a history of legal problems, or a diagnosis of a mental health condition, the risk of substance abuse is increased (4).

18.2 Screening and diagnosis

When screening for substance abuse in pregnant teens, validated screening tools are recommended. Some of the usual substance abuse questionnaires may not be appropriate because it is important to know if any substances are being used during the pregnancy. The 4P's Plus Screen is a screening tool used in pregnancy to determine past or current substance use (5). If this screening tool elicits a positive response, further assessment should be done. A limitation of this screening tool is that it is copyrighted and may not be reproduced. Another screening tool is the CRAFFT Substance Abuse screen, and this is available to be used without restriction. Some research has been done on this tool, and it has been found to have a better response than the medical record and the T-ACE alcohol screen (6). This is also a preliminary screening tool, and if there are two or more positive responses, further investigation should be performed. Other screening tests that have been used in this population with varying results are the T-ACE, TWEAK, and AUDIT-C screening tools (7). It is important that with any screening tool there is a question regarding any substance use.

When asking pregnant teenagers about substance use, it is best to ask questions about legal substances, such cigarettes and alcohol, first, though depending on the age of the adolescent, these may be illegal as well. The questioning can then progress to use/misuse of over-the-counter, prescription, and herbal drugs and finally to the use of illegal substances. The questions should be asked in a neutral, respectful tone, and the provider should be sensitive in the wording of these questions. The patient may also be asked if she has any history of participation in substance abuse programs, such as Alcoholics Anonymous or Narcotics Anonymous, or participation in rehabilitation programs. If the history is positive for substance use, it is then important to find out all the substances used, the frequency of the usage, the duration of the usage, and the last time the substance(s) was used. It is also important to find out the quantity of the substance used.

Laboratory testing for drug use can be used following a positive screen, but laboratory tests have their limitations. Universal laboratory screening of pregnant adolescents is not recommended, and random testing in which the adolescent did not give consent is unethical. Although there is no consensus as to who should undergo laboratory testing, there are some clinical situations that would indicate testing. These situations would include a previous positive drug test, late prenatal care or frequently missed prenatal appointments, an unstable social environment, monitoring for methadone use, or previous involvement with child protective services.

Additional medical complications that would potentially indicate a need for testing include placental abruption, idiopathic preterm labor, idiopathic intrauterine growth restriction (IUGR), or an unexplained fetal demise. It is important to receive consent from the pregnant adolescent before performing this testing, and it is important to follow the state's requirements for testing and reporting of the test results. The adolescent should be made aware of the legal and economic implications of the testing. Consent is not needed when a pregnant adolescent presents unconscious or under the influence of a substance and that substance needs to be identified for further medical management (4).

The most common mode of testing is via the mother's urine. Blood, hair, and saliva may also be used for drug testing. Screening can be performed for a single substance or for multiple substances. The common substances tested are opiates, marijuana, amphetamines, and cocaine, although other specific substances can be tested for, based on history. Maternal urine drug testing does have limitations, most notably that it can only be used to detect recent drug use. Amphetamines and cocaine can be detected for 2–3 days, opiates can be detected for 1–3 days, phencyclidine can be detected for 7–14 days, and marijuana can be detected for 1–7 days for light use and up to 1 month for chronic moderate to heavy use (4). Alcohol is hard to screen for in a urine or blood test due to its short half-life.

In addition, there are other medications and foods that can create a false-positive drug screen. If drug testing does come back positive for a specific substance, it may be worthwhile to look for concomitant drug use at that time. Studies show that half of mothers who use illicit drugs are also using tobacco and/or alcohol (8). Drug testing can also be performed on the infant after birth. A neonatal urine drug screen can be easily obtained, and, unlike maternal testing, most times consent is not needed to test the neonate. Both hair and meconium can provide information on longer-term substance use during pregnancy.

18.3 Alcohol

Alcohol is one of the leading preventable causes of birth defects. Women who may be pregnant or may become pregnant are urged to abstain from alcohol for this reason. The Centers for Disease Control and Prevention (CDC) reports that 7.6% of pregnant women have used alcohol during pregnancy and 1.4% admitted to binge drinking during pregnancy. This is based on 2006–2010 Behavioral Risk Factor Surveillance System data (9).

There is no known safe level of alcohol use in pregnancy; therefore, women should not drink any alcohol while pregnant. Yet, binge drinking while pregnant appears to have a greater negative effect than comparable consumption of smaller amounts more frequently (9,10). A good history during the first prenatal visit that includes the use of alcohol is important. Screening tools are available to investigate the mother's level of alcohol use, as described previously. Screening tools assess for such things as the mother's alcohol tolerance, if she feels the need to cut back on drinking, how many drinks are consumed, and how often drinks are consumed. If a mother's initial screen comes back positive, intervention will be needed. Intervention includes counseling on the risks of alcohol intake during pregnancy, increasing the amount of prenatal visits, informing the pediatrician of the risk for neonatal withdrawal (11).

Alcohol crosses the placenta and is known to be damaging to the fetus. The damage ranges from short-term withdrawal symptoms to long-term chronic disorders. Withdrawal typically begins within the first 3–12 hours after delivery. Initially, the symptoms include hyperactivity, irritability, tremors, sleep disturbances, and seizures. These initial symptoms can last approximately 72 hours. During this time, the pediatrician must also watch for hypoglycemia and acidosis. After the initial 72 hours, the infant may experience up to 48 hours of a lethargic phase. Soon after, the infant may return back to normal. Treatment during this time includes symptomatic care. Infants benefit from low stimulation including dim lights, swaddling, and keeping the room quiet. Good nutrition is also important because the infant's metabolic needs are increased. Also, monitor for and correct any metabolic derangements. Benzodiazepines may be needed for treatment of seizures (11).

The long-term effects of alcohol are placed into a spectrum, termed fetal alcohol spectrum disorder, with fetal alcohol syndrome (FAS) being the most severe end of the spectrum. FAS is the most common identifiable cause of mental retardation (11) (see chapter 15). It is estimated that FAS affects anywhere from 0.2 to 2.0 cases per 1,000 live births (12). Abnormalities in several areas are required for diagnosis of FAS: poor growth, central nervous system (CNS) abnormalities, and dysmorphic facies. The infant may face poor growth starting in utero and continuing into childhood. CNS abnormalities include irritability, jitteriness, and increased response to noise, as well as permanent brain damage with resulting adverse effects to the child's neurodevelopmental outcome. The characteristic facial features include a smooth philtrum, thin vermillion boarder, and small palpebral fissures (11). The effects even extend into adolescence with significant cognitive impairment, attention-deficit/hyperactivity disorder (ADHD) symptoms (hyperactivity, impulsivity, and poor concentration), poor memory, and reasoning. Prenatal exposure to alcohol does not have to be confirmed for a diagnosis of FAS to be diagnosed.

Other less severe forms of the fetal alcohol spectrum disorder exist as well. Like FAS, the following syndromes and defects have been confirmed with prenatal alcohol exposure. Infants with partial FAS have the same facial dysmorphisms and either poor growth or CNS disturbances. Alcohol-related birth defects include the abnormal facies with structural anomalies in other organs (renal and cardiac involvement) without poor growth or CNS abnormalities. Alcohol-related neurodevelopmental disorders occur in patients without the facial abnormalities and normal growth. They do, however, show behavioral and cognitive impairment with risk for diminished memory skills and lower IQ (12). One study showed that consuming two or more drinks per day during pregnancy resulted in a 7-point decrease in IQ at 7 years of age (13).

Per the American Academy of Pediatrics (AAP), alcohol is compatible with breast-feeding, yet adverse effects (such as drowsiness, diaphoresis, weakness, a decrease in linear growth, and abnormal weight gain) may occur in infants of mothers with a high alcohol intake (14). In addition, with ingestions larger than 1 g/kg per day, the milk ejection reflex is decreased and may cause a decrease in breast milk supply (15). Yet, there are some studies suggesting that beer ingestion can increase milk production due to an increase in serum prolactin (16,17).

18.4 Tobacco

It is reported by the CDC that 13% of pregnant women reported smoking during the last 3 months of pregnancy. Of those who try to quit smoking during pregnancy, about half will relapse by the time the infant is 6 months of age (18). Screening the mother for cigarette smoking in addition to other drug use is an important part of the first prenatal visit. Cigarette smoking has been proved over time to be detrimental to the fetus. Smoking increases the risk of placental abnormalities (abruption and previa), premature rupture of membranes, preterm labor resulting in preterm delivery, low-birth-weight infants, and sudden infant death syndrome (SIDS). These complications are of concern as they increase the risk of neonatal mortality (18). In addition, studies have shown that infants exposed to tobacco in utero show increased signs of stress, hypertonicity, excitability, and irritability (19). It is uncertain if these effects are from nicotine toxicity or withdrawal.

Maternal smoking also increases the infant's risk of type 2 diabetes later in life (20). Prenatal exposure to nicotine has also been linked to an increased risk of psychiatric problems later in life including substance abuse (21). Cognitive ability has been suspected to be affected by cigarette smoke as well, but when studies were adjusted for maternal IQ and education levels, there was no significant affect on IQ. Behavioral issues increased when children were exposed to tobacco in utero, and there is an increased incidence of ADHD and conduct disorder in males. It has also been shown that the female offspring are at a greater risk of smoking later in life (22).

It has been noted that prenatal smoking is associated with other drug use. Second hand smoke is a problem as well, in utero and after birth. It has been shown that pregnant women exposed to second hand smoke were at greater risk of delivering a low birth weight infant. After the mother has delivered it is important to encourage her to continue to abstain from smoking and to decrease the infant's exposure to smoking. Secondhand smoke exposure after delivery increases the infant's risk of SIDS, upper respiratory infections, ear infections, and asthma attacks (18). In order to preserve the health of the child, as well as the mother, it is important encourage smoking cessation.

Per the AAP, breast-feeding while smoking is recommended, although under consideration. Nicotine is present in breast milk in concentrations between 1.5 and 3.0 times the simultaneous maternal blood concentration, and its elimination half-life is 60 to 90 minutes in both milk and plasma. There is no evidence to document whether this amount of nicotine presents a health risk to the nursing infant (15). Mothers who smoke have a lower breast milk supply and a lower milk fat content, and they tend to supplement with formula and wean sooner (16). A mother who wants to breast-feed is an excellent opportunity to discuss smoking cessation.

18.5 Marijuana

Marijuana is a commonly used substance worldwide with about 4% of the world's population reporting use of cannabis at least once in 2004 (23) (see chapters 8 and 16). It is also the most common illegal substance used during pregnancy in the United States (4). Even though it is a commonly used substance in pregnancy, the outcomes to the neonates are not clear. Research has shown associations but no strong evidence of adverse effects related to marijuana use in utero. One confounding factor is that there are not many people using cannabis alone (4). The Avon Longitudinal Study of Pregnancy and Childhood surveyed mothers asking about cannabis use and neonatal outcomes including late fetal and perinatal death, special care admission of the newborn infant, birth weight, birth length, and head circumference.

Results suggested that the use of cannabis during pregnancy was not associated with a greater risk of neonatal morbidity or mortality (24). Yet, infants of mothers who abused marijuana while pregnant can have neurobehavioral effects such as a decreased ability to self soothe, increased fine tremors, increased startle reflex, sleep disturbances, and increased hand-to-mouth activity (3). In addition, mothers who use marijuana may sleep heavily after use and may be unresponsive to the infant's needs. Secondhand smoke, or passive smoke, is a significant issue to the infants, though (17).

Per the AAP, breast-feeding is contraindicated with marijuana use (15). A case-control study looking at maternal marijuana use and breast-feeding found that infants exposed to marijuana in breast milk during the first month postpartum appeared to have a decrease in motor development at 1 year of age (25). An article published in the *Journal of Reproductive Medicine* looked at the transition of tetrahydrocannabinol (THC) through pregnancy and breast milk in rhesus monkeys. It was found that THC readily crossed the placenta and was also transferred in the breast milk. The infant receives 0.8% of the mother's dose per kilogram from one joint (26). Significant depressant effects were seen in the mother and the neonates if THC was ingested 1 hour prior to either birth or breast-feeding (27), although data are limited.

18.6 Opioids

Opioids are a class of natural, endogenous, and synthetic compounds that activate μ-opioid receptors in the CNS (see chapter 10). The term *opiate* refers to a subclass of alkaloid opioids. Morphine is one of the natural opioids, while endorphins, enkephalins, and endomorphone are endogenous opioids. Synthetic opioids include codeine, heroin, hydromorphone (Dilaudid), fentanyl, and methadone (28).

Opioids acutely inhibit the release of noradrenaline at synaptic terminals. Tolerance develops with chronic opioid exposure as the rate of noradrenaline release over time increases toward normal. Abrupt discontinuation of exogenous opioids results in supranormal release of noradrenaline and causes withdrawal (28).

Opioid abuse during pregnancy results in high obstetric complications and increased perinatal morbidity and mortality. Heroin and methadone are the two most commonly abused opioids in pregnancy. Fluctuations in daily opioid use due to voluntary abstinence or lack of access to the drug during pregnancy can affect the fetus as well. Abrupt blood drug level changes can result in fetal abstinence syndrome, fetal demise, premature delivery, stillbirth, and low birth weight (28,29). If a mother is abusing certain opioids, such as heroin, it is important that this is not stopped abruptly.

Prenatal opioid exposure has been associated with low birth weight and length, low head circumference at birth, and SIDS. Opioid use during pregnancy has been associated with obstetric complications including toxemia of pregnancy and antepartum hemorrhage. It also increases risk of postpartum hemorrhage (3,29). It has been shown that 55%–94% of neonates exposed to opioids in utero can suffer from opioid withdrawal syndrome (28). The constellation of clinical findings associated with opioid withdrawal has been termed the neonatal abstinence syndrome (NAS). These clinical findings are mentioned in detail figure 18.1 (28).

The clinical presentation of NAS varies with the type of opioids, the maternal drug history including last use of the drug, maternal metabolism, infant metabolism, and placental metabolism. It also depends on the use of concomitant substances such as cocaine, barbiturates, sedatives, and nicotine. NAS is more common and severe with methadone exposure in comparison to those exposed to heroin or buprenorphine (28). The onset of withdrawal symptoms depends on the half-life of the drug. Withdrawal from heroin usually begins within 24 hours of birth, while withdrawal from methadone usually begins around 24–72 hours of age. Sometimes, withdrawal effects may be delayed up to 5–7 days with both opioids (28).

NEONATAL ABSTINENCE SCORING SYSTEM

SYSTEM	SIGNS AND SYMPTOMS	SCORE		AM						PM					COMMENTS
CENTRAL NERVOUS SYSTEM DISTURBANCES	Continuous High Pitched (or other) Cry	2													
	Continuous High Pitched (or other) Cry	3													
	Sleeps <1 Hour After Feeding	3													
	Sleeps <2 Hours After Feeding	2													
	Sleeps< 3 Hours After Feeding	1													
	Hyperactive Moro Reflex	2													
	Markedly Hyperactive Moro Reflex	3													
	Mild Tremors Disturbed	1													
	Moderate-Severe Tremors Disturbed	2													
	Mild Tremors Undisturbed	3													
	Moderate-Severe Tremors Undisturbed	4													
	Increased Muscle Tone	2													
	Excoriation (Specific Area)	1													
	Myoclonic Jerks	3													
	Generalized Convulsions	5													
METABOLIC/VASOMOTOR/ RESPIRATORY DISTURBANCES	Sweating	1													
	Fever 100.4°–101°F (38°–38.3°C)	1													
	Fever> 1 01°F (38.3°C)	2													
	Frequent Yawning (>3–4 times/interval)	1													
	Mottling	1													
	Nasal Stuffiness	1													
	Sneezing (>3–4 times/interval)	1													
	Nasal Flaring	2													
	Respiratory Rate >60/min	1													
	Respiratory Rate >60/min with Retractions	2													
GASTRO-INTESTIONAL DISTURBANCES	Excessive Sucking	1													
	Poor Feeding	2													
	Regurgitation	2													
	Projectile Vomiting	3													
	Loose Stools	2													
	Watery Stools	3													
	TOTAL SCORE														
	INITIALS OF SCORER														

Figure 18.1: Modified Finnegan's neonatal abstinence scoring tool (Hudak ML, et al. Pediatrics 2012;129:e540–60). Source: Finnegan LP. Neonatal abstinence. In: Nelson NM (ed). Current Therapy in Neonatal-Perinatal Medicne. 2nd Ed. Toronto, Ontario: BC Decker, Inc, 1990.

Pregnant women addicted to heroin specifically benefit from opioid agonist therapy such as methadone maintenance treatment (MMT). It should be the standard of care for all opioid-dependent women during pregnancy (3). MMT can sustain a stable serum opioid concentration in the mother and fetus in ranges that minimizes fetal abstinence and decreases perinatal mortality. MMT also provides several additional benefits including reduction in use of illegal heroin and optimization of prenatal care and maternal health (3,28,29). But, there are few disadvantages to MMT. NAS is more severe and prolonged after methadone exposure in comparison to heroin exposure, and it is extremely unlikely to achieve successful detoxification after delivery (28).

Other slow-release opioid preparations like bupronorphine may be considered if methadone is not available. Antenatal planning for intrapartum and postpartum analgesia may be offered for all women in consultation with appropriate health care providers. Opioid detoxification should be reserved for selected women because of the high risk of relapse to opioids. Few studies have showed that opioid detoxification in the second and third trimester of pregnancy is not linked to increased adverse perinatal events if done under close observation (3,30). Thus, due to high relapse rate to opioids, detoxification is not advisable during pregnancy (3).

It is also critical to provide psychosocial support and treat comorbid medical problems including STIs and mental disorders for better pregnancy outcomes (26). Opioid-dependent women should be informed that neonates exposed to heroin, prescription opioids, methadone, or buprenorphine during pregnancy are monitored closely for symptoms and signs of neonatal withdrawal after birth.

Newborns exposed to opioids prenatally should be observed closely for withdrawal symptoms and scored based on their clinical pictures. The modified Finnegan Neonatal Abstinence Scoring System is commonly used in the United States. Neonates consistently scoring high on that scale benefit from pharmacotherapy. Morphine and methadone are first-line treatments for moderate to severe NAS followed by second-line treatment of phenobarbital in unresponsive neonates. Mild NAS can be managed by nonpharmacological interventions. Supportive care includes an environment with low stimulation such as being placed in a dark and quiet room and swaddled carefully to avoid any autostimulation (28).

The risks and benefits of breast-feeding should be weighed on an individual basis. Per the AAP, methadone is compatible with breast-feeding, but heroin is contraindicated (15). Heroin is excreted in breast milk in quantities sufficient to cause addiction. All opiates have been documented in breast milk in small amounts, and some clinical effects that may be seen include tremors, restlessness, vomiting, and poor feeding (31). Lactating mothers should use codeine with caution as some women have a genetic predisposition to convert codeine to morphine at a faster rate (3). Mothers who are enrolled in a supervised methadone maintenance program should be encouraged to breast-feed, as long as their HIV status is negative. They should abstain from breast-feeding 2–4 hours after their methadone dose (32).

Women on methadone maintenance should only breast feed for up to 5 months, after which the volume of milk consumed by the baby is large enough to supply a sedating dose of methadone to the baby and may produce NAS when breast-feeding is ceased. Chaotic substance use by a breast-feeding mother may result in the infant receiving fluctuating doses of opioids. Fluctuating levels may mean that breast-feeding is not reliable enough to be used as a method for preventing withdrawal.

18.7 Cocaine

Cocaine is an addictive CNS stimulant that prevents uptake of extracellular dopamine into the presynaptic cell by blocking its transporter, resulting in excess stimulation of dopamine receptors in the synaptic cleft (33) (see chapters 11 and 16). It is also known as "coke," "C," "snow," "flake," or "blow." A combination of cocaine and heroin is known as a "speedball" (34).

There are several research studies showing that cocaine abuse during pregnancy can increase the risk of IUGR, placental abruption, premature rupture of membrane, and premature deliveries. It also increases the risk of spontaneous abortion and precipitous delivery. Due to its vasoconstrictive effects, its abuse can increase the risk of pregnancy-induced hypertension (3,29). Cocaine abuse during pregnancy has also been associated with genitourinary malformations, fetal demise, and intracranial bleeding in neonatal period. In addition, it has associated with low birth weight and length and microcephaly (3,29,35).

An abstinence syndrome after intrauterine exposure to CNS stimulants like cocaine and amphetamine has not been clearly defined. Several studies have showed that cocaine-exposed infants had no clinically significant withdrawal signs (28).

Cocaine abuse is a complex problem like any other substance abuse. Management of cocaine abuse should be systematic and should be focused on medical management as well as psychosocial aspects. There are two main phases to the management for cocaine abuse during pregnancy. The first phase includes treatment of withdrawal symptoms with the cessation of the drug. Sometimes, women may benefit from a supportive admission to a nonmedical withdrawal management center (3). The second phase focuses on prevention of a relapse by providing psychosocial support for abstinence in addition to treating comorbid medical problems including STIs and mental disorders. (3) Currently, there are no U.S. Food and Drug Administration–approved pharmacological treatment options available to treat cocaine abuse and to help with cessation and withdrawal symptoms. A few medications including vigabatrin, tiagabine, topiramate, modafinil, and disulfiram have shown reduction in cocaine use in controlled clinical trials (34).

Behavioral interventions are the mainstay of management for cocaine abuse. Contingency management or motivational incentives have proved to be an effective treatment for cocaine dependence, especially during the achievement of initial abstinence. Cognitive behavior therapy (CBT) is also a very effective approach to prevent relapse (34).

Per the AAP, cocaine is contraindicated in breast-feeding due to its vasoconstrictive effects (15). Cocaine is excreted into breast milk in fairly high concentrations and has been detected in the serum of breast-fed babies. Effects on the infant include irritability, vomiting, diarrhea, tremors, and seizures (31). Mothers should be advised that it is best to abstain from cocaine use while nursing (3).

18.8 Methamphetamine/amphetamines

Amphetamines are also CNS stimulants (see chapters 10 and 11). They are different from cocaine in terms of mechanism and have a prolonged half-life up to 12 hours. They reverse the actions of monoamine transporters and enhance the release of dopamine, norepinephrine, and serotonin into the synaptic cleft, increasing their availability to act on postsynaptic receptors. Ampetamines can also block the reuptake and degradation of these neurotransmitters, further increasing their concentrations in the synaptic cleft (33). Methamphetamine is commonly known as "speed," "meth," "chalk," "ice," "crystal," "crank," and "glass" (36).

There are very few studies showing the consequences of prenatal methamphetamine abuse. However, methamphetamine abuse during pregnancy has been associated with IUGR, fetal demise, and placental abruption at the same rate as cocaine abuse (28). Due to its vasoconstrictive effects, its abuse can increase the risk of pregnancy-induced hypertension. Methamphetamine abuse during pregnancy has been associated with several congenital anomalies involving the CNS and cardiovascular systems, oral clefts, and limb anomalies (3,29). Prescription amphetamines should also be avoided during pregnancy due the pregnancy-related complications and the risk of perinatal mortalities (29).

Behavioral therapies like CBT and contingency management are also very effective for the management for amphetamine abuse. Currently, there are no specific pharmacological options available that help to reduce abuse and prevent relapse. Bupropion has shown some effectiveness in clinical trials by reducing the methamphetamine-induced "high" and drug cravings (36).

An abstinence syndrome after intrauterine exposure to CNS stimulants like cocaine and amphetamines has not been clearly defined. One study showed that only 4% of infants exposed to methamphetamine in utero were treated for drug withdrawal, but concomitant abuse of other drugs could not be excluded (28). Breast-feeding should be evaluated on an individual basis because amphetamines have been shown to cross through breast milk (37). Effects on the infant from the contaminated breast milk include irritability and a poor sleeping pattern (31). Breast-feeding is contraindicated when the mother is taking in high doses of the drug, due to the vasoconstrictive properties (15).

18.9 Benzodiazepines

Benzodiazepines are one of the most common classes of anxiolytic drugs used in the United States and are commonly prescribed to women of reproductive age and to pregnant women (see chapter 10). When benzodiazepines are used in pregnancy and lactation, the benefits to the mother have to be weighed against the risks to the fetus and neonate. These drugs are classified into three different groups: long acting, intermediate acting, and short acting. The effects of these drugs, although not fully described physiologically, appear to be mediated through the inhibitory neurotransmitter gamma-aminobutyric acid. The drugs appear to act on the CNS to produce sedative and hypnotic effects, reduction of anxiety, anticonvulsant effects, and skeletal muscle relaxation (38).

All benzodiazepines diffuse readily through the placenta and pass through breast milk. The amount that passes through depends on the specific drug. Among the whole drug class, the most studied drug is diazepam. Several studies have shown an increased risk of oral clefts in fetuses of mothers who used diazepam in the first trimester of their pregnancy, although the results of this connection are not universally accepted. Studies also have shown an increased risk of low birth weight and microcephaly (38,39). A neonatal withdrawal syndrome has been reported among infants exposed to diazepam during labor for preeclampsia, eclampsia, and sedation in the mother and has also been seen with more prolonged use of the lower dosages that are commonly prescribed for anxiety disorders. This syndrome can present a few days to a few weeks after birth and can last up to several months. Symptoms of neonatal withdrawal include hypertonia, hyperreflexia, restlessness, irritability, abnormal sleep patterns, inconsolable crying, tremors or jerking of the extremities, bradycardia, cyanosis, suckling difficulties, apnea, risk of aspiration of feeds, diarrhea and vomiting, and growth retardation (39). In addition, acute use of diazepam during labor and delivery can lead to "floppy baby syndrome," which includes hypothermia, lethargy, respiratory problems, and feeding difficulties, in addition to other withdrawal symptoms.

Per the AAP, the risk of breast-feeding while taking benzodiazepines is unknown and it may be of concern (15). Published data regarding these drugs are highly variable. Neonatal withdrawal symptoms have been noted after exposure to alprazolam (Xanax) during breast-feeding, but the drug has a relatively short half-life. Long-acting benzodiazepines such as diazepam and its metabolites can accumulate in infants and have the potential to cause lethargy, sedation, and weight loss in infants. If an infant is abruptly weaned or the mother has rapid cessation of long-term treatment/use, this may cause infant withdrawal symptoms. If breast-feeding is going to be accomplished while a mother is taking a benzodiazepine, it is best to wait 6–8 hours after a single dose of the drug before nursing.

18.10 Inhalants

Inhalant abuse is prevalent in the adolescent population, particularly in younger adolescents. Nearly 20% of middle school and high school students have experimented with inhalants. Abused substances include fuels, solvents, propellants, glues, adhesives, and paint thinners (40). Inhalant abuse can produce a wide variety of physical and psychiatric side effects and when used during pregnancy can lead to fetal abnormalities. There is an increased risk of spontaneous abortion in pregnant adolescents who abuse inhalants. In addition, it can cause fetal solvent syndrome, which includes symptoms of low birth weight, microcephaly, abnormal brain development, dysmorphic facies, and muscle tone abnormalities (41). These symptoms are similar to those seen in FAS. Studies have also shown long-term residual deficits in speech, motor, and cognitive delays (42).

Management of inhalant abuse includes strict abstinence from the substance and supportive care. Counseling and support groups can also be offered. It is important to screen for other substance use because inhalants are often a gateway to other illicit drugs. Withdrawal symptoms in the neonate are still being studied, but tremors, malaise, and gastrointestinal symptoms have been documented (3). It is important for these infants to be closely monitored for alcohol-like withdrawal symptoms.

The AAP has not thoroughly reviewed inhalants and breast-feeding, but many solvents that are used as inhalants will readily cross over into the breast milk, and they do have short half-lives. An infant's nervous system continues to develop after birth, and nursing infants may be more sensitive to the neurotoxic effects of solvents (43).

18.11 Conclusions

It is important to thoroughly screen all pregnant adolescents for substance use and abuse. It is also important to develop a trusting relationship with the adolescent so that an honest and complete history can be obtained. Depending on the substance that is being abused, the effects on the mother, fetus, and neonate can vary widely. Substance-using women need additional support from their health care providers during the postpartum period to address their complex medical and psychosocial needs. They need support with breast-feeding, follow-up of medical problems including mental problems and STIs, support with child protective services involvement, and assessment of substance use and encouragement to continue attending a drug treatment program.

References

1. Hamilton BE, Ventura SJ. Birth rates for U.S. teenagers reach historic lows for all age and ethnic groups. NCHS data brief, no 89. Hyattsville, MD: National Center Health Statistics, 2012.

2. Substance Abuse and Mental Health Services Administration. Results from the 2011 National Survey on Drug Use and Health: Summary of national findings. NSDUH Series H-44, HHS Publication No. (SMA) 12–4713. Rockville, MD: Substance Abuse Mental Health Services Administration, 2012.
3. Chasnoff IJ, McGourty RF, Bailey GW, Hutchins E, Lightfoot SO, Pawson LL et al. The 4P's Plus screen for substance use in pregnancy: Clinical application and outcomes. J Perinatol 2005;25(6): 368–74.
4. Chang G, Orav EJ, Jones JA, et al. Self-reported alcohol and drug use in pregnant young women: A pilot study of associated factors and identification. J Addict Med 2011;5:221.
5. Burns E, Gray R, Smith LA. Brief screening questionnaires to identify problem drinking during pregnancy: A systemic review. Addiction 2010;105:601.
6. CDC. Alcohol use and binge drinking among women of childbearing age. United States, 2006–2010. MMWR 2012;61(28):534–8.
7. Sielski LA. Infants of mothers with substance abuse. In: Basow DS, ed. UpToDate. Waltham, MA: UpToDate, 2012.
8. CDC. Fetal alcohol spectrum disorder. Accessed January 2, 2013. URL: http://www.cdc.gov/ncbddd/fasd/index.html
9. Streissguth AP, Barr HM, Sampson PD. Moderate prenatal alcohol exposure: Effects on child IQ and learning problems at age 7 1/2 Years. Alcohol Clin Exp Res 1990;14(5):662–9.
10. Ebrahim SH, Gfroerer J. Pregnancy-related substance use in the United States during 1996-1998. Obstet Gynecol 2003;101:374.
11. CDC. PRAMS and smoking. Accessed Jan 2, 2013. URL: http://www.cdc.gov/prams/Tobaccoand-Prams.htm
12. Montgomery SM, Ekbom A. Smoking during pregnancy and diabetes mellitus in a British longitudinal birth cohort. BMJ 2002;324(7328):26–7.
13. Ernst M, Moolchan E, Robinson M. Behavioral and neural consequences of prenatal exposure to nicotine. J Am Acad Child Adolesc Psychiatry 2001;40(6):630–41.
14. Chang G. Overview of illicit drug use in pregnant women. In: Basow DS, ed. UpToDate. Waltham, MA: UpToDate, 2012.
15. Bailey JA, DuPont RL, Teitelbaum SA. Cannabis use disorders: Epidemiology, comorbidity and pathogenesis. In: Basow DS, ed. UpToDate. Waltham, MA: UpToDate, 2012.
16. Fergusson DM, Horwood LJ, Northstone K, et al. Maternal use of cannabis and pregnancy outcome. BLOG 2002;109(1):21.
17. Astley SJ, Little RE. Maternal Marijuana use during lactation and infant development at one year. Neurotoxicol Teratol 1990;12(2):160–8.
18. Asch RH, Smith CG. Effects of delta 9-THC, the principal psychoactive component of marijuana, during pregnancy in the rhesus monkey. J Reprod Med 1986;31(12):1071–81.
19. Hudak ML, Tan RC. Neonatal drug withdrawal. Am Acad Pediatrics 2012;101(6):540–60.
20. Luty J, Nikolaou V, Bearn J. Is opiate detoxification unsafe in pregnancy? J Subst Abuse Treat 2003;24(4):363–7.
21. Minnes S, Lang A, Singer L. Prenatal tobacco, marijuana, stimulant, and opiate exposure: Outcomes and practice implications. J Natl Inst Drug Abuse 2011;6(1):57–70.
22. National Institute on Drug Abuse. Cocaine: Abuse and addiction. National Institute on Drug Abuse Research Report Series, 10(4166). Accessed January 2, 2013. URL: http://www.drugabuse.gov/publications/research-reports/cocaine-abuse-addiction
23. National Institute on Drug Abuse. Methamphetamine abuse and addiction. National Institute on Drug Abuse Research Report Series, 06(4210). Accessed January 2, 2013. URL: http://www.drugabuse.gov/publications/research-reports/methamphetamine-abuse-addiction
24. Slutsker L. Risks associated with cocaine use during pregnancy. Obstet Gynecol 1992;79(5, Pt1): 778–89.

25. Thompson BL, Levitt P, Stanwood GD. Prenatal exposure to drugs: Effects on brain development and implications for policy and education. Nat Rev Neurosci 2009;10:303–12.
26. Wong S, Ordean A, Kahan M. Substance use in pregnancy. J Obstet Gynaecol Can 2011;33(4):367–84.
27. Steiner E, Villen T, Hallberg M, Rane A. Amphetamine secretion in breastmilk. Eur J Clin Pharmacol 1984;27:123–4.
28. Shor S, Nulman I, Kulaga V, Koren G. Heavy in utero ethanol exposure is associated with the use of other drugs of abuse in a high-risk population. Alcohol 2010;44:623.
29. American Academy of Pediatrics Committee on Drugs. Transfer of drugs and other chemicals into human milk. Pediatrics 2001;108:776.
30. Section of Breastfeeding. Breastfeeding and the use of human milk. Pediatrics 2012;129:e827.
31. Law KL, Stroud LR, LaGasse LL, et al. Smoking during pregnancy and newborn neurobehavior. Pediatrics 2003;111:1318.
32. Maier SE, West JR. Drinking patterns and alcohol-related birth defects. Alcohol Res Health 2001;25:168.
33. Anderson CE, Loomis GA. Recognition and Prevention of Inhalant Abuse. Am Fam Physician 2003;68(5):869–74.
34. Jones HE, Balster RL. Inhalant abuse in pregnancy. Obstet Gynecol Clin North Am 1998;25:153–67.
35. Howard MO, Bowen SE, Garland LE, et al. Inhalant use and inhalant use disorders in the United States. Addict Sci Clin Pract 2011;6(1):18–31.
36. American Academy of Pediatrics Committee on Drugs. Transfer of drugs and other chemicals into human milk. Pediatrics 2001;108(3):776–89.
37. Ho E, Collantes A, Kapur BM, Moretti M, Koren G. Alcohol and breast feeding: Calculation of time to zero level in milk. Biol Neonate 2001;80(3):219–22.
38. Hale TW. Medications and mother's milk: A manual of lactational pharmacology, 11th ed. Amarillo, TX: Pharmasoft Medical, 2004.
39. Royal Women's Hospital Drug Information Centre. Misuse of drugs in pregnancy and breastfeeding. Carlton, Victoria: Royal Women's Hospital, 2003.
40. Anderson PO. Drugs and breastfeeding. In: Anderson PO, Knoben JE, Troutman WG, eds. Handbook of clinical drug data, 10th ed. New York: McGraw-Hill, 2002.
41. Liston J. Breastfeeding and the use of recreational drugs-alcohol, caffeine, nicotine and marijuana. Breastfeed Rev 1998;6(2):27–30.
42. McElhatton PR. The effects of benzodiazepine use in pregnancy and lactation. Reprod Toxicol 1994;8(6):461–75.
43. Iqbal MM, Sobhan T, Ryals T. Effects of commonly used benzodiazepines on the fetus, the neonate, and the nursing infant. Psychiatr Serv 2002;53(1):39–49.

Section IV: **New challenges and policy**

19 New drugs of abuse in the 21st century

Joseph L. Calles, Jr.

There has been an increased awareness by health care providers that today's youth are purchasing and using drugs that are synthesized and marketed specifically to circumvent current drug laws. This chapter provides an overview of several such compounds, including synthetic cannabinoids, nonamphetamine stimulants, dissociative anesthetics, and hallucinogens, that may be used by adolescents and young adults. The information presented should help to inform clinical assessment and facilitate earlier referrals for treatment.

19.1 Introduction

There is evidence that psychoactive substances have been used by humans for millennia (1). The original sources of mind-altering drugs were – and still are – found in the natural environment, with the majority being plant based. It can be argued that the current, worldwide problem with drug abuse has its origins in three interactive factors: our inherent neurochemical makeup (i.e., neurotransmitters, such as dopamine and serotonin), the availability of purer and more potent forms of drugs (e.g., morphine derived from opium), and more efficient delivery systems (e.g., intravenous needles vs. oral ingestion) (2).

What has complicated and exacerbated the contemporary drug problem is the development of multiple synthetic substances that mimic the actions of the traditional drugs of abuse (e.g., marijuana, stimulants, hallucinogens, etc.), but in a much more powerful – and potentially dangerous – manner. As will be described in the chapters that follow, the production of constantly evolving variants of abusable drugs carries with it untold human costs and creates a myriad of legal issues. This chapter will focus on the descriptions of several of the synthetic drugs of abuse that currently are, or may be, used by adolescents, as well as the implications for future drug development and availability.

19.2 Cannabinoids

It should come as no surprise that marijuana remains the most commonly abused drug by adolescents, with daily use in a U.S. sample by 1.3%, 3.6%, and 6.6% of 8th, 10th, and 12th graders, respectively (3) (see chapter 8). What is surprising, and very concerning, is that 11.4% of adolescents, from that same sample, had also tried synthetic marijuana (3). Synthetic cannabinoids (CBs) were developed to further explore the structures and functions of the CB receptors, not as drugs of abuse. Unfortunately, the chemical formulas became available on the Internet,

Table 19.1: Chemical classes of cannabinoids (7) and representative compounds*

1. Tetrahydrocannabinols (classical cannabinoids) – natural or synthetic analogues (e.g., HU-210, nabilone)
2. Naphthoylindoles (e.g., JWH-015, JWH-018, JWH-019, JWH-073, JWH-081, JWH-122, JWH-200, JWH-210, JWH-387, JWH-398, AM-1220, AM-2201)
3. Naphthylmethylindoles (e.g., JWH-175, JWH-184)
4. Naphthoylpyrroles (e.g., JWH-146, JWH-147)
5. Naphthylmethylindenes (e.g., JWH-176)
6. Phenylacetylindoles (e.g., JWH-250, JWH-251, JWH-253)
7. Cyclohexylphenols (e.g., cannabicyclohexanol [CP 47,497-C8]; CP 47,497; CP 55,940)
8. Benzoylindoles (e.g., AM-694, RCS-4)
9. WIN 55,212–2 (an aminoalkylindole)

*See text for the descriptions of the letters associated with the individual compounds.

with subsequent production of the actual compounds, by amateur chemists, for recreation and/or profit. The concerns regarding the use of synthetic CBs include the lack of testing in humans for long-term effects, their greater potency when compared to natural marijuana, and emerging reports of serious toxic reactions, including psychosis (4), seizures (5), and myocardial infarction (6).

One of the inherent problems in monitoring the use of, and the adverse effects from, the synthetic CBs is that they are sold as incense under various names, including Spice and K-2, the brand names of which (especially Spice) have come to be generically used to refer to any "incense" blend that contains synthetic CBs. It is obvious that these blends are not incense in the traditional sense, as they are not burned to scent the air, but are smoked to "get high." An important task for clinicians is to try and determine which type of CB has been used by their patients, given the variety of chemical compounds, and their varying strengths of cannabimimetic activity, that are readily available for retail purchase. Table 19.1 lists the nine categories of CBs that were banned by the state house of representatives in Kansas, the first U.S. state to ban CBs by broad chemical classes, rather than by individual compounds (7).

The active component of marijuana (cannabis) is Δ9-tetrahydrocannabinol (Δ9-THC). Its analogues include the antiemetics/appetite enhancers (for those receiving cancer chemotherapy) (-)-Δ9-THC (dronabinol; Marinol) and its analogue nabilone (Cesamet), both of which have low abuse potential (8,9). Another Δ9-THC analogue, HU-210, is at least 100 times more potent than the natural chemical, has great potential for causing abuse and addiction, and has been found in some Spice blends. This molecule was synthesized in 1988 by Mechoulam, and colleagues, at the Hebrew University (thus the "HU" designation) (8,10).

Several synthetic CBs are designated as "JWH" molecules because they were synthesized by John W. Huffman, a research chemist at Clemson University, in the 1980s (10). The most extensively studied compound from that laboratory is the naphthoylindole JWH-018, which continues to appear in Spice blends, despite its illegal status in many countries (5). The Spice manufacturers have liked using JWH-018 in their blends because it is very potent when compared to Δ9-THC. Unlike Δ9-THC, which is a partial agonist at the CB1 receptor, JWH-018 is a full agonist and has a four times greater affinity for the receptor than does Δ9-THC (10). Two newer naphthoylindole cannabimimetic molecules, AM-1220 and AM-2201, were synthesized by Alexandros Makriyannis (therefore the "AM" designation), a bioorganic chemist at Northeastern University. They have recently been showing up in some Spice blends, and AM-2201 was one of the four synthetic CBs identified in the mixture that caused seizures in a young adult male (5). As can be seen in table 19.1, Drs. Huffman and Makriyannis have synthesized cannabinoid agonist compounds in several other chemical classes.

Another group of research cannabinoids are the cyclohexylphenols, such as CP 47,497, its C8 homologue CP 47,497-C8 (cannabicyclohexanol) and CP 55,940 (8,10). These were developed by the Charles Pfizer ("CP") company (now Pfizer Inc.) in the 1970s but have only recently found their way into Spice blends. These compounds are also very potent when compared to the natural Δ9-THC.

Two other compounds of note are the benzoylindole RCS-4 (an analogue of JWH-018) and the aminoalkylindole WIN 55,212–2. The original source of the RCS series of synthetic CBs is unclear, but it may have been the company named Research Chemical Supplier. Due to its potential hazards to health, the use of RCS-4 has been banned in several countries. The origin of the WIN series is well-known, that being the former Sterling Winthrop Pharmaceuticals company, which is now a part of Sanofi S.A. WIN 55,212–2 is a potent full agonist of the CB1 receptor (9).

In summary, there are numerous CBs that have been synthesized (e.g., there about 60 compounds in the JWH series and about 40 in the AM series). Given the complexity of the chemical compounds that are discussed in this section, and the multiple ways in which those molecules can be modified, there will undoubtedly be many more cannabimimetic compounds in the future. One of the obvious concerns is the potential for acute and long-term adverse effects, especially given that many of these compounds are several times more powerful than naturally occurring cannabis, which already contributes to the risk of adolescent users developing neuropsychiatric disorders (11).

19.3 Stimulants

In the recently published Youth Risk Behavior Surveillance, researchers found that 3.8% of students had used methamphetamines at least once during their lifetime (12) (see chapters 9, 10, 11, and 16). A positive aspect of the report is that from 1999 through 2011, among U.S. high school students, there was a significant linear decrease in the prevalence of use of methamphetamines (9.1%–3.8%). Unfortunately, methamphetamines are not the only stimulant drugs that can be abused. Comparable to the

Table 19.2: Chemical classes of stimulants (19) and representative compounds

1. Piperazines
   a) Benzylpiperazines (e.g., BZP, MBZP)
   b) Phenylpiperazines (e.g., mCPP, pFPP, TFMPP)
2. Phenethylamines
   a) Methyl derivatives (e.g., amphetamine, methamphetamine, phentermine)
   b) Hydroxyl derivatives (e.g., phenylpropanolamine, ephedrine/pseudoephedrine)
   c) Ketone derivatives (e.g., cathinone and methcathinone, which are derived from the Khat plant, *Catha edulis*, and are naturally occurring analogues of amphetamine. Synthetic versions include methedrone and methylone.)
   d) Methylenedioxy derivatives (e.g., MDA, MDMA ["Ecstasy"])
   e) Methoxy derivatives (e.g., mescaline*)
3. Pyrovalerones (e.g., MDPV)
4. Naphthylpyrovalerones (e.g., naphyrone, Bromo-Dragonfly*)
5. Cocaine and synthetic cocaines (e.g., pFBT, dimethocaine)

*These are also hallucinogens.

increased availability of synthetic CBs, in recent years several amphetamine-like compounds have been manufactured abroad and sold legally as "party pills," or as "bath salts," which are not put into bathwater but instead are ingested, inhaled, smoked, or injected. Also comparable to the use of synthetic CBs, the use of "bath salts" can produce several toxic reactions, including agitation, tachycardia, psychosis, and even death (13). Table 19.2 lists the chemical classes of stimulants and some representative compounds.

The piperazine stimulants first appeared in Europe, sold as "party pills" commonly containing benzylpiperazine (BZP) or trifluoromethylphenylpiperazine (TFMPP) (14,15). In New Zealand, a product called "the Good Stuff" contained both BZP and TFMPP (16), which together have demonstrated pharmacological effects similar to 3,4-methylenedioxy-N-methylamphetamine (MDMA or "Ecstasy") (17). Another piperazine, meta-chlorophenylpiperazine (mCPP), also has effects similar to MDMA and, in Europe, has been sold in combination with MDMA or in some cases has totally replaced MDMA, in pills sold as Ecstasy (18). Other drugs of abuse in this family include MDBP (the methylene dioxy analogue of BZP) and 1-(4-methoxyphenyl)piperazine (MeOPP) (19), with the potential for several other analogues to be synthesized. One obvious concern about the use of these drugs is that young people who are purchasing them (often via the Internet) may be getting chemical compounds that can have unintended consequences, including agitation, anxiety, confusion, tremor, insomnia, seizures, and even severe multiorgan toxicity (15).

The phenethylamines are a diverse group of stimulatory compounds that includes common drugs of abuse, such as the amphetamines, MDMA (Ecstasy), and mescaline (20). One particular subgroup is the ketone derivatives, which includes cathinone, the major psychoactive alkaloid from the Khat plant (*Catha edulis*) and a naturally occurring analogue of amphetamine. There are many synthetic cathinones that have been produced, several of which have found their way into "bath salts" (21). Another synthetic cathinone group, the pyrovalerones, can be modified to produce the pyrrolidine derivative 3,4-methylenedioxypyrovalerone (MDPV) (22), which was the active compound found in the "bath salts" used in Michigan and the "primary factor contributing to (the) death" of one of its users (13). Given the potential dangers associated with their use, in late 2011 the U.S. Drug Enforcement Administration temporarily placed the synthetic cathinones mephedrone, methylone, and MDPV into Schedule I of the Controlled Substances Act (23). There is no doubt that illegal labs will continue to produce variants of these drugs for profit.

19.4 Dissociative anesthetics

The dissociative anesthetics were developed for use during surgical procedures, but their use has been limited by serious adverse effects, including psychosis. One of the popular dissociative drugs has been phencyclidine (PCP; "angel dust"), the use of which had its heyday in the 1970s, but which never went away completely. The use of PCP has enjoyed a slight resurgence in recent years as young people have rediscovered its mind-altering properties (see chapter 12). In the national Monitoring the Future survey, in 2011, 2.3% of 12th graders reported having used PCP at some point during their lifetime (3). Of equal concern is that 17.2% of those same respondents said that PCP was "fairly easy" or "very easy" to obtain. Other data are somewhat more reassuring, as the trend for first-use of PCP by young people (aged 12 years or older) is decreasing, from 123,000 individuals in 2002 to 45,000 in 2009 and 2010 (24). However, analogues of PCP have been synthesized (table 19.3), and more are likely to be available in the future, to be used by those who are always looking for "the next high."

Ketamine ("Special K") is a dissociative agent that has legitimate medical uses in humans and in nonhuman species (25) (see chapter 12). It has also become a drug of abuse. In 2011, 1.7% of 12th graders reported having used ketamine at some point during the year preceding the survey (3). Ketamine offers some advantages over PCP in that it has a wide margin of safety, even in cases of overdose, because it does not appreciably alter respiratory functions (25). It should not, however, be considered a benign drug, because it can cause depression, psychosis, and cognitive dysfunction (25). Recently, in Europe, there have been reports of a ketamine analogue, methoxetamine (MXE), which is available through Internet vendors (26). Although little is known about this drug, MXE appears to be similar in its effects to ketamine, but with a longer duration of action.

Table 19.3: Dissociative anesthetics and representative compounds

1. Phencyclidine (PCP) and analogues (e.g., 4-methoxyphencyclidine [methoxydine, 4-MeO-PCP], 3-methoxyphencyclidine [3-MeO-PCP])
2. Ketamine and analogues (e.g., methoxetamine)
3. Dextromethorphan (DXM)

Dextromethorphan (DXM) is used clinically as an antitussive agent but is included in this section because it, along with PCP and ketamine, derives its psychotropic effects from antagonism of the glutamate N-methyl-D-aspartate receptor (see the chapter 10).

19.5 Hallucinogens

The hallucinogens have traditionally been classified by their chemical structures into two broad categories, the tryptamines and the phenethylamines (27) (see chapter 12). The tryptamines can be further subdivided into "simple" tryptamines (e.g., psilocybin) and the ergolines (e.g., lysergic acid diethylamide [LSD]) (table 19.4). Compared to other psychoactive drugs, the hallucinogens are unique in that the pharmacological effects are very dependent on the expectations (i.e., the mindset) of the user and on the environment (setting) in which the drug is used. Anticipating a negative experience and/or being in negative surroundings can lead to the proverbial "bad trip." Despite that possibility, many youth continue to use hallucinogens, from the 1960s-era classics LSD, mescaline, and psilocybin to newer synthetic drugs. By 2005–2006, youth in Los Angeles were already using a myriad of tryptamine and phenethylamine compounds (28).

Recently there have been reports of new hallucinogenic drugs becoming available for use in Europe. The drugs 4-HO-MET (4-hydroxy-N-methyl-N-ethyltryptamine) (29) and Bromo-Dragonfly [1-(8-bromobenzo[1,2-b;4,5b'] difuran-4-yl)-2-aminopropane] (30) are described as producing the same mind-altering effects as LSD. Given that activation of the 5-HT2A receptor seems to be crucial for the clinical effects of the hallucinogens (31), and that other serotonin receptors (5-HT2C for the phenethylamines and 5-HT1A for the tryptamines), as well as other chemical systems (e.g., glutamatergic), are involved, it is anticipated that more hallucinogenic compounds will be synthesized in the years to come.

Table 19.4: Chemical classes of hallucinogens (27,28) and representative compounds

1. Tryptamines
   a) "Simple" tryptamines (e.g., DMT, AMT, DiPT, 5-MeO-DMT, 5-MeO-AMT, 5-MeO-DiPT, DPT, 5-MeO-DPT, 4-ACO-MiPT, 4-HO-MiPT, 4-HO-DiPT, 4-HO-DPT, 4-HO-MET, ibogaine, psilocybin [the prodrug of the biologically active psilocin])
   b) Ergolines (e.g., LSD and a few very closely related compounds)
2. Phenethylamines*
   a) Phenethylamines (e.g., mescaline, 2C-B, 2C-E, 2C-P, 2-CT-7, 2-CT-2, DOI, DOB)
   b) Amphetamine (e.g., MDMA, DOM)
   c) "FLY" drugs (e.g., 2C-B-FLY, 3C-B-FLY, Bromo-Dragonfly ["B-fly"])

*These are also included in the stimulants (see table 19.2); most are not hallucinogenic.

19.6 Conclusions

The diversity and availability of newer drugs of abuse is increasing. The chemistry of the compounds is complex, but not so much that it hinders their production by clandestine laboratories and amateur chemists. Laws controlling the possession and use of drugs of abuse are being circumvented by modifying them enough to be "legal." By the time that legislation is amended to outlaw certain compounds, untold youth have tried them and placed themselves at risk for experiencing adverse effects, some of which may be serious or permanent. During that same lag in time, drug producers will have come up with other compounds to get around the law – and the cycle will continue. There are at least two ways that this problem can be addressed. Legally, the passage of laws that outlaw broad categories of drugs should slow down the production of compounds that are modifications of previously banned drugs. Clinically, the early identification of, and intervention with, youth who are at high risk for drug use and dependence needs to be incorporated into our daily practice lives. It is hoped that the information presented in this chapter will lead to a greater awareness, and better treatment, of drug-using youth in the 21st century.

References

1. Sullivan RJ, Hagen EH. Psychotropic substance-seeking: Evolutionary pathology or adaptation? Addiction 2002;97(4):389–400.
2. Nesse RM, Berridge KC. Psychoactive drug use in evolutionary perspective. Science 1997;278 (5335):63–6.
3. Johnston LD, O'Malley PM, Bachman JG, Schulenberg JE. Monitoring the Future national results on adolescent drug use: Overview of key findings, 2011. Ann Arbor: Institute Social Research, University Michigan, 2012. Accessed January 3, 2013. URL: www.monitoringthefuture.org/pubs/monographs/mtf-overview2011.pdf
4. Pierre JM. Cannabis, synthetic cannabinoids, and psychosis risk: What the evidence says. Curr Psychiatry 2011;10(9):49–57.
5. Schneir AB, Baumbacher T. Convulsions associated with the use of a synthetic cannabinoid product. J Med Toxicol 2012;8(1):62–4.
6. Mir A, Obafemi A, Young A, Kane C. Myocardial infarction associated with use of the synthetic cannabinoid K2. Pediatrics 2011;128(6):e1622–7.
7. Committee on Corrections and Juvenile Justice, Kansas House Bill 2049. Accessed January 3, 2013. URL: www.kslegislature.org/li/b2011_12/. . ./hb2049_01_0000.pdf
8. Thakur GA, Nikas SP, Makriyannis A. CB1 cannabinoid receptor ligands. Mini Rev Med Chem 2005;5(7):631–40.
9. Seely KA, Prather PL, James LP, Moran JH. Marijuana-based drugs: Innovative therapeutics or designer drugs of abuse? Mol Interv 2011;11(1):36–51.
10. Fattore L, Fratta W. Beyond THC: The new generation of cannabinoid designer drugs. Frontiers Behav Neurosci 2011;5:60.
11. Rubino T, Zamberletti E, Parolaro D. Adolescent exposure to cannabis as a risk factor for psychiatric disorders. J Psychopharmacol 2012;26:177–88.

12. Eaton DK, Kann L, Kinchen S, Shanklin S, Flint KH, Hawkins J, et al. Youth risk behavior surveillance – United States, 2011. MMWR Surveill Summ 2012;61(4):1–162.
13. Centers for Disease Control and Prevention (CDC). Emergency department visits after use of a drug sold as "bath salts" – Michigan, November 13, 2010–March 31, 2011. MMWR Morb Mortal Wkly Rep 2011;60(19):624–7.
14. Cohen BM, Butler R. BZP-party pills: A review of research on benzylpiperazine as a recreational drug. Int J Drug Policy 2011;22(2):95–101.
15. Schep LJ, Slaughter RJ, Vale JA, Beasley DM, Gee P. The clinical toxicology of the designer "party pills" benzylpiperazine and trifluoromethylphenylpiperazine. Clin Toxicol (Phila) 2011;49(3):131–41.
16. Sheridan J, Butler R, Wilkins C, Russell B. Legal piperazine-containing party pills – A new trend in substance misuse. Drug Alcohol Rev 2007;26(3):335–43.
17. Baumann MH, Clark RD, Budzynski AG, Partilla JS, Blough, BE, Rothman RB. N-substituted piperazines abused by humans mimic the molecular mechanism of 3,4-methylenedioxymethamphetamine (MDMA or 'Ecstasy'). Neuropsychopharmacol 2005;30(3):550–60.
18. Bossong MG, Brunt TM, Van Dijk JP, Rigter SM, Hoek J, Goldschmidt HM, et al. mCPP: An undesired addition to the ecstasy market. J Psychopharmacol 2010;24(9):1395–401.
19. Maurer HH, Kraemer T, Springer D, Staack RF. Chemistry, pharmacology, toxicology, and hepatic metabolism of designer drugs of the amphetamine (Ecstasy), piperazine, and pyrrolidinophenone types, a synopsis. Ther Drug Monit 2004;26(2):127–31.
20. Khan JI, Kennedy TJ, Christian DR Jr. Phenethylamines. In: Khan JI, Kennedy TJ, Christian DR Jr, eds. Basic principles of forensic chemistry. New York: Humana Press, 2012:157–76.
21. Prosser JM, Nelson LS. The toxicology of bath salts: A review of synthetic cathinones. J Med Toxicol 2012;8(1):33–42.
22. Coppola M, Mondola R. 3,4-methylenedioxypyrovalerone (MDPV): Chemistry, pharmacology and toxicology of a new designer drug of abuse marketed online. Toxicol Lett 2012;208(1):12–5.
23. Drug Enforcement Administration, Department of Justice. Schedules of controlled substances: Temporary placement of three synthetic cathinones in Schedule I. Final Order. Fed Regist 2011;76(204):65371–5.
24. Substance Abuse and Mental Health Services Administration. Results from the 2010 National Survey on Drug Use and Health: Summary of national findings. NSDUH Series H-41, HHS Publication No. (SMA) 11–4658. Rockville, MD: Substance Abuse and Mental Health Services Administration, 2011.
25. Morgan CJ, Curran HV, Independent Scientific Committee on Drugs. Ketamine use: A review. Addiction 2012;107(1):27–38.
26. Corazza O, Schifano F, Simonato P, Fergus S, Assi S, Stair J, et al. The phenomenon of new drugs on the Internet: The case of the ketamine derivative methoxetamine ('MXE'). Hum Psychopharmacol Clin Exp 2012; 27:145–49.
27. Nichols DE. Hallucinogens. Pharmacol Ther 2004;101(2):131–81.
28. Sanders B, Lankenau SE, Bloom JJ, Hathazi D. "Research chemicals": Tryptamine and phenethylamine use among high-risk youth. Subst Use Misuse 2008;43(3–4):389–402.
29. Kjellgren A, Soussan C. Heaven and hell – A phenomenological study of recreational use of 4-HO-MET in Sweden. J Psychoactive Drugs 2011;43(3):211–9.
30. Corazza O, Schifano F, Farre M, Deluca P, Davey Z, Torrens M, et al. Designer drugs on the internet: A phenomenon out-of-control? The emergence of hallucinogenic drug Bromo-Dragonfly. Curr Clin Pharmacol 2011;6(2):125–9.
31. Fantegrossi WE, Murnane KS, Reissig CJ. The behavioral pharmacology of hallucinogens. Biochem Pharmacol 2008;75(1):17–33.

20 Estimating the societal burden of substance abuse: Advantages and limitations of current methodologies

Jonathan P. Caulkins, Anna Kasunic, and Michael A. C. Lee

This chapter discusses efforts to quantify the societal burden of substance abuse (illicit drugs, alcohol, and cigarette smoking) in the United States. The literature finds that the social costs of substance abuse are very high, with monetized estimates of indirect and direct costs exceeding $700 billion per year (in 2011 dollars). Despite media focus on illicit drugs, the estimates for alcohol and tobacco are each separately at least as high, if not higher. Premature death and the indirect costs of productivity and crime-related losses drive the totals. For cigarettes, medical care expenditures are also substantial. The chapter breaks down specific cost components and considers key factors in estimating the damage from alcohol consumption and cigarette smoking. In its conclusion, the chapter illustrates how these estimates can be used in policy formation, focusing on prevention and treatment services.

20.1 Introduction

Substance abuse kills hundreds of thousands of people every year in the United States, and sends hundreds of thousands more to the emergency room; for illegal drugs, black market violence adds to the toll. Billions are spent on drug treatment and on treating associated medical complications, including HIV/AIDS. Substance abuse is implicated in a large proportion of child abuse and neglect cases and is common among youth and young adults; the 2010 National Survey of Drug Use and Health (NSDUH) estimates that of youth aged 12–17, 25% have used tobacco, 35% have used alcohol, and 26% have used illicit drugs in their lifetime, with 43% of 18-year-olds having used marijuana at least once (1).

Common sense says the societal costs of substance abuse are large, but how large are they? Studies vary on the specific figures, but all agree that the costs are high. Harwood et al. (2) produced the most frequently cited figures in the United States for alcohol and drug abuse (3), and the Centers for Disease Control and Prevention (CDC) provided a related estimate for cigarettes, which excluded cigar smoking, pipe smoking, and smokeless tobacco (4). Figure 20.1 shows all three adjusted to 2011 dollars, totaling more than $700 billion. Throughout this chapter, all dollar amounts have been inflated to 2011 dollars for ease of comparison using annual averages from the Consumer Price Index from the Bureau of Labor Statistics.

Corresponding estimates for other countries (5,6) reveal that the United States is not alone in experiencing a high societal burden of substance abuse. Among peer

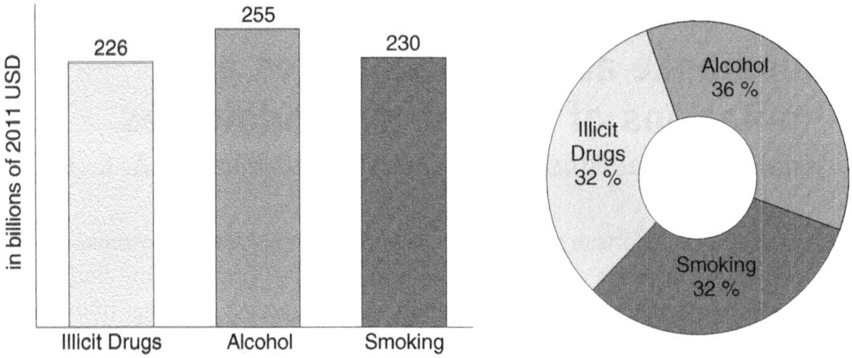

Figure 20.1: Costs of substance abuse and costs as percents of total. Sources: Illicit drugs (3), alcohol (2), smoking (4)

countries, the United States has higher rates of abuse of illegal drugs but lower rates of alcohol and tobacco consumption. This article delves into the US figures in detail, rather than dispersing attention on estimates from multiple countries, because the focus is on understanding how to interpret the figures, not on international comparisons.

20.2 The cost-of-illness (COI) approach

Monetizing social costs is tricky, as is properly interpreting the resulting figures (7). Policy makers want a number, and analysts oblige, but the numbers come with endless footnotes and more than a little controversy. What do the figures really mean? What is included? What is excluded?

Most studies take a COI approach. COI studies estimate the net value of resources a health condition makes unavailable for other purposes. They have been conducted for conditions such as heart disease, cancer, diabetes, stroke, and Alzheimer's. Studies typically include "direct" and "indirect" costs but often ignore "intangibles" such as diminished quality of life.

The COI approach has become the standard in substance abuse studies, but it is not the only or even necessarily the best method available. Economists regularly employ other valuation techniques in other areas of social policy, such as crime, education, gambling, and the environment.

To give an example of a difference, where other frameworks value illness and death in terms of lost quality of life, COI studies use productivity losses. Not all economists agree with this valuation method, but its logic is easy enough to understand. When workers go on disability leave, either someone else has to do their work or society goes without the fruits of their labor. For example, if the patient were a writer, society would be made poorer by the loss of the short story that didn't get written because the writer was too sick to work during that time.

Embedded in this view is an assumption that the economy is functioning near full employment, so lost labor leads to lost output. Someone who thought the economy offered a fixed number of jobs, with unemployment implying that there are "too many" workers relative to the number of jobs, wouldn't worry about this cost. One person's illness would create a job opening for someone else who would otherwise have been idle. Most COI scholars have a more optimistic view that the economy will always expand to take advantage of talent, and, conversely, when sickness sidelines some of that talent, total economic output shrinks.

This "human capital approach" views death as essentially equivalent to an illness that lasts until what would have been the age of retirement. If a smoking-related ailment strikes down a worker at age 50, society loses the benefit of that person's labor services for the 17 remaining years until they would have reached the retirement age of 67. COI studies ignore the fact that premature death implies that this person also does not consume resources from their own savings or from taxpayer-funded programs like Medicare and Social Security. When a disease imposes a high societal cost through premature death, it does not necessarily make survivors poorer, but it does make overall national economic output smaller, which is the focus of COI estimates.

There remains the question of how to monetize lost work time. For sickness, COI studies might view the person's current salary as a good measure, on the principle that Adam Smith's invisible hand drives salaries up or down to the point where they equal the societal value of the worker's labor (a view that can please investment bankers but distress social workers).

That approach becomes awkward in the case of premature death. As a purely technical matter, it is hard to forecast how any given individual's career would have progressed. The larger problem, though, is moral. It would mean valuing the death of a high-income individual more than the death of someone with less marketable skills; by this cruel logic, the deaths of those who were already permanently disabled are of no consequence. Instead, COI scholars assign to every life-year lost a cost equal to the national average of workers' income.

Some might still object that while this treats everyone equally, all are treated not as humans, but as mere cogs in the great industrial machine. No account is made for the pain someone suffers from cancer or from the radiation or chemotherapy that treats it. And no account is made of the sorrow dying people feel for not getting to see their children achieve various life milestones, or of family and friends who are left mourning lost loved-ones. These costs are deemed "intangibles." COI scholars are not senseless to such pain, and they are working to include intangible costs via willingness-to-pay (WTP) and quality-adjusted life year (QALY) models, but at this point, it is common to restrict estimates to direct and indirect costs on the grounds that they are more reliably quantified and so provide a more consistent yardstick for comparing across diseases.

We want to close this section by stressing that, despite our at times critical tone, we think COI studies are valuable, and that their limitations flow from the difficulty of the task, not any failings of the scholars who undertake them. Even if COI studies are imprecise by nature, we discourage readers from dismissing their worth altogether. As Erasmus noted, in the land of the blind, the one-eyed man is king; having some numbers, however imperfect, can ground analyses, allow for comparisons among substances, and highlight particular areas of concern.

20.3 What components drive the costs of abuse for each substance?

20.3.1 Cigarette smoking

Although the total estimated social costs are similar for alcohol, cigarettes, and illegal drugs, their compositions vary dramatically. For ease of exposition, we will refer to "three substances" (cigarettes, alcohol, and illicit drugs), even though the third is obviously a category of substances, not literally one drug. Likewise, the literature on the social costs of tobacco focus almost exclusively on cigarette smoking due to the small number of regular users of cigars and chewed tobacco. Working through the components of each substance uncovers additional insights. We begin with cigarettes (see chapter 7).

The costs of smoking are largely medical, unlike those of alcohol and illicit drugs. Figure 20.2 shows that the total combined social costs for illicit drugs, alcohol, and cigarettes approach those of cancer and diabetes, but their direct medical expenditures fall widely short. While the medical costs of cigarette smoking are quite high – roughly comparable to the medical costs of cancer, with which they overlap considerably – the medical costs of illicit drugs and alcohol are appreciably smaller; they even fall below direct expenditures for older adults' falls.

Smoking is also a mortality problem. Although cigarette use among young adults has declined, tobacco remains the leading cause of preventable death in the United States, averaging 443,000 deaths annually during 2002–2004 (4). To give a sense of scale, there were an estimated 39,701 alcohol-induced deaths in 2009, which includes alcoholic liver disease deaths but excludes accidents and homicides (8); 10,228 alcohol-impaired traffic fatalities in 2010 (9); and 38,371 drug-induced deaths (includes deaths from illicit, prescription, and over-the-counter drugs) in 2007 (10). Hence, estimates of the relative social cost of cigarettes versus alcohol or illegal drugs are sensitive to methodological choices concerning how one monetizes the value of a premature death.

While direct medical expenditures accounted for half of the CDC's estimated costs of smoking, the other half is indirect costs – namely, productivity losses from tobacco-related deaths (see figure 20.2). Dividing the CDC estimate of $115 billion for 2004 (4) by 443,000 deaths gives an average social cost per premature death of only about $250,000. There are reasons why the figure is so low, including that the average age at premature death from smoking is considerably older than for, say, heroin overdose. Nevertheless, the arithmetic highlights the idea that different and equally defensible approaches to monetizing things for which there is no market and, hence, no true market-based "price," can have important effects on social cost estimates.

Furthermore, the CDC estimates only the productivity losses from mortality, not morbidity, so it is an understatement of the total productivity losses. Inasmuch as the alcohol study by Harwood et al. calculates the indirect costs of morbidity as more than three times those of premature death, the CDC's exclusion of indirect morbidity losses would have quite significant effects on the total cost estimate. This is by no means to discredit the CDC's estimate, which is valuable and informative in its own right. But understanding how methodological differences that only surface upon careful reading can greatly shift where the numbers lie cautions against paying attention only to the grand total reported in the press release. It is important to "look under the hood" to appreciate the nuances involved.

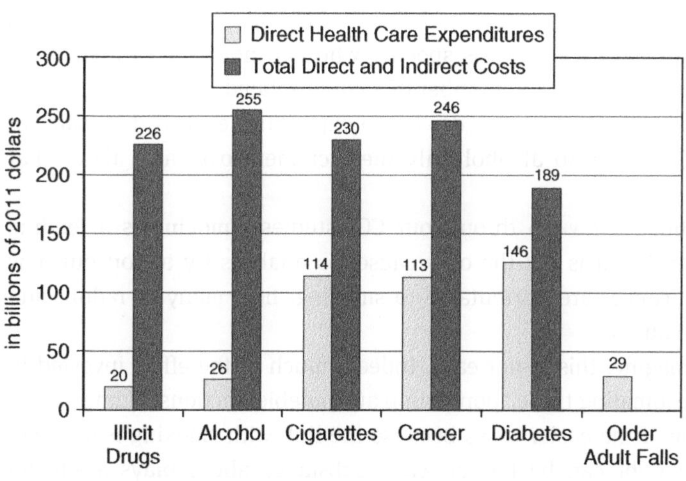

Figure 20.2: Total direct and indirect costs and direct health care expenditures associated with substance abuse and other health care problems in the United States (inflated to 2011 dollars). Sources: Illicit drugs (3), alcohol (2), cigarettes (4), cancer (11), diabetes (12), falls (13)

20.3.2 Alcohol

Alcohol is such an integral part of US culture that many have become inured to its harms (see chapters 9 and 16). Yet it wreaks awesome havoc through dependence, decreased productivity, unemployment, alcohol-related illness such as cirrhosis, and premature death. Additionally, the behavioral effects of alcohol can result in "bar brawls" and other violent crime, family strife, and motor vehicle crashes.

Youth alcohol use can be particularly deleterious. Heavy alcohol use can permanently damage the developing brain, and those who start drinking early are more likely to become alcohol-dependent adults (14). Drunk driving is a special concern; for those under 21 years, driving under the influence of alcohol results in fatal crashes two times more than for adults (14). The Institute of Medicine estimated that the 2002 social costs of underage drinking alone were $77.4 billion in inflation-adjusted 2011 dollars (14).

According to the estimate by Harwood et al. (see figure 20.3), lost earnings dominate the total costs of alcohol abuse, at 73% of the total. The wedge for fetal alcohol syndrome is small but raises a general issue. Some of the societal costs are borne by those who consume the substance; others are not. COI studies pay no attention to that difference, but it matters from some other perspectives.

Alcohol's next largest wedge pertains to traffic crashes. In 2010, according to the National Highway Transportation Safety Administration, 10,228 people perished in crashes involving a driver with a blood alcohol content of 0.08 or higher (9).

Those are alcohol-related crashes, but COI studies focus on costs of crashes that are not only related but also actually attributable to alcohol. The distinction is that in some crashes involving alcohol-impaired drivers, the alcohol-impairment in no way caused the crash. For example, an alcohol-impaired driver stopped at a light might be rear-ended by a reckless speeder who had not been drinking. COI studies try to subtract from the total number of alcohol-related crashes the number one would have expected the drinking drivers to experience even if they had not been drinking and attribute to alcohol only the increment over and above that baseline.

Similar calculations show up throughout COI studies. Smoking is a leading cause of lung cancer, but it is not the only cause. So analysts try to sort out how many cases of lung cancer are attributable to smoking, how many to radon, and how many to other causes.

As one might imagine, this is not easy. Indeed, much of the effort invested in COI studies goes to estimating these "population attributable fractions." Lung cancer is in some sense one of the easier cases because the link with smoking is so clear. Getting the fraction right can be harder when substance abuse plays a smaller role. For example, the CDC reports that there are about the same number of smoking-attributable fatalities each year for pneumonia and influenza (10,423) as for

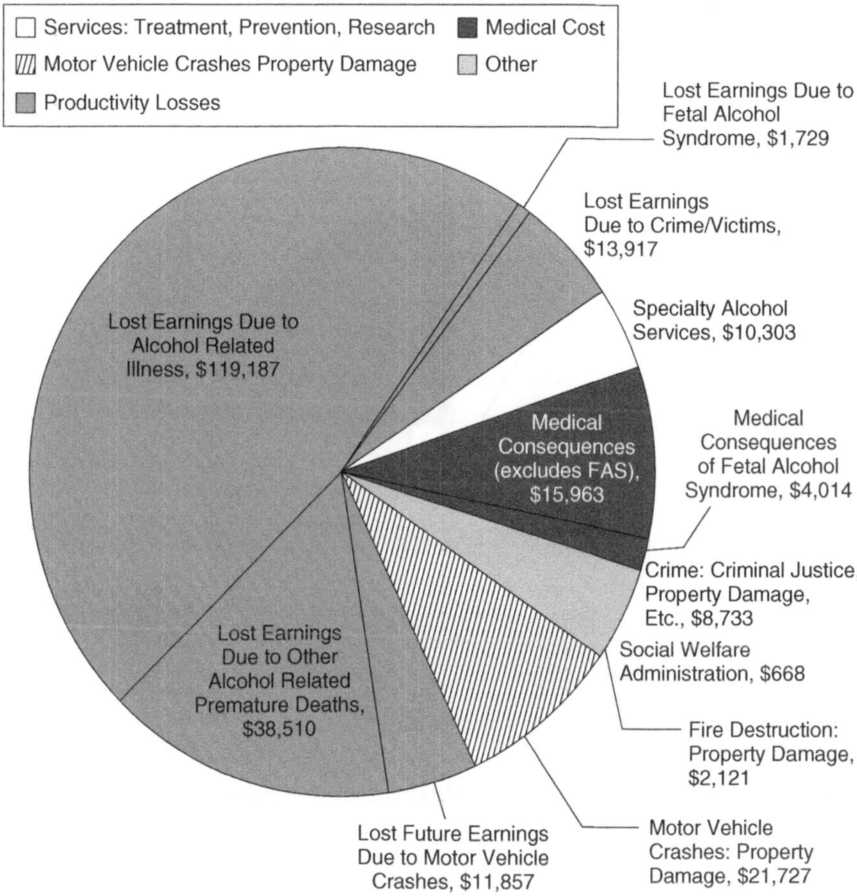

Figure 20.3: Costs of alcohol in the United States in 1998 (in millions of 2011 dollars) (2)

bronchitis and emphysema (13,927) (using data for 2000–2004). However, inasmuch as five out of six deaths from bronchitis and emphysema were attributed to smoking, the attribution may be less uncertain than it is for pneumonia and influenza, for which those 10,423 were just 17% of the total of 62,525 deaths (4).

20.3.3 Illegal drugs

While the social costs of illegal drugs are comparable in magnitude to those of alcohol and tobacco, the breakdown by component is entirely different, as shown in figure 20.4. Harwood et al. estimated a total of $226 billion (in 2011 dollars) in direct and indirect (but not intangible) costs of all illicit drugs, including marijuana,

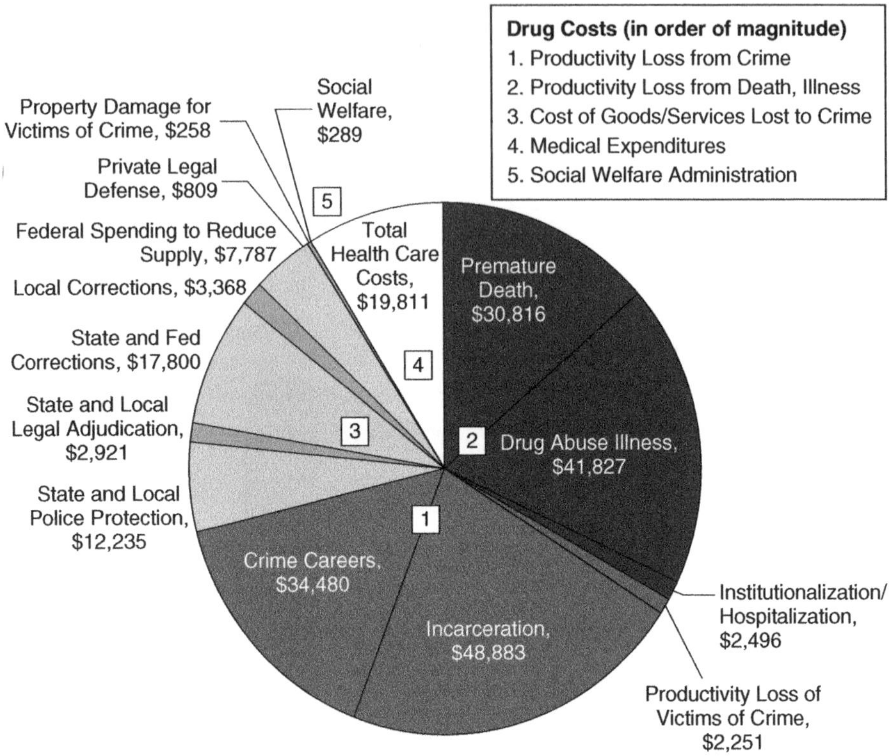

Figure 20.4: Costs of drug abuse in the United States in 2002 (in millions of 2011 dollars) (3)

cocaine, heroin, amphetamines, methamphetamines, and nonprescribed use of legal psychoactive medications and other substances (i.e., sedatives and solvents) (see chapters 8 and 16).

Costs attributable to premature death are smaller, largely since chronic use of illegal drugs is less directly associated with organ failure, such as lung cancer for smoking or cirrhosis for alcohol. The bulk of deaths that the CDC associates with illegal drugs are overdose/poisonings, infections (HIV/AIDS and hepatitis), and a proportion of homicides attributed to illegal drugs. The counts ignore drugged driving and the consequences of the long-term poverty that often accompanies addiction to expensive illegal drugs.

The categories specific to illicit drugs pertain to drug control, crime, and their interaction. Of these, the single biggest wedge is for incarceration-related productivity losses. It reflects primarily incarceration for violation of drug laws, but also considers other crimes, prorated by the proportions thought to be attributable to illegal drugs (roughly 30% of property crimes, 15% of homicides, 5% of sexual assaults, etc.). This is not, as one might first imagine, what taxpayers pay to build and operate the prisons and jails; that is accounted for by separate wedges labeled state, federal, and local corrections.

Rather, the social cost of incarceration represents the lost productivity of working age people who languish behind bars instead of contributing to the workforce.

The third largest wedge, for "crime careers," represents the value of the time that criminals spend committing crimes – including both distributing drugs and stealing things to buy drugs – rather than working in legitimate occupations. Essentially, this is the opportunity cost of their criminal behavior.

Recall that COI scholars prefer to value high- and low-income people equally when estimating lost earnings from premature death. The same principle applies to time. The lost labor time is valued at the average national income; that is generous, since criminals, in economic estimations, tend to possess less human capital than the national average. So if those hundreds of thousands of people were freed from incarceration and their criminal careers, they might not be able to contribute as much to the economy as the Harwood et al. estimates credit them.

Correctly interpreting the "incarceration" wedge shows that there is more commonality across substances than one might at first suppose. For cigarettes, alcohol, and illegal drugs, lost productivity accounts for a large proportion of social costs. For cigarettes, the productivity is lost primarily through premature death; for illegal drugs, time spent in incarceration and criminal careers incurs similarly high productivity losses.

The cost category that is prominent only for illegal drugs is taxpayers' costs of trying to suppress use. Corrections – paying to build and operate jails and prisons – is the largest chunk ($21 billion per year), followed by policing ($12 billion), federal spending to reduce the drug supply ($8 billion, including border control and operations in source countries), and adjudication ($3 billion).

That description makes it seem as if law enforcement is the only form of drug control, but the accounting conventions place treatment and prevention spending within the health care wedge ($20 billion per year overall).

Although health costs make up a relatively small portion of the Harwood cost estimates (8.7%), they are still sizable at about $19.8 billion (in 2011 dollars). Figure 20.5 breaks that wedge into constituent parts; the largest costs are community-based specialty treatment and expenditures to treat HIV/AIDS.

The prevention bar is a bit misleading because it does not reflect in-kind donations. For example, mentoring programs may help restrain adolescent drug use, but COI studies place no value on the volunteers' time; other methods value volunteers' time at their current wage rate, reasoning that is a good measure of the opportunity cost.

In-kind donations are an acute issue for school-based prevention. The teachers' salary and costs of the school building do not show up in prevention's accounting statements, even though from a societal perspective, the largest cost of school-based prevention programs is the opportunity cost of not using that class time to teach academic subjects (15).

Not all illegal drugs are equally dangerous. Marijuana is by far the most frequently used – a recent NSDUH shows that 17.4% of those 12 and older are

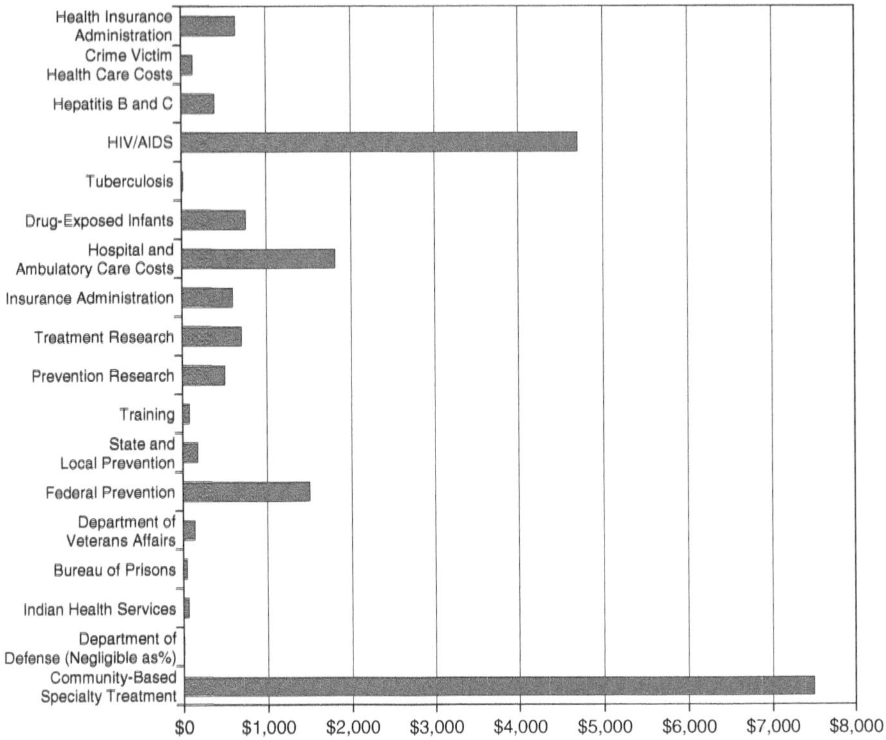

Figure 20.5: Drug abuse–related medical expenditures (in millions of 2011 dollars) (3)

past-month marijuana users, while 7.0% used psychotherapeutics and 1.5% used cocaine in the past month (16) (see chapters 8 and 16). However, it would be wrong to estimate marijuana's social cost by prorating the Harwood et al. total for all illegal drugs according to the number of marijuana users. Marijuana is not injected, so it is not implicated in the spread of HIV/AIDS or hepatitis; it is rarely involved in fatal overdose, and despite accounting for half of all drug arrests, it plays a relatively minor role in drug-related incarceration (17). Furthermore, marijuana habits are rarely so expensive as to prompt the commission of property crimes to finance purchases. Ideally, COI studies would separately estimate the social cost of each substance, but unfortunately, a RAND study of methamphetamine is one of the few substance-specific analyses (18).

20.4 Variations and controversies

The COI approach is something of an "industry standard," but it is not the only way to sum social costs. This section discusses outcomes excluded by COI studies that some might argue could be included.

20.4.1 Revisiting costs of crime

COI studies' approach to the costs of crime has been particularly controversial. Suppose a dependent heroin user robs you by sticking a gun in your ribs and forcing you to turn over your wallet, which contains $40 in cash. After you do so, the robber swats you in the face with the butt of the gun, an injury for which you need stitches. Once safely away, the robber pockets the $40 and throws your wallet in a garbage bin.

What societal cost would a COI study assign to this event?

That depends on what the robber buys with the $40. If the robber buys a new pair of shoes, the entire event is ruled not drug-related. The robbery is only attributed to drug dependence if the proceeds are spent on illegal drugs.

Even if the crime is deemed drug-related, the $40 never enters into a COI study's estimate of social cost. It is irrelevant whether the robber stole $40, $0.40, or $400, as long as a portion was spent on drugs. COI studies view theft as a frictionless transfer of goods from one individual to another. Since both the criminal and the victim are members of society, that transfer is a wash; it does not reduce society's aggregate wealth.

On the other hand, the wallet is a loss because the robber didn't keep it. It would be included under "property damage of victims of crime." The loss estimates tend to be larger when physical goods, rather than cash, are stolen. You may not consider parting with your TV for anything less than $500, but a robber will sell it for much less on the black market. Collins and Lapsley (5) assess this drop in value as a loss to the community and assume that 40% of the value of stolen property is lost. Other analysts may use different percent values. Regardless, as figure 20.4 shows, such property damage is a minor share of social cost ($258 million, or roughly 0.1% of the total).

COI studies would count the cost of the stitches under "Crime Victim Health Care Costs" (which total $138 million for illicit drugs, see figure 20.5), but the pain of getting hit in the face and any ensuing psychological damage would be dismissed as "intangible."

If the victim were on the way to work, and getting stitches took 4 hours, this lost work time would count under "Productivity Losses of Victims of Crime." If the victim were on the way home from work, and getting stitches made the victim miss an evening out with friends, then COI studies would assign no social cost to that lost time.

Suppose the robbery was so traumatic that the victim couldn't sleep well for weeks. In COI studies, that only counts as a cost if the victim sought professional help, in which case the doctor's charges and the cost of any sleeping pills would count. Any subsequent measures the victim took to avoid further victimization such as staying home, carrying mace, or moving to a safer neighborhood would not factor in.

To some, these rules seem perfectly sensible; to others, they seem capricious and divorced from common sense. How could a methodology with such a long and esteemed history make such an odd collection of distinctions? The simple answer is that COI methods were invented for conditions such as diabetes and cancer, for which crime costs are largely irrelevant.

Other methods for crime cost estimations exist that dwarf the costs considered by COI studies. Methods developed by criminal justice researchers including Mark Cohen (of Vanderbilt), Ted Miller (of PIRE), and their colleagues tend to (1) exclude any benefits accruing to the criminal and (2) count the victim's intangible pain and suffering, often measured by WTP to avoid victimization. Cohen et al. (19) estimate the WTP to avoid a burglary in the United States at $31,000 ($36,900 in 2011 dollars) compared to direct costs of just $1,300 (about $1,550 in 2011). Other methods use QALYs to quantify crime victims' psychological suffering.

Applying alternative methods would portray crime as a much more important contributor than standard substance abuse cost estimates suggest. Using a QALY-based approach, Miller et al. revised the 1992 Harwood estimates by adjusting certain factors and including the intangible costs of pain, suffering, and lost quality of life from crime involving illicit drugs and/or alcohol (20). They found a total cost in 1999 (when adjusted to 2011 dollars) of $277.5 billion. Notwithstanding the media's focus on illicit drugs and crime, Miller et al. found that alcohol-attributable crime costs are double those of drugs, with alcohol-only crimes costing four times what drug-only crimes do, in part because alcohol is so often involved in violent altercations (see figure 20.6). Note, though, that per regular user, illicit drugs probably have higher crime costs (20, p. 340).

Including the intangible costs of crime makes little difference to estimates of the social cost of smoking. But higher crime cost estimates for alcohol and illicit drugs would reduce smoking's proportionate share of the total combined costs of substance abuse.

20.4.2 Including domestic violence, child abuse, and neglect

COI studies ignore most domestic violence and child abuse and neglect. Data limitations make causal attribution difficult, so omitting domestic-related costs is perhaps a safer choice. But historians remind us that the social costs of family pain from substance abuse are very important; the Women's Christian Temperance Union was a driving force behind alcohol prohibition, activism motivated in no small part by the damage alcoholism wrought on families.

A simple calculation can give a sense of perspective. The Substance Abuse and Mental Health Services Administration (21) estimates that more than 8.3 million children live with a parent who abused or depended on alcohol or an illicit drug. The average social cost per instance of child abuse is very high; Miller et al. (22) estimate

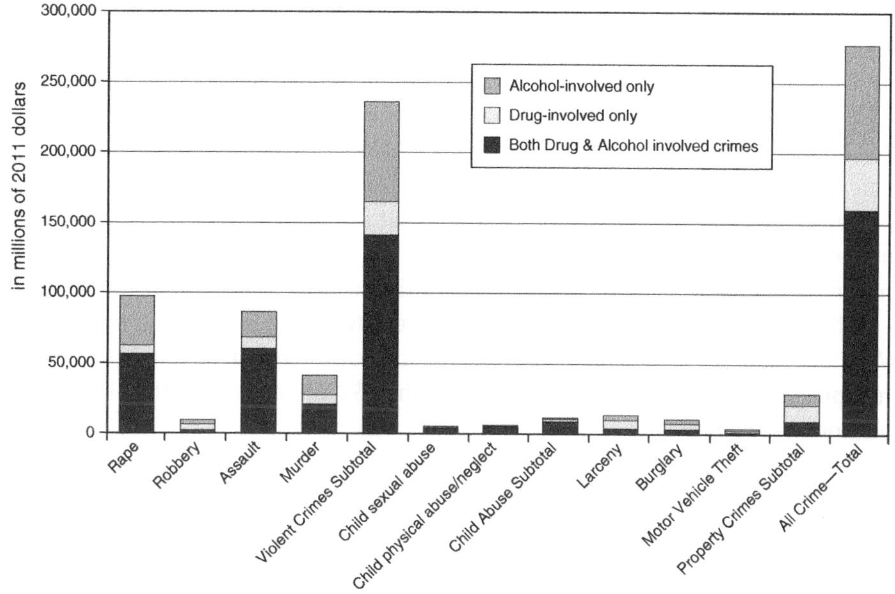

Figure 20.6: Costs of alcohol- and drug-involved crime (20)

$60,000 in 1993 dollars ($93,400 in 2011 dollars). However, not all cases of abuse or neglect committed by parents who are dependent should be causally attributed to substance abuse – intuitively, some of this abuse would have still occurred without drugs. But even if only 10% of cases could be causally attributed to parents' substance abuse, the social cost would be $49.8 billion (8.3 million * 10% * $60,000) in 1993 US dollars per year (equivalent to $77.5 billion per year in 2011 US dollars).

20.4.3 Including intangible costs of dependence and death

There are other intangible costs of consequence, notably the psychological cost of dependence itself. Most people who are substance dependent do not wish to be; if they could snap their fingers and wipe away the dependence, they would happily do so. That means there is some WTP to be rid of addiction, over and above its direct medical costs and indirect effects on productivity and earnings.

Kleiman (23) offers a simple, illustrative calculation. If at any given time about 10% of the US adult population is suffering from a substance abuse disorder and they and/or their families dislike that situation so much that on average they would be willing to pay $10,000 to be rid of it, then "the total willingness-to-pay to avoid addiction itself, as distinct from the financial losses it generates, would total $200 billion per year in the United States, nearly as much as the Harwood et al. estimate of $246 billion" (for alcohol and drugs combined, 1992 dollars, or $394 billion in 2011 dollars) (23, p. 640).

Nicosia et al. (18) reach a similar conclusion in a different way when producing the first national estimate of the societal costs of methamphetamine use. They measure quality of life lost from dependence via QALYs and use the standard WTP estimate of $5.2 million (inflation-adjusted to 2011 dollars) for the intangible cost of premature death. Their calculations suggest that the highest costs of methamphetamine abuse stem from lost quality of life and premature mortality. They judge that these intangibles could make up 71% of the costs.

The intangible costs of tobacco-related premature deaths could be staggering. With that value of $5.2 million per premature death, the annual intangible costs from premature tobacco death would be more than $2 trillion, not just the $115 billion mentioned previously.

20.4.4 Cost offsets

Recall that for alcohol-impaired automobile crashes, COI studies estimate how many crashes would have occurred in the absence of intoxication, and then only "charge" to alcohol abuse the increment between that "baseline" number of crashes and the number that actually occurred. That analysis can be quite difficult to pull off in practice, but the principle is entirely sensible.

Yet parallel logic is not applied to medical costs associated with end-of-life care. The issue is most pertinent to cigarettes, so we discuss it in that context, but the principle applies to all substances.

Suppose a smoker dies from lung cancer that is known to be attributable to smoking, not radon, asbestos, or some other cause. COI studies count all of the associated medical costs as social costs of smoking. They make no effort to estimate how much would have been spent on medical care for the patient had he or she never smoked and, hence, not died then of lung cancer, but instead died later of something else. So the social cost reported by COI studies is greater than the increment in health care spending caused by smoking. This would be analogous to the increment in costs associated with the extra traffic crashes due to alcohol intoxication.

Although it may seem coldhearted, COI calculations could recognize that premature deaths bring not only medical costs but also cost savings by avoiding future medical expenditures or leaving more in the pot for Social Security. Paying attention to these "cost offsets" may be a political nonstarter within the tobacco control community, so it is unlikely that they will be factored into COI studies in the near or even long-term future. However, studies that pay attention to "cost offsets" find that they are not insubstantial. Notably, a 1989 RAND study of excise taxes on cigarettes and alcohol that considered the costs of financed health insurance, pensions, disability insurance, group life insurance, fires, motor vehicle accidents, and the criminal justice system found that smokers do "pay their own way," while excise taxes on alcohol only cover about half of indirect costs to society (24).

20.4.5 Imperfect rationality

Standard economic theory assumes that consumers rationally act in their own self-interest and so presume that drug users must benefit from their drug use; the pleasures derived from consumption must fully offset any personal pain or risks of substance use (addiction, behavioral effects, illness, and premature death). But several drug policy scholars – notably Mark Kleiman in *Against Excess* (25) – question that assumption and suggest thinking of drug users themselves, particularly those who are dependent, as among the victims who suffer from substance abuse.

In Kleiman's favor, we should not trust children – nor even adult drug users, in many cases – to be responsible for their own welfare. Inasmuch as teens are not seen as capable of acting consistently in their own self-interest, substance abuse among youth may be exempt from the standard rational consumer assumption. This distinction matters enormously because while most drugs are consumed by adults, most decisions to start using drugs are made by youth and young adults, with mean ages at first use for different substances ranging from 16.3 to 24.6 (shown in figure 20.7). Furthermore, some unknown proportion of adult consumption comes from people who not only initiated as youth but also became dependent before reaching adulthood.

20.5 Conclusions

Monetizing the societal burden of substance abuse is a difficult task fraught with uncertainties and difficult choices. No estimates should be viewed as precise. Nonetheless, the literature provides salient insights.

- The societal burdens of illicit drugs, alcohol, and tobacco are very large.
- Many estimates judge the burdens of alcohol or tobacco as higher than for all illicit drugs combined.
- Medical expenditures constitute a substantial chunk of cigarette smoking costs, but a small fraction of the costs of alcohol and illicit drug abuse.
- Productivity losses and crime-related costs are important drivers of economic costs as reflected in COI studies.

A skeptical view is that these COI estimates are used primarily as "policy props" to champion specific causes or programs (7); many problem domains compete for

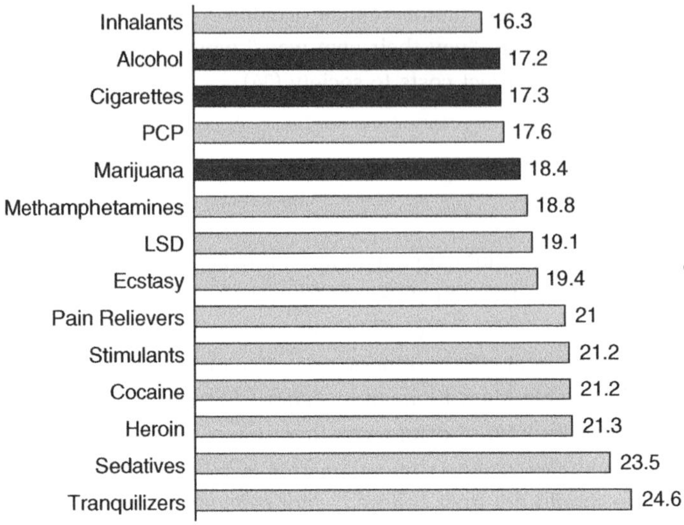

Figure 20.7: Mean age at first use for alcohol, cigarettes, marijuana, and other specific drugs, 2010 (1)

attention in the crowded public policy arena by trumpeting cost estimates that run to the hundreds of billions of dollars, including not just conventional diseases (diabetes and heart disease) but also broader public health concerns (obesity and inadequate sleep) and more eclectic domains (cybersecurity breeches and bailing out banks).

However, having a sense of magnitude can produce meaningful insights. We close by sketching one example. Even high-quality substance abuse treatment programs suffer high relapse rates – by some sources ranging from 50% to 90% (26). Skeptics jump to the conclusion that high relapse rates imply that funding drug treatment is a bad investment for taxpayer dollars. The modern view is that addiction is a chronic relapsing condition that must be managed over an extended period, not thought of as something treatment can "cure" in the way that doctors can fix a broken bone. But COI studies can rebut the skeptics on their own terms by showing that treatment can be cost-effective despite high relapse rates.

A "back-of-the-envelope" calculation captures the idea, although a full analysis would be much more detailed. If the total social costs from illegal drugs are more than $200 billion per year, then the social cost per person-year of dependent use of cocaine/crack, heroin, or methamphetamine is at least $25,000 per year. This can be derived in a variety of ways. But consider that most of the social costs are associated with cocaine/crack, heroin, and meth, not marijuana. Most of the use of those drugs, and hence the social costs, comes from the minority of users who consume frequently, and there are "only" at most about 4 million people in need of treatment for those drugs, so the $25,000 figure is likely if anything conservative.

Now suppose that a person enters a 3-month drug treatment program that costs $2,000, cuts the person's substance abuse during treatment by 50%, and has no effect whatsoever on long-term use. Is it in taxpayers' interest to fund such a program? Instinctively most people would say "no." There is zero long-term benefit, and the program didn't even produce abstinence while the client was in the program.

But simple arithmetic suggests otherwise. To determine if the program breaks even from a "return on investment" perspective, a policy analyst might calculate as follows:

Annual societal cost of drug abuse × *Length of treatment in years*
× *Fraction of use rate during treatment*

$$\$25,000 \times \frac{3}{12} \times \frac{1}{2} > \$3,000$$

A benefit of more than $3,000, in the form of averted social costs, exceeds the program cost of $2,000, suggesting that the treatment program is a good social investment.

That illustration is painfully oversimplified, but its basic conclusion is echoed by much more refined analyses. For example, a 1992 study by the California Drug and Alcohol Treatment Assessment using a sample of 150,000 participants found that the cost-savings generated by alcohol and other drug treatment services outweighed the program costs at ratios from 4:1 to more than 12:1 (27). Rydell and Everingham's (28) oft-cited RAND report reached a similar conclusion.

Parallel analyses have been done on prevention. Of course there must be some effectiveness to achieve any cost-effectiveness, and the Institute of Medicine (14) notes that certain efforts geared toward youth are simply not effective – in particular, information distribution, or programs about improving self-esteem or resisting peer pressure. However, well-designed school-based programs have been shown in randomized control trials to have beneficial effects, at least in delaying initiation (which is associated with lower long-term use) (29,30). Policy analyses suggest that those model programs can be good societal investments (31,15).

The point for present purposes, though, is not to endorse this or that intervention, but to illustrate the idea that however imperfect COI studies' estimates are, having even a rough sense of the magnitude of the social costs of substance abuse can be valuable for policy analysis and resource allocation.

Acknowledgments

The authors of this chapter are indebted to Emel Atkas and Stephen Davenport, who provided valuable comments during the revision and editing process.

References

1. Substance Abuse and Mental Health Services Administration. Results from the 2010 National Survey on Drug Use and Health: Detailed tables [Internet]. US Department of Health and Human Services. Accessed January 3, 2013. URL: http://www.samhsa.gov/data/NSDUH/2k10ResultsTables/NSDUHTables2010R/HTM/TOC.htm#TopOfPage
2. Harwood H, Fountain D, Livermore G. Updating estimates of the economic costs of alcohol abuse in the United States: Estimates, update methods, and data. Rockville, MD: National Institutes Health, Department Health Human Services, 2000;98–4327:13.
3. Harwood H, Bouchery E, The Lewin Group, Office of National Drug Control Policy. The economic costs of drug abuse in the United States, 1992–2002. Washington, DC: Executive Office of the President, 2004;207303:102.
4. Center for Disease Control. Smoking attributable mortality, years of potential life lost, and productivity losses: United States, 2000–2004. MMWR 2008;57(45):1226–8.
5. Collins DJ, Lapsley HM. Counting the cost: Estimates of the social costs of drug abuse in Australia in 1998–99. Canberra: Commonwealth Australia, 2002:113.
6. Fenoglio P, Parel V, Kopp P. The social cost of alcohol, tobacco and illicit drugs in France, 1997. Eur Addict Res 2003;9(1):18–28.
7. Reuter P. Are calculations of the economic costs of drug abuse either possible or useful? Addiction 1999;94(5):627–30.
8. Center for Disease Control and Prevention. Alcohol use: CDC FastStats. Accessed January 3, 2013. URL: http://www.cdc.gov/nchs/fastats/alcohol.htm/
9. National Highway Traffic Safety Information. Traffic safety facts 2010 data: Alcohol-impaired driving. US Department of Transportation. Accessed January 3, 2013. URL: http://www-nrd.nhtsa.dot.gov/Pubs/811606.pdf
10. Centers for Disease Control and Prevention. Drug-induced deaths: United States, 2003–2007. MMWR 2011;60(1):60–1.
11. American Cancer Society. Economic impact of cancer. Accessed January 03, 2013. URL: http://www.cancer.org/Cancer/CancerBasics/economic-impact-of-cancer
12. American Diabetes Association. Economic costs of diabetes in the US in 2007. Diabetes Care 2008;31(3):596–615.
13. Centers for Disease Control and Prevention. Costs of falls among older adults. Injury prevention and control: Home and recreational safety. Accessed January 3, 2013. URL: http://www.cdc.gov/HomeandRecreationalSafety/Falls/fallcost.html
14. Bonnie RJ, O'Connell ME. Reducing underage drinking: A collective responsibility. Washington, DC: The National Academies Press, 2004:740.
15. Caulkins JP, Pacula RL, Paddock S, Chiesa J. School-based drug prevention: What kind of drug use does it prevent? Santa Monica, CA: RAND, 2002:174.
16. Substance Abuse and Mental Health Services Administration (SAMHSA). Results from the 2010 National Survey on Drug Use and Health: Summary of national findings. HHS Publication (SMA) 11–4658 Vols. NSDUH Series H-41. Rockville, MD: SAMHSA, 2011.
17. Caulkins JP, Hawken A, Kilmer B, Kleiman M. Marijuana legalization: What everyone needs to know. New York: Oxford University Press, 2012:288.
18. Nicosia N, Pacula RC, Kilmer B. The economic cost of methamphetamine use in the United States, 2005. Santa Monica, CA: RAND, 2009:147.
19. Cohen MA, Rust RT, Steen S, Tidd ST. Willingness-to-pay for crime control programs. Criminology 2004;42(1):89–110.
20. Miller TR, Lew DT, Cohen MA, Cox KL. Costs of alcohol and drug-involved crime. Prev Sci 2006;7(4):333–42.

21. Substance Abuse Mental Health Services Administration (SAMHSA), Office of Supplied Studies. Children living with substance-abusing or substance-dependent parents: 2002–2007. National Survey on Drug Use and Health Report, 2009. Accessed January 3, 2013. URL: http://www.samhsa.gov/data/2k9/SAparents/SAparents.htm
22. Miller TR, Cohen MA, Wiersema B. Victim costs and consequences: A new look. NCJ155282:28. Washington, DC: National Institute Justice, 1996.
23. Kleiman MA. "Economic cost" measurements, damage minimization and drug abuse control policy. Addiction 1999;94(5):638–41.
24. Manning WG, Emmett B, Keeler JP, Newhouse EM, Sloss JW. The costs of poor health habits. Cambridge: Harvard University Press, 1991:240.
25. Kleiman M. Against excess: Drug policy for results. New York: Basic Books, 1993:496.
26. Caron Pennsylvania. Current statistics. Caron Treatment Centers, 2012. Accessed January 3, 2013. URL: http://www.caron.org/current-statistics.html
27. Gerstein DR, Johnson RA, Harwood HJ, Suter N, Malloy K, et al. Evaluating recovery services: The California drug and alcohol treatment assessment (CALDATA) general report. Sacramento, CA: National Opinion Research Center, California Dept Alcohol Drug Programs, 1994.
28. Rydell CP, Everingham SS. Controlling cocaine: Supply versus demand programs. Santa Monica, CA: RAND, 1994:120.
29. Gottfredson DC, Wilson DB. Characteristics of effective school-based substance abuse prevention. Prev Sci 2003;4(1):27–38.
30. Faggiano F, Vigna-Taglianti FD, Versino E, Zambon A, Borraccino A, Lemma P. School-based prevention for illicit drugs' use. Cochrane Database Syst Rev 2005;2:CD003020.
31. Caulkins JP, Everingham SS, Rydell CP, Chiesa J, Bushway S. An ounce of prevention, a pound of uncertainty: The cost-effectiveness of school-based drug prevention programs. MR-923-RWJ. Santa Monica, CA: RAND, 1999.

21 The pros and cons of legalization

Jonathan P. Caulkins, Anna Kasunic,
Mark Kleiman, and Michael A. C. Lee

The immense harms that drugs (illicit drugs, prescription drugs, alcohol, and tobacco) cause both users and nonusers have prompted many governments to impose strictly enforced bans on production and possession of some of these substances. Such bans can help constrain drug use. However, prohibition also causes its own harms, including harms from black-market crime and violence. Drug legalization would ameliorate the black-market harms, and perhaps reduce harm-per-use by improving product reliability and consumer information, but increase other harms by decreasing price and thus increasing use and dependence. This chapter offers a framework for understanding the pros and cons of legalization, and some of its complexities, including the differences between state- and national-level legalization, the monetary and human costs of regulation and enforcement, and effects of different policies on youth. It also discusses "middle path" policy options, such as decriminalization, policy changes under prohibition, and harm reduction. The aim is to inform by peeling away the rhetoric of the drug legalization/prohibition debate, not to argue for any specific policy.

21.1 Introduction

In a sense, drugs are just consumer goods, like doughnuts and dietary supplements. But *caveat emptor* is no longer the rule for even routine consumer goods. Doughnut shops must comply with public health inspections, and nutraceutical manufacturers must follow good manufacturing practices, eschew false labeling, and report the adverse effects of their products. Regulation is not the same as prohibition, though. Governments generally do not block the open market from catering to consumer desires.

There are exceptions, often rooted in cultural or religious mores. Both Judaism and Islam proscribe pork, a ban that several Muslim-majority states have incorporated into their national laws. Prohibitions of consumer goods are less common in contemporary secular societies but still occur. Health, quality of life, ethics, and human rights concerns (as well as what is sometimes called the "'ick!' factor" – disgust and moral disapprobation beyond concerns about measurable harm) motivate laws forbidding prostitution, child pornography, and human organ markets. Other bans protect nonhumans, such as rules against the ivory and tropical hardwood trades. In 2006, Congress effectively banned eating horse meat by withholding federal funds for required slaughterhouse inspections. The prohibition remained in place for 5 years until the Obama administration lifted it, even though in many countries eating horse meat is no more controversial than eating beef.

Historically, intoxicants have been a frequent target of prohibitions. England's King James I tried to prohibit tobacco in the 17th century, and alcohol has been subject to numerous bans. Neither tobacco nor alcohol are prohibited in the United States today, but the Controlled Substance Act places scores of other psychoactive chemicals into one of five "schedules" depending on their potential for abuse and their potential value in medicine. Schedule I substances include heroin and marijuana (high potential for abuse, no recognized medical value). Cocaine is in Schedule II, despite high potential for abuse, because it has medical uses (as a topical anesthetic).

The fact that drug use can harm users is, for some, sufficient justification for market intervention. Consumers are usually left to deal with their own odd choices, but overdoses of pet rocks and low-rider pants are not fatal. Drugs are different, so the argument goes, because they are so seductive and dangerous. Drug-induced behavior can impair decision-making processes through dependence or intoxicated reasoning; the "choice" to continue abusing drugs is something less than completely free. Users may not fully understand the risks before initiating use. After all, the great bulk of initiation is by adolescents and young adults, for whom immediate pleasures can cloud judgments involving probabilistic risks of adverse outcomes that are mostly in the future. Precocious use is also a strong risk factor predicting subsequent dependence. Once users become dependent, it can be psychologically and/or physically painful to abstain. Furthermore, the minority of heavy users account for a disproportionate share of all drug consumption, which means that a goodly share of all "decisions" to imbibe are made while intoxicated by earlier doses.

While drugs can harm users, so can other unhealthy consumer goods or high-risk activities. Yet few laws forbid eating artery-clogging foods, competing in mixed martial arts, or bungee jumping. (Though two states, Michigan and Florida, have introduced temporary bans on bungee jumping, and others highly regulate the activity).

What makes drugs – legal and illegal – different from those examples though, is their capacity to harm nonusers, including people completely uninvolved in the market. Nonusers suffer when passersby breathe secondhand smoke, when drug use during pregnancy causes congenital defects in newborns, or when impaired drivers smash their cars into other cars, pedestrians, or property. More diffuse damage arises when drug use reduces worker productivity or creates health care costs others in the same insurance pool must bear. Such "externalities" make otherwise private consumption decisions a matter of public concern.

However, these facts merely argue for drug policies that are distinct from, and perhaps more assertive than, polices toward consumer goods generally. It does not imply that the policy must be to ban all nonmedical use. Still, given the problems that drug use creates, prohibition has obvious appeal.

21.1.1 Difficult policy choices

Public policies often create unintended consequences, or side effects. Abolishing the legal market for drugs may reduce drug use, but it doesn't eradicate all use, and the residual consumption sustains black markets that generate other social problems including crime, violence, and corruption. Enforcement of prohibition can cause still other problems. The United States incarcerates about 500,000 people for drug-law violations at any given time, more people than all but three other countries each incarcerate for all types of crime combined. The burden falls disproportionately on minorities and the poor. Human Rights Watch, among other groups, sharply criticizes the United States on this point, noting that black adults are sentenced to state prisons for drug offenses at 10 times the corresponding rate for white adults (1).

Formulating drug policy is not easy. Enormous social costs follow from abuse of both illegal and legal drugs (see chapter 20), so neither legalization nor prohibition is a panacea. In addition, new psychoactive chemicals are appearing with a frequency that tests the capacity of the current framework for "scheduling" substances (see chapter 19). Given the complexities of the social problem of drug use and the various interests at stake, it should come as no surprise that the policy outcomes leave some people dissatisfied.

Prohibitions are not unchangeable. In 1930, the United States prohibited alcohol, but not marijuana. Ten years later, the positions were reversed. Some might wonder if all problems can be solved by changing a drug's legal status, either legalizing a drug that is now prohibited or prohibiting one that is now legal, such as tobacco. This seems unlikely. Underground markets produce one set of problems, and legal markets another. Changing the legal status of a drug is no silver bullet; it's more "trading the devil you know for the devil you don't know."

Nevertheless, thinking hard about prohibition and legalization is valuable for three reasons: the devil you don't know might not be as bad; the exercise can inspire ideas for improving the current legal regime; and, as a practical matter, policy changes are happening regardless of whether or not one wants them.

Some jurisdictions are tightening regulations on legal drugs. Atlanta's recent ban on smoking in public parks is backed by fines of up to $1,000 and sentences of up to 5 months in jail (2). Virginia's penalties for first-time driving-while-intoxicated offenses already included fines of up to $2,500 and jail sentences of up to a year. But as of July 1, 2012, those with restricted licenses were also required to install an ignition interlock system (a breathalyzer-like tool that prevents a car engine from starting if blood alcohol concentration is over a certain level) (3).

Other jurisdictions are relaxing laws pertaining to marijuana. US states started decriminalizing marijuana in the 1970s, and more are considering it now. California already treated possession of less than 1 ounce of marijuana as only a "citable" misdemeanor (typically leading to the equivalent of a traffic ticket) before California

SB 1449 went into effect in January 2011, which downgraded the offense to a mere infraction. Seventeen states and the District of Columbia have implemented medical marijuana programs, and six more are actively considering it. In November 2012, Colorado, Oregon, and Washington voted on full legalization – and those propositions passed in Colorado and Washington.

Other countries are also considering liberalization. President of Uruguay José Mujica recently proposed that the government supply marijuana to registered users. Current and former leaders of a number of countries, particularly in South and Central America, want open discussion about legalizing "hard" drugs like cocaine and heroin.

Legalizing marijuana and legalizing "hard" drugs are very different choices, with significantly different stakes and likely outcomes. Marijuana is special for at least four reasons (see chapters 8 and 20). First, marijuana markets are associated with much less violence; one reason why is that marijuana rarely dominates the budgets of its users, so its consumption is much less associated with income-generating crime. Second, regardless of the merits of the matter, there is essentially no prospect of the United States legalizing cocaine/crack, heroin, or methamphetamine in the near or even medium-term future. Such proposals would have almost no public support. In contrast, marijuana prohibition is under active attack now. Third, 17 million Americans use marijuana in any given month, a figure that far exceeds use of any other class of illegal drugs (except diverted pharmaceuticals). Finally, and perhaps most importantly, marijuana use is simply much less dangerous, in terms of risk of overdose, risk of disastrous intoxicated behavior, and risk of dependence coming to dominate one's life.

Unfortunately, much of the literature on legalization comes from advocates committed more to their cause than to objectivity. The following two sections attempt to give a more balanced overview of the merits, detriments, and important considerations of first, prohibition, and second, legalization. [Space limitations necessitate an abbreviated discussion. MacCoun and Reuter (4) remains the single best book on legalization, and we highly recommend it to those interested in further reading.] The subsequent sections ask whether middle path options exist that could cherry-pick the best attributes of the two extremes.

This chapter does not advocate one position or another. Our aim is not to sway readers, but to caution them against the hyperbolic statements that both prohibitionists and legalization advocates sometimes make.

21.2 Current policy: Prohibition

Prohibition constrains the number of users and quantity consumed in four ways. First, prohibition probably reduces demand, on net. While there can be so-called "forbidden fruits" effects, meaning that the very act of prohibiting something can increase its allure, those are counterbalanced by factors that discourage the consumption of prohibited substances: the black market's poor production quality control, minimal labeling information, and social disapprobation, not to mention the risk of arrest and other sanctions, such as loss of scholarships or opportunities to compete in interscholastic athletics (5,6).

Second, prohibition reduces availability. While the Monitoring the Future survey famously finds that the proportion of high school students reporting that marijuana is fairly or very easy to obtain (82%) is nearly as high as the corresponding proportion for alcohol (89%), marijuana is the exception. Those same surveys find much lower rates of availability for cocaine (31%), MDMA (3,4-methylenedioxy-N-methylamphetamine) (37%), and heroin (21%) (7). Indeed, even long-term daily heroin users often report search times approaching an hour in order to "score" their drug of choice (8).

Third, prohibition backed by even modest enforcement raises production costs by imposing what Peter Reuter has called "the structural consequences of product illegality": illegality forces suppliers to operate covertly, which creates inefficiencies. Black-market producers cannot invest in bulky machinery that would be hard to hide and easy for police to confiscate. As a result, crack dealers' staff can package crack vials at a rate of about 100 per hour; by contrast, sugar-packaging machines fill the sugar packets you see in restaurants at a rate of about 1,000 per minute (9). Likewise, drug dealers cannot resolve business disputes in courts, and while lawyers are expensive, resolving disagreements with knives and guns is even more costly.

Fourth, drug dealers must pay extra to compensate employees for incurring the considerable risks of experiencing arrest or violence, what economists call "compensating wage differentials" (10). Drug distributors and dealers don't make a lot of money because they are unusually skilled; they make a lot of money to compensate them for the risks they incur.

Together these factors have spectacular effects on the cost of production and distribution, which manifest in enormous price markups from one distribution level to the next. Traffickers demand $10,000 to move a kilogram of cocaine from Colombia to New York. FedEx will ship a kilogram of anything else for $60. While prohibition cannot seal the borders, it does make drugs – which are really nothing more than semirefined agricultural commodities – extraordinarily expensive, costing users many times their weight in gold. Figure 21.1, which is adapted from a similar figure in the United Nations' *World Drug Report*, illustrates how large the markups are, especially when crossing national borders.

High prices reduce use because drug users are sensitive to price changes (12). Economists evaluate price responsiveness by measuring different "price elasticities." The total price elasticity of demand measures the percent change in total consumption produced by a 1% increase in price. This is composed of the participation elasticity, which measures the percent change in the number of users, and the conditional elasticity, which measures the percent change in the average amount a given consumer purchases.

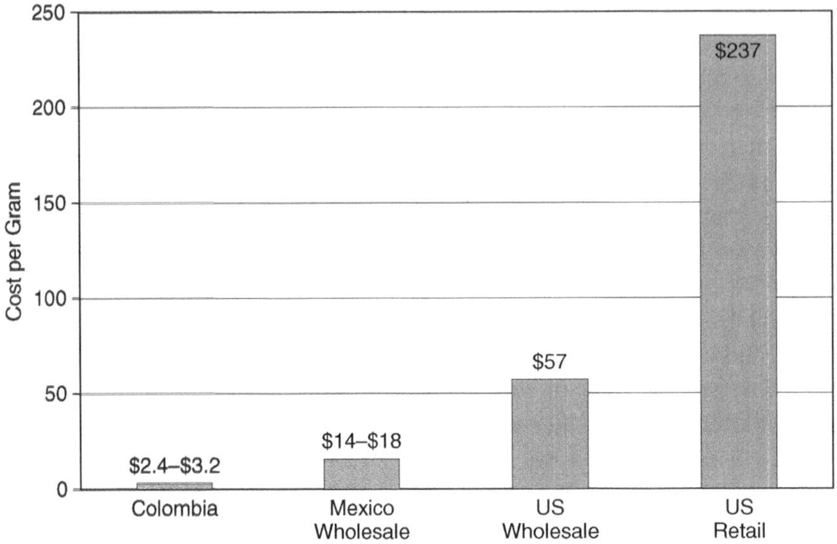

Figure 21.1: Purity-adjusted cost of cocaine per gram down the supply chain in 2009. The price shown for cocaine in Colombia is the price in major cities. The United Nations Office of Drugs and Crime also reports that the price for cocaine in Peru (the world's second-largest producer behind Colombia) in the producing regions is only $1.10 to $1.50. Source: United Nations Office of Drugs and Crime (11)

In 1977, Silverman and Spruill were among the first to study the price sensitivity of drug users (13). They found that even users of heroin – a notoriously addictive drug – consume less when it is more expensive. Since then, a growing literature has reinforced that basic conclusion: lower prices lead to more total drug use, more drug users, and more emergency department visits associated with that use. Youth can be particularly sensitive to price changes. For example, in her review of the literature on price elasticities in marijuana markets, Pacula notes that a 10% drop in the price of marijuana could lead to a 3% to 5% increase in new marijuana users under the age of 18 (14). Chaloupka et al. found estimates that a 10% increase in the price of cocaine would lead to a 9% to 10% decrease in youth use (15).

Prohibition may help suppress use, but the resulting underground markets bring crime, violence, and incarceration, and the public costs of controlling these markets can be great – an oft-cited estimate is $41.3 billion in enforcement costs per year (16). These considerations, along with libertarian concerns, are prompting increasing calls to "end the war on drugs."

Stopping the "war on drugs" can refer to either of two quite different propositions. When President Nixon created the Drug Enforcement Administration (DEA) to fight "an all-out global war on the drug menace," prohibition was already in place. So "ending the war on drugs" could simply mean retaining prohibition but pursuing enforcement less zealously. There is ample opportunity for improving US drug policy while retaining overall prohibition; for example, the Affordable Care

Act dramatically expanded access to treatment, and there is great excitement about "mandated abstinence" programs such as Hawaii's Opportunity Probation with Enforcement (HOPE) and South Dakota's 24/7 Sobriety programs (17,18).

For other people, the "war on drugs" is equivalent to prohibition itself, which they would like to replace with some form of legal drug production and distribution. Their argument is that total social harm under prohibition surpasses what it would be if drug markets were legal, because while prohibition reduces the number of users, it exacerbates harm per user or per dose. Indeed, that is why alcohol and tobacco are legally available (albeit substantially regulated) in most jurisdictions even though they are the two most problematic drugs in terms of the magnitude of their social costs. The harms of alcohol abuse prompted the nation to attempt the "Noble Experiment," but then the harms of Prohibition prompted a reversion to legal markets 14 years later (see chapter 9).

21.3 The effects of drug legalization

Many of the effects of legalization are simply the inverse of those of prohibition. Over time, legalization would lead to sharp declines in production costs and, hence, (pretax) drug prices. That in turn would increase drug use and dependence. But legalization would also eliminate black-market crimes and violence, save the public the cost of having to enforce prohibition, and allow the government to institute market regulation (e.g., requiring accurate labeling and forbidding harmful additives). Still, there are many particulars of legalization that advocates and opponents often gloss over.

Legalization could take different forms. One question is which drug, or drugs, to legalize. The options are not limited to either legalizing everything or prohibiting everything. Policy is already substance-specific (with alcohol, tobacco, and caffeine legal), and there is no reason not to pick and choose among the currently illicit drugs if some of them are to be permitted.

Another question is how much of a role, if any, the government wants to play in the market for the drug it is legalizing. Even some of the staunchest advocates of legalization balk at pure *laissez-faire* markets. The government might want to impose taxes, penalize public use, restrict sales from minors, mandate product testing and labeling, or require licenses for suppliers and vendors.

21.3.1 Product regulation

Illicit markets have no regulation, so the products can be impure and unsafe – unsafe even relative to the intrinsic risks stemming from the chemicals that the user intended to buy and use. This can result in users unwittingly consuming a more dangerous or potent substance than intended. One issue is impurities. For example, in the early

1980s, underground chemists trying to produce a synthetic substitute for heroin called MPPP (1-methyl-4-phenyl-4-propionoxypiperidine) created batches contaminated with another chemical, MPTP (1-methyl-4-phenyl-1,2,3,6-tetrahydropyridine), which apparently caused permanent Parkinson's-like symptoms after even one use (19).

Another problem associated with lack of regulation is dilution. Dealers routinely dilute drugs such as cocaine and heroin. Superficially, dilution with inactive ingredients would seem to reduce the risk of overdose, but one theory hypothesizes that high variance may matter more than high potency, with users always at a risk of that leads to overdose, with users always at risk of being surprised by a bag with higher-than-expected purity.

A third issue is lack of labeling. Cocaine is a simple chemical; the quality of a bag of powder containing cocaine is pretty well captured by its purity (percent by weight that is cocaine), at least as long as the other materials are just fillers, like lactose, not toxins or adulterants (adulterants are other psychoactives; diluents just add bulk) (see chapter 11). Cannabis is different. Depending on the plant, highgrade marijuana could contain more than 20% tetrahydrocannabinol (THC), while the same weight of low-grade would contain less than 5%. Also, while THC potency was once thought of as a sufficient statistic for the quality of marijuana, marijuana plants contain many other psychoactive chemicals, and it is increasingly recognized that other cannabinoids matter (see chapters 8 and 19). Some believe that cannabidiol (CBD) helps relieve anxiety created by THC (20), so that high ratios of THC to CBD, not just high THC potency, might trigger adverse reactions. A few dispensaries operating under state medical-marijuana laws report both the THC and CBD content of their products (21); this is almost unheard of among black-market dealers.

Illegality also creates harm associated with certain methods of drug administration. Injecting heroin is more cost-efficient than "chasing the dragon" (smoking), in the sense that a larger proportion of the (expensive) heroin ends up in the user's bloodstream (see chapter 10). However, users who share needles risk transmitting blood-borne diseases like HIV/AIDS and hepatitis C. If legalized, heroin would be cheaper, possibly reducing the incentive for intravenous use.

Advocates of legalization suggest it could bring other beneficial shifts in mode of administration. For example, marijuana vaporization may be less toxic than smoking a joint; if marijuana were legalized, regulations could be put in place to encourage vaporization and discourage smoking.

21.3.2 Availability to youth

Most proposals to legalize drugs would continue to ban use by youth, just as alcohol is only legal in the United States for those over the age of 21. This distinction is important because adolescents' brains are still developing, minors are not generally trusted to consistently make choices that are in their long-run interests, and quite

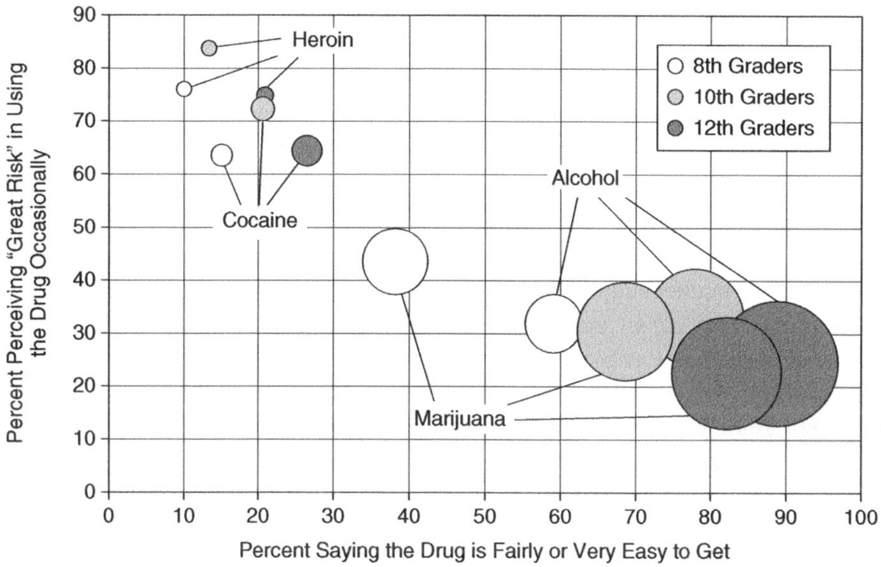

Figure 21.2: Rates of past-year drug use by grade level compared to availability and perceived risk. The question for perceived risk of drug use has to do with using the drug "occasionally" except in the case of alcohol. Here, we used the students' perceived risk of having one or two alcoholic drinks per day. The rates of drug use shown are for past-year use except for alcohol, where it is the rate of students reporting they had been drunk in the past year. Source: Monitoring the Future (7)

simply, most drug use starts when people are young. If an individual has not initiated use of a drug by around their mid-twenties, there is strong likelihood the person will never use it. (So, if a 50-year-old proclaims, "Legalization wouldn't affect drug use. It's not as if it'd make me go out and start using!" one should ask, "Yes, but the real question is, would you have been more likely to use the substance when you were 18 if it had been legal then?")

However, it is hard to prevent 20-year-olds from getting access to what their 21-year-old friends can buy legally. It is instructive to look at perceptions of availability and risk for different substances, legal and illegal, and how those vary with age. Such comparisons are not dispositive, since correlations do not imply causality, but without data from experimental trials that vary the legal status of drugs, cross-sectional data may be better than none.

Figure 21.2 illustrates the relationship between drug use and two of its risk factors. The Monitoring the Future survey asks youths in 8th, 10th, and 12th grades how difficult it would be to obtain various substances if they wanted them. The horizontal axis measures the percent that answered that it would be either fairly easy or very easy for them to get the substance. Another question asks what degree of health risks students perceive in occasional use of various substances. The vertical axis shows the percent of students that perceive a "great risk" in occasional use. The scatter plot has circles for each drug (heroin, cocaine, marijuana, and alcohol), one per grade (8th, 10th, and 12th). The size of each circle indicates what proportion of students reported having used that drug at some point in the past year, with larger circles indicating higher rates of use.

All four substances are illegal for these respondents, since they are under 21 years, but there is variation in enforcement intensity. Possession of heroin and cocaine are punished most severely, alcohol least, with marijuana somewhere in between. That ranking applies both to personal possession by the respondents and to sanctions for market suppliers.

Not surprisingly, heroin and cocaine are used the least, perceived as being the least available, and perceived as being the most dangerous. Conversely, alcohol is the most readily available, is generally not seen as especially dangerous, and is used the most.

For 8th graders, marijuana is intermediate between heroin and cocaine on the one hand, and alcohol on the other. For 10th and 12th graders, marijuana's circles almost coincide with the circles for alcohol, being just slightly to the left (indicating slightly lower availability).

21.3.3 The monetary and human costs of enforcement

Legalization would save taxpayers money by reducing both the number of criminals put in prison or jail and the time officers spend enforcing prohibition. ("Reducing," not "eliminating," because many legalization proposals would retain prohibition for those under the age of 21 and all would require enforcement to prevent tax evasion and regulatory violations.) Marijuana accounts for fully half of all drug arrests, so prorating total enforcement costs in proportion to marijuana arrests would make marijuana legalization appear to be a big money saver. However, a more careful analysis would recognize the lower rates of incarceration for marijuana arrests; this means that, even in a state the size of California, the cost of enforcing marijuana prohibition on adults is probably below $200 million (22). The big savings in law enforcement costs would come from legalizing cocaine/crack, heroin, and methamphetamine.

Legalization would entail some regulatory enforcement costs, probably rising with the stringency of the regulations. However, the costs for alcohol and tobacco regulation today are quite minor compared with what is now spent trying to control illegal drugs. It is surprisingly difficult to provide a precise figure for drug control spending. Even the federal drug control budget, which is reported annually, is tricky to interpret, but the bigger challenge is that state and local governments account for the majority of drug control spending, and they do not follow on any common reporting system. It therefore seems reasonable to conclude that the costs of regulating legalized drugs would be significantly less than the current costs of enforcing prohibition.

There is also a human cost to mass incarceration. The 500,000 person-years spent behind bars for drug-law violations each year (23) is on a par with the number of life-years lost due to premature death caused by street drugs, or roughly 10–15,000 deaths per year times 30–50 life-years lost per death. (The equation would not hold if premature deaths from prescription drugs were included, but controlling diversion of pharmaceuticals is also not responsible for much imprisonment.) Indeed, the scale of incarceration in the United States and of community-based sanctions, such as probation and parole, is so large as to be antidemocratic. Significant numbers of well-defined subpopulations have lost voting rights as a result of felony convictions (24), with drug-law enforcement contributing substantially to the overall effect.

21.3.4 State-level versus nationwide legalization

When discussing the effects of legalization, it is also important to distinguish state legalization from national legalization. Three US states voted on and two approved. However, one state legalizing is very different from the nation legalizing, because even if a state were to attempt to end prohibition, federal law would remain in effect. State-level legalization does not protect anyone from arrest by a DEA agent, not even a medical user with a single joint.

That does not mean state-level legalization is irrelevant. State and local enforcement agencies are responsible for 97% of marijuana arrests (25). Removing those arrests would greatly reduce the risks of punishment faced by dealers as well as users, unless the federal government dramatically expanded its focus and stepped up its efforts. (Traditionally, federal prosecutors focus on cases involving a few hundred pounds of marijuana or more, unless there are special circumstances.) Even if federal enforcement does not change, federal prohibition alone would prevent marijuana production and distribution from getting too brazen. Kilmer et al. speculate that unobtrusive grow houses might be able to operate below federal enforcement radar (26), but completely outdoor farming or even large-scale greenhouse production might provide targets too easy to detect and too tempting to seize for federal enforcement agencies to ignore.

While many advocates of legalization favor regulating rather than banning drug sales, the ongoing federal ban might stymie certain regulatory structures. For example, permitting sales in state-run stores only (analogous to state liquor stores) might be impossible because the operation of state stores would be judged to positively conflict with the federal Controlled Substances Act.

Yet there is nothing to stop a state from simply repealing its laws against drugs, as the state of New York did in 1923 when it repealed its laws against alcohol prohibition, a full decade before federal repeal.

21.4 Middle paths and alternative approaches

Thinking about prohibition versus legalization as a binary choice is useful because a fairly sharp line can be drawn based on whether or not it is legal to produce and distribute a substance for nonmedical use. However, seeing policy choices as existing somewhere along a continuum can also be useful (27). From that perspective, there are many options in the territory between the extremes of (A) aggressively enforcing full prohibition and (B) legalizing all drugs without any rules or regulations beyond what would apply to any other article of commerce.

21.4.1 Decriminalization

Decriminalization and legalization are not synonyms (28). Decriminalization retains criminal sanctions on production and sale but replaces criminal penalties for the possession of drugs in small amounts with civil penalties. Several US states have decriminalized marijuana, beginning in the 1970s. Other countries have too, and some extend decriminalization to other drugs as well. Colombia's Constitutional Court recently voted to decriminalize small amounts of marijuana and cocaine, Portugal decriminalized possession of all drugs in 2001, and Brazil's legislature is revising the penal code to possibly include the decriminalization of small amounts of narcotics (29).

The majority of academics judge the empirical evidence as suggesting that decriminalization has only very modest effects on prices and use (30). That noneffect is good news for drug reformers in final market countries, but decriminalization in final market countries will do nothing to alleviate the burden those markets create on source and transshipment countries, where the (sometimes violent) trade would be undiminished and remain wholly illegal.

21.4.2 A kinder, gentler prohibition

Some negative effects of prohibition are not really the consequence of prohibition per se, but rather of how prohibition is implemented. Legalization may not be necessary to address those concerns. For example, opponents of current drug policy are right to criticize the disproportionate share of punishment that poor and minority communities face, but reducing the overall intensity of enforcement and shifting its focus rather than fully legalizing a drug could reduce the degree and importance of that disparity. However, as long as drug dealing is illegal, sales activity will take place in higher-crime neighborhoods, which tend to be predominantly minority. For this reason, a shift in enforcement focus may only reduce the degree of this disparity, not eliminate it altogether.

Mandatory minimum sentences are particularly decried, but the question of determinate sentencing versus judicial discretion is orthogonal to the question of prohibition or legalization. Some nondrug offenses carry mandatory minimum sentences too, notably gun law violations, and there are many countries and even US states that prohibit drugs without using mandatory sentences.

Sometimes objections to mandatory minimum sentences are really objections to excessive average sentence length, not to the removal of judicial discretion. Again, there is nothing intrinsic to prohibition that requires long sentences. No one would accuse Ronald Reagan of having legalized drugs, but when he was in office, there were only 10%–20% as many people incarcerated for drug-law violations as there are today (23).

21.4.3 Embracing harm reduction

For better and for worse, a principal goal of drug policy in the United States since the late 19th century has been to discourage, or minimize, drug use. While the official rhetoric speaks of "drug use and related consequences," the emphasis is on reducing use, and on reducing consequences by reducing use. We can conceptualize drug harm via some very basic arithmetic:

total harm = total number of users × dosages per user × harm per dose

While US policy has focused on ways to reduce use (both number of users and dosage per user), other countries prioritize reducing the third term in the harm equation. Such so-called harm reduction strategies focus on minimizing the consequences of drug use and embrace policies that reduce consequences even if they do not reduce use. MacCoun (31) has offered an insightful discussion of the distinction between "use reduction" and "harm reduction."

In official US drug policy circles, favoring harm reduction has about the same status that favoring Communism had during the McCarthy era. However, for many, harm reduction merely entails taking a pragmatic public-health approach within an overall framework that continues to ban commercial production and distribution.

Harm reduction advocates believe that many dire consequences of our current prohibition can be reversed without legalizing drugs. Notably, some nations, such as Australia, have embraced syringe-exchange programs early and aggressively and have largely avoided the HIV/AIDS epidemic that has plagued drug users in the United States. These programs are less successful at constraining hepatitis because that virus is so much more virulent. Likewise, Australia, Canada, and a number of European countries operate, or at least tolerate, "supervised injection facilities." These are rooms where proctors permit and oversee drug injections so that they can detect and respond to any overdoses as quickly as possible.

Information campaigns that inform and encourage responsible use can substitute for programs that preach abstinence. In a study in Washington State, death rates for former inmates in the first 2 weeks after release are elevated by more than a factor of 10 as compared with other state residents (adjusted for age, sex, and race), with drug overdose being the leading cause (32). While incarceration can force users to abstain and thus largely reverse their acquired tolerance to large doses, abstinence alone may not eliminate long-term craving. A variety of ways to promote responsible use in lieu of abstinence have been suggested. One could try to prevent some of those deaths by warning inmates before release not to return immediately to their preincarceration dosages. Weeks et al. (2006) suggest training active drug users to be "Peer/Public Health Advocates" who promote safer forms of drug taking.

21.5 Conclusions

From a consequentialist perspective, prohibiting drugs is good policy only if prohibition reduces use enough to reduce total harm (compared to legalization) despite greater harm per dose. Prohibition imposes very visible harms on a minority of identifiable individuals, most notably those whom it incarcerates and victims of black-market crime. Its benefits are invisible, consisting primarily of all the people who are not drug dependent now, but who would have been if drugs had been cheaper, less stigmatized, and more available when they were younger.

There is widespread dissatisfaction with the US approach to prohibition, but the government has alternatives other than outright legalization. Indeed, since no country (not even the Netherlands) has yet legalized any of the important "controlled" drugs (not even cannabis), the wide range of policies around the world are all variants of prohibition. And US policy is changing. Voters in Washington State and Colorado approved state marijuana legalization measures. Some mandatory minimum sentences are being repealed, the Affordable Care Act greatly expands access to treatment, and "testing with consequences" approaches such as Hawaii's HOPE and South Dakota's 24/7 Sobriety are achieving promising results. Yet there is more continuity than change, which leaves many people impatient to try something more radical: commercial availability of one or more currently illicit drugs.

For marijuana, "many people" means about half of all Americans. Fundamental change in the US prohibition of marijuana in the not-too-distant future is a distinct possibility, with state-level legalization already approved in Washington and Colorado. For hard drugs, "many people" means only about 10% of voters. Changes in the legal regimes for those drugs may be more likely to come from source and/or transit countries further up the supply chain.

Either one of these fundamental changes would have myriad consequences, both good and bad, that are essentially impossible to forecast with any precision. And even if everyone agreed on what would happen, people could still disagree on whether those changes are, on balance, good or bad. There is inevitably a question of personal values when thinking about whether the benefits of fewer people incarcerated justify the harms from having more drug-dependent people. And there are distributional issues. Prohibition helps parents who mistrust their teenagers' self-restraint by preventing large corporations from marketing marijuana and cocaine as aggressively as they now promote tobacco and alcohol. Legalization would help residents of inner-city neighborhoods plagued by open-air drug markets if it let convenience store chains outcompete violent gangs on price and service quality.

Drugs and drug policy offer choices, and few are more complicated than the fundamental question of whether we want to ban or allow production and distribution of one or more of the currently banned drugs for nonmedical use by a larger fraction of the population.

Acknowledgments

We are sincerely indebted to Marjorie Carlson, who provided valuable comments in the editing of the chapter, as well as to the members of the Spring 2012 Policy Modeling Workshop at Carnegie Mellon University's Heinz College, who provided analysis that guided the discussion of state versus national marijuana legalization.

References

1. Fellner J. Race, drugs, and law enforcement in the United States. Stanford Law Policy Rev 2009;20(2):257–92.
2. Brown R. Atlanta curbs smoking, part of southern wave of bans. New York Times, July 21, 2012. Accessed January 3, 2013. URL: http://www.nytimes.com/2012/07/21/us/atlanta-curbs-smoking-part-of-southern-wave-of-bans.html?_r=1
3. Smith RE. Tougher DWI penalties set to take effect in Virginia. FindLaw KnowledgeBase, April 24, 2012. Accessed January 3, 2013. URL: http://knowledgebase.findlaw.com/kb/2012/Mar/487778.html
4. MacCoun RJ, Reuter P. Drug war heresies: Learning from other vices, times, and places. Cambridge: Cambridge University Press, 2001:496.
5. MacCoun RJ. Drugs and the law: A psychological analysis of drug prohibition. Psychol Bull 1993;113(3):497–512.
6. MacCoun RJ. Estimating the non-price effects of legalization on consumption. WR-767-RC. Santa Monica, CA: RAND, 2010:10.
7. Johnston LD, O'Malley PM, Bachman JG, Schulenberg JE. Monitoring the Future national survey results on drug use, 1975–2011. Vol. 1, Secondary school students. Ann Arbor: Institute Social Research, University Michigan, 2012:760.
8. Roddy J, Steinmiller CL, Greenwald MK. Heroin purchasing is income and price sensitive. Psychol Addict Behav 2011;25(2):358–64.
9. Babor T, Caulkins J, Edqards G, Fischer B, Ubot I, Rehm J, et al. Drug policy and the public good. New York: Oxford University Press, 2010:369.
10. Reuter P, Kleiman M. Risks and prices. In: Tonry M, Morris N, eds. Crime and justice. Vol. 7, An annual review of research. Chicago, IL: University Chicago Press, 1986.
11. United States Office on Drugs and Crime. World drug report 2011. New York: United Nations Office Drugs Crime, 2011:111.
12. Grossman M. Individual behavior and substance use: The role of price. Adv Health Econ Health Serv Res 2005;16:15–39.
13. Silverman LP, Spruill NL. Urban crime and the price of heroin. J Urban Economics 1977;4(1): 80–103.

14. Pacula RL. Examining the impact of marijuana legalization on marijuana consumption. RAND Corporation, 2010. Accessed January 3, 2013. URL: http://www.rand.org/pubs/working_papers/WR770.html
15. Chaloupka FJ, Grossman M, Tauras JA. The demand for cocaine and marijuana by youth. In: Chaloupka FJ, Grossman M, Bickel WK, Saffer H, eds. The economic analysis of substance use and abuse: An integration of econometrics and behavioral economic research. Chicago, IL: University Chicago Press, 1999:133–56.
16. Miron JA, Waldock K. The budgetary impact of ending drug prohibition. Washington, DC: Cato Institute, 2010.
17. Hawken A, Kleiman M. Managing drug involved probations with swift and certain sanctions: Evaluating Hawaii's HOPE. Submitted to the US Department of Justice, 2009. Accessed January 3, 2013. URL: https://www.ncjrs.gov/pdffiles1/nij/grants/229023.pdf
18. Kilmer B, Nicosia N, Heaton P, Midgette G. Efficacy of Frequent Monitoring with Swift, Certain, and Modest Sanctions for Violations: Insights from South Dakota's 24/7 Sobriety Project. American Journal of Public Health 2013;103(1):e37–e43.
19. Baum RM. New variety of street drugs poses growing problem. Chem Eng 1985;7–16.
20. Zuardi AW, Shirakawa I, Finkelfarb E, Karniol. Action of cannabidiol on the anxiety and other effects produced by D9-THC in normal subjects. Psychopharmacology 1982;76:245–50.
21. Harborside Health Center. Menu of products. Oakland, CA: Harborside Health Center, 2011.
22. Caulkins JP, Kilmer B. Criminal justice costs for prohibiting marijuana for those aged 21 and older in California. In: Tate K, Taylor JL, Sawyer MQ, eds. Something's in the Air: Race, Crime, and the Legalization of Marijuana. Routledge. Forthcoming.
23. Caulkins JP, Chandler S. Long-run trends in incarceration of drug offenders in the US. Crime Delinquency 2006;52(4):619–41.
24. Uggen C, Manza J. Democratic contraction? Political consequences of felon disenfranchisement in the United States. Am Sociol Rev 2002;67(6):777–803.
25. US Department of Justice. Crime in the United States 2010. Washington, DC: Federal Bureau of Investigation, 2012.
26. Kilmer B, Caulkins J, Bond B, Reuter P. Reducing drug trafficking revenues and violence in Mexico: Would legalizing marijuana in California help? Santa Monica, CA: RAND, 2010:72.
27. MacCoun RJ, Reuter P, Schelling T. Assessing alternative drug control regimes. J Policy Analysis Manage 1996;15(3):330–52.
28. Pacula R, MacCoun R, Reuter P, Chriqui J, Kilmer B, Harris K, et al. What does it mean to decriminalize marijuana? A cross-national empirical examination. Adv Health Econ Health Serv Res 2005;16:347–70.
29. Glickhouse R. Brazil, Colombia, and Uruguay consider drug decriminalization. Americas Society/Council of the Americas, 2012. URL: http://www.as-coa.org/articles/brazil-colombia-and-uruguay-consider-drug-decriminalization
30. Room R, Fischer B, Hall W, Lenton S, Reuter P. Cannabis: Moving beyond the stalemate. Oxford: Oxford University Press, 2010:300.
31. MacCoun RJ. Toward a psychology of harm reduction. Am Psychol 1998;53(11):1199–208.
32. Binswanger IA, Stern MF, Deyo RA, Heagerty PJ, Cheadle A, Elmore JG, et al. Release from prison: A high risk of death for former inmates. N Engl J Med 2007;356(2):157–65.

22 Internet resources and treatment facilities

Jeffrey Berman and Michael Paolello

Today, there is a wealth of information on substance abuse, especially with the introduction of the Internet. In order to guide the reader, we have compiled various websites and Internet resources in addition to a list of treatment centers. This list of resources is offered as a comprehensive, although not all-inclusive, guide. None of the sites mentioned carries a specific endorsement by the authors, editors, or publisher.

22.1 Informational websites

http://findtreatment.samhsa.gov/

This site provides a database to search for alcohol and drug abuse treatment and mental health treatment services.

http://nationalsubstanceabuseindex.org/new-york/facilities.php

This site offers comprehensive information about recreational drugs, treatment facilities, local resources, and substance abuse statistics for each state.

http://www.soberrecovery.com/links/adolescenttreatment.html

This website lists a number of residential rehab programs for adolescents around the country. It also includes therapeutic communities, drug rehab centers, and boot camp rehabilitation programs.

http://www.bhddh.ri.gov/serviceproviders/bh_sa_agencylist.htm

The website gives a list of detoxification programs, residential rehab services, outpatient services, narcotic treatment services, and in-hospital services in Rhode Island for both adults and adolescents.

http://www.drug-rehabs.com/adolescent-substance-abuse.htm

This website provides a brief overview on teen substance abuse. The website also has information on recreational drugs, articles about high school drug use and teen alcoholism, and links for addiction treatment programs.

http://www.theagapecenter.com

The Agape Link Collection provides links for Alcoholics Anonymous (AA), Al-Anon, Cocaine Anonymous (CA), and Narcotics Anonymous (NA) meetings for each state.

http://www.hopelinks.net/drug-rehab/teen.html

This provides links to adolescent substance abuse and addiction services by each state and city.

http://www.lifelineinterventions.net/resources.htm

http://www.treatmentsolutions.com/families/

These two sites list treatment programs for adolescent drug rehabilitation.

22.2 Treatment center websites

http://www.visionsteen.com/
Visions is a psychiatric center for adolescents based in California. It provides residential and outpatient services as well as family programs.

http://www.acadiahealthcare.com/locations-by-state/

Acadia Healthcare is a nationwide psychiatric program that has inpatient and outpatient facilities for children, adolescents, and adults.

http://www.tarzanatc.org/

Tarzana Treatment Centers are located in California and provide various levels of addiction programs for adolescents such as detoxification, residential rehabilitation, day treatment, and intensive outpatient treatment programs.

http://www.rosecrance.org/substance-abuse/adolescent-services

Rosecrance offers different tiers of services for adolescent addiction services in Illinois.

http://www.hptc.org/

This website lists six treatment centers in Massachusetts. The Castle is a short-term treatment center for teens with a substance abuse problem. In addition to an inpatient unit, it has after-school and outpatient adolescent programs.

http://www.caron.org/locations.html

Caron Treatment Centers provide both short-term and long-term addiction services for teens with addiction. Family programs are incorporated into care. Caron Treatment Centers are located in Pennsylvania, Texas, and Florida.

http://www.pyramidhealthcarepa.com/

These centers offer residential and partial hospitalization programs for the treatment of addiction in adolescents. Outpatient services are also offered.

http://www.sharp.com/mcdonald/chemical-dependency-services.cfm

This is an addiction treatment center that offers both inpatient and outpatient programs for children and teens.

http://yakima.backpage.com/HealthServices/affordable-yakima-wa-adult-adolescent-addiction-treatment-center/4664156

Yakima WA Affordable Drug Rehab Treatment Center for Adults/Adolescents in Washington provides several aspects of drug rehab programs for adolescents including inpatient, outpatient, and family treatments.

http://www.bridgeinc.org/programs

On the website, one can find a list of addiction programs for adolescents in Alabama. The Bridge offers residential programs, outpatient programs, and community-based programs. The website also has links for resources regarding substance abuse.

http://www.capstonetreatmentcenter.com/assessment/index.html

Capstone Treatment Center offers an online assessment to determine the appropriate level of care for teens with addiction. There is also information regarding warning signs of addiction and 12-step treatment.

http://www.lakesidemilam.com/

Lakeside-Milam Recovery Centers are located in western Washington. The programs for adolescents include an inpatient residential program, an outpatient program, and a family program. The website also provides links for AA, NA, and locations for AA meetings in the Seattle and Tacoma area.

http://www.newportacademy.com/about/

Newport Academy is an addiction treatment center for adolescents located in California. It offers gender-specific treatment programs, a residential program, a family program, an intensive family program, an equine-assisted therapy program, a day school, an outpatient program, and individual and group therapies. There are also links for teen drug abuse facts and treatments.

http://www.hazelden.org/

Hazelden provides substance abuse treatment programs for both adults and adolescents in various locations. For adolescents, there is a rehab program in Minnesota, as well as a sober housing program in New York City. There are also family programs available. Through the website, there are also links for books on addiction and articles for patients and families.

http://www.inspirationsyouth.com/

Inspirations Youth offers an inpatient rehab program for teens in Florida. In addition, the website provides information on marijuana, alcohol, teen prescription addiction, ecstasy/club drugs, cocaine, methamphetamine, inhalants, heroin, Xanax, Oxycontin, and phencyclidine (or PCP). It also contains data about substance abuse among teens and addiction treatment programs in different states.

http://www.lawlispeavey.com

The Lawlis Peavey PsychoNeuroPlasticity (PNP) center provides treatment for those with an addiction problem.

http://www.twintowntreatmentcenters.com/

Twin Town Treatment Centers is an outpatient treatment center for adolescents. On the website, one can learn more about the disease model of addiction and recreational drugs and take screening tests.

http://www.summersky.us/

Summersky offers an adolescent addiction treatment program. The website also provides information about alcohol, heroin addiction, methamphetamines, cocaine addiction, marijuana addiction, prescription drug abuse, hallucinogens, and inhalants.

http://www.altabatessummit.org/clinical/thunderroad.html

Thunder Road Adolescent Treatment Centers provide short-term inpatient programs, long-term residential programs, outpatient services, and weekly support recovery services. In addition, the website also provides a link for a health information library, which covers a vast number of health topics.

http://fullcircletreatmentcenter.org/

Full Circle Treatment Center provides services for teens with addiction. Its website lists Q&A links with scenarios to help parents deal with children who may be abusing substances.

http://www.mountainmanor.org/

Mountain Manor Treatment Center offers residential and outpatient programs for adolescents with substance abuse.

http://www.rushford.org/

Rushford provides both residential and outpatient adolescent outpatient programs. In addition, the website lists an addiction quiz, a few Q&A's that teens can read about drug abuse, and Q&A's for parents on various topics including drug facts and cyberbullying.

http://www.mntc.org/

Minnesota Teen Challenge offers both short-term and long-term treatment programs for teens with addiction.

http://www.phoenixhouse.org

Phoenix House offers short term outpatient and long term residential programs for teens and young adults in 10 States.

Section V: **Acknowledgments**

23 About the editors

Donald E. Greydanus, MD, Dr. HC (Athens), FAAP, FSAM (Emeritus), FIAP (HON) is Professor and Founding Chair of the Department of Pediatric and Adolescent Medicine, Western Michigan University School of Medicine (WMED), Kalamazoo, Michigan, USA. He is also Professor of Pediatrics and Human Development at Michigan State University College of Human Medicine (East Lansing, Michigan, USA) and Director of the Pediatrics Residency Program at Michigan State University/Kalamazoo Center for Medical Studies (Kalamazoo, Michigan, USA). He received the 1995 American Academy of Pediatrics' Adele D. Hofmann Award for "Distinguished Contributions in Adolescent Health"; the 2000 Mayo Clinic Pediatrics Honored Alumnus Award for "National Contributions to the Field of Pediatrics"; and the 2003 William B. Weil, Jr., MD Endowed Distinguished Pediatric Faculty Award from Michigan State University College of Medicine for "National and international recognition as well as exemplary scholarship in pediatrics." He received the 2004 Charles R. Drew School of Medicine (Los Angeles, California, USA) Stellar Award for contributions to pediatric resident education and was awarded an honorary membership in the Indian Academy of Pediatrics – an honor granted to only a few pediatricians outside of India. He was the 2007–2010 Visiting Professor of Pediatrics at Athens University, Athens, Greece, and received the Michigan State University College of Human Medicine Outstanding Community Faculty Award in 2008. In 2010, he received the title of Doctor Honoris Causa from the University of Athens (Greece) as a "distinguished scientist who through outstanding work has bestowed praise and credit on the field of adolescent medicine (Ephebiatrics)."

In 2010, he received the Outstanding Achievement in Adolescent Medicine Award from the Society for Adolescent Medicine "as a leading force in the field of adolescent medicine and health." He is Past Chair of the National Conference and Exhibition Planning Group (Committee on Scientific Meetings) of the American Academy of Pediatrics and a member of the Pediatric Academic Societies' (SPR/PAS) Planning Committee (1998 to present). In 2011, he was elected to the Alpha Omega Alpha Honor Society (faculty member) at Michigan State University College of Human Medicine. He is a former member of the Appeals Committee for the Pediatrics' Residency Review Committee (RRC) of the Accreditation Council for Graduate Medical Education (Chicago, Illinois, USA) in both adolescent medicine and general pediatrics. He has numerous publications in adolescent health and lectureships in many countries on adolescent health. E-mail: Donald.Greydanus@med.wmich.edu

Dilip R. Patel, MD, FAAP, FSAM, FAACPDM, FACSM, CPHQ, CMQ, CPE, is a professor in the Department of Pediatric and Adolescent Medicine, Western Michigan University School of Medicine, Kalamazoo, Michigan, USA; and Department of

Pediatrics and Human Development at the Michigan State University College of Human Medicine, East Lansing, Michigan, USA. He is a full-time teaching faculty member in the Pediatric Residency Program at Western Michigan University School of Medicine and has subspecialty training and interests in neurodevelopmental disabilities, developmental-behavioral pediatrics, adolescent medicine, and sports medicine. He has published numerous papers on wide-ranging topics in these areas and has edited several special symposia and books. E-mail: Dilip.Patel@med.wmich.edu

Gabriel Kaplan, MD, DFAPA, is a clinical associate professor of psychiatry at the Rutgers New Jersey Medical School, Newark, New Jersey, USA: a board-certified adult and child psychiatrist; and a Distinguished Fellow of the American Psychiatric Association. A graduate of the University of Medicine of Buenos Aires, Argentina, he completed his adult and child psychiatric training at New York Hospital-Cornell Medical Center in New York. As a researcher, he has published work in the fields of suicide, attention-deficit/hyperactivity disorder, substance abuse, and violence, and he is well known in the United States and international medical education fields, having chaired multiple continuing medical education courses and symposia since 1997. He has served on several New Jersey State committees dealing with child psychiatry treatment issues and is the recipient of awards granted by Cornell Medical College, UMDNJ, and the New Jersey Mental Health Association. He has been featured in the Castle Connolly guide *Top Doctors: New York Metro Area* since 2001, and as a frequent guest on local cable and radio broadcasts, he comments on issues of impact to the community. He is also the Director of Behavioral Health Services at Bergen Regional Medical Center in Paramus, the largest hospital in New Jersey. E-mail: drgkaplan@gmail.com

Joav Merrick, MD, MMedSc, DMSc, is a professor of pediatrics, child health and human development affiliated with Kentucky Children's Hospital, University of Kentucky, Lexington, USA, and the Division of Pediatrics, Hadassah Hebrew University Medical Center, Mt. Scopus Campus, Jerusalem, Israel; the medical director of the Health Services, Division for Intellectual and Developmental Disabilities, Ministry of Social Affairs and Social Services, Jerusalem; and the founder and director of the National Institute of Child Health and Human Development in Israel. He has numerous publications in the field of pediatrics, child health and human development, rehabilitation, intellectual disability, disability, health, welfare, abuse, advocacy, quality of life, and prevention. He received the Peter Sabroe Child Award for outstanding work on behalf of Danish Children in 1985 and the International LEGO-Prize ("The Children's Nobel Prize") for an extraordinary contribution toward improvement in child welfare and well-being in 1987. E-mail: jmerrick@zahav.net.il

24 About the Department of Pediatric and Adolescent Medicine, Western Michigan University School of Medicine

The Department of Pediatric and Adolescent Medicine, Western Michigan University School of Medicine (WMED) was developed in 2012 with the formation of a new medical school in Kalamazoo, Michigan. The WMED residency programs have more than 200 residents and include residents in pediatrics.

24.1 Mission and service

The WMED Department of Pediatric and Adolescent Medicine has a unique balance between behavioral science and clinical pediatrics. The department has a commitment to a comprehensive approach to the health and development of the child, the adolescent, and the family.

The mission of the WMED includes training of medical students and residents. The WMED residency program in pediatrics is a fully accredited, three-year program preparing physicians for board certification in pediatrics.

The values of the WMED Department of Pediatric and Adolescent Medicine include compassionate service, leadership training, commitment to lifelong learning, emphasis on teamwork, and commitment to excellence in health care. Trainees at the WMED Department of Pediatric and Adolescent Medicine become skilled at providing patient care that is compassionate, appropriate, and effective for the treatment of health problems and the promotion of health. They learn to demonstrate interpersonal and communication skills that result in the effective exchange of information and collaboration with patients, their families, and health professionals. They are taught to develop a commitment to carrying out professional responsibilities and an adherence to ethical principles throughout their training with a goal of these values becoming a lifelong habit that reveals professional compassion, integrity, and respect for others. Kalamazoo is the home of the Kalamazoo Promise, a truly unique program that guarantees college education for students who graduate from the Kalamazoo public schools.

24.2 Research activities

The WMED Department of Pediatric and Adolescent Medicine has a variety of research projects in adolescent medicine, neurobehavioral pediatrics, adolescent gynecology, pediatric diabetes mellitus, asthma, and cystic fibrosis.

The department has recently published a number of medical textbooks: *Essential Adolescent Medicine* (McGraw-Hill Medical Publishers); *The Pediatric Diagnostic Examination* (McGraw-Hill); *Pediatric and Adolescent Psychopharmacology* (Cambridge University Press); *Behavioral Pediatrics, 2nd Edition* (New York and Lincoln, Nebraska: iUniverse Publishers); *Behavioral Pediatrics, 3rd Edition* (New York: Nova Biomedical Books); *Pediatric Practice: Sports Medicine* (McGraw-Hill); *Handbook of Clinical Pediatrics* (Singapore: World Scientific); and *Neurodevelopmental Disabilities: Clinical Care for Children and Young Adults* (Dordrecht: Springer). Other books include *Tropical Pediatrics* (New York: Nova); *Pediatric Psychodermatology* (Berlin, Germany: De Gruyter); *Adolescent Medicine: Pharmacotherapeutics in General, Mental, and Sexual Health* (Berlin, Germany: De Gruyter); and *Adolescent Medicine: Pharmacotherapeutics in Medical Disorders* (Berlin, Germany: De Gruyter).

The department has published in journals covering pulmonology (*State of the Art Reviews: Adolescent Medicine* [*AM:STARs*]), genetic disorders in adolescents (*AM:STARs*), neurological/neurodevelopmental disorders (*AM:STARs*), behavioral pediatrics (*Pediatric Clinics of North America*), pediatric psychopharmacology in the 21st century (*Pediatric Clinics of North America*), nephrologic disorders in adolescents (*AM:STARs*), college health (*Pediatric Clinics of North America*), adolescent medicine (*Primary Care: Clinics in Office Practice*), behavioral pediatrics in children and adolescents (*Primary Care: Clinics in Office Practice*), adolescents and sports (*Pediatric Clinics of North America*), and developmental disabilities (*Pediatric Clinics of North America*). The department has also edited a journal issue on musculoskeletal disorders in children and adolescents for the American Academy of Pediatrics' *AM:STARs* as well as an AM:STARs issue on Update in Subspecialty in Adolescent Medicine (2013;24:1–355).

The department has developed academic ties with a variety of international medical centers and organizations, including the Queen Elizabeth Hospital in Hong Kong; National Taiwan University Hospital (Taipei, Taiwan); the Indian Academy of Pediatrics (New Delhi, India); the University of Athens Children's Hospital (First and Second Departments of Paediatrics) in Athens, Greece; and the National Institute of Child Health and Human Development in Jerusalem, Israel.

24.3 Contact

Professor Donald E. Greydanus, MD, and Professor Dilip R. Patel, MD
Department of Pediatric and Adolescent Medicine
Western Michigan University School of Medicine
1000 Oakland Drive, D48G
Kalamazoo, MI 49008–1284, USA
E-mail: Donald.Greydanus@med.wmich.edu
E-mail: Dilip.Patel@med.wmich.edu

25 About the National Institute of Child Health and Human Development in Israel

The National Institute of Child Health and Human Development (NICHD) in Israel was established in 1998 as a virtual institute under the auspices of the Medical Director, Ministry of Social Affairs and Social Services in order to function as the research arm for the Office of the Medical Director. The establishment of the NICHD was endorsed by the National Council for Child Health and Pediatrics, Ministry of Health in 1998 and by the Director General and Deputy Director General of the Ministry of Health in 1999.

25.1 Mission

The mission of the NICHD in Israel is to provide an academic focal point for the scholarly interdisciplinary study of child life, health, public health, welfare, disability, rehabilitation, intellectual disability, and related aspects of human development. This mission includes research, teaching, clinical work, information, and public service activities in the field of child health and human development.

25.2 Service and academic activities

Over the years, many activities became focused in the south of Israel due to collaboration with various professionals at the Faculty of Health Sciences (FOHS) at the Ben Gurion University of the Negev (BGU). Since 2000, an affiliation with the Zusman Child Development Center at the Pediatric Division of Soroka University Medical Center has resulted in collaboration around the establishment of the Down Syndrome Clinic at that center. In 2002, a full course on disability was established at the Recanati School for Allied Professions in the Community, FOHS, BGU, and in 2005, collaboration was started with the Primary Care Unit of the faculty, and disability became part of the master-of-public-health course Children and Society. In the 2005–2006 academic year, the one-semester course Aging with Disability was started as part of the master-of-science program in gerontology in our collaboration with the Center for Multidisciplinary Research in Aging. In 2010, collaborations began with the Division of Pediatrics, Hadassah Medical Centers, Hebrew University, Jerusalem, Israel.

25.3 Research activities

The affiliated staff have over the years published their work from projects and research activities in many peer-reviewed international journals and also published books with several international known publishers.

25.4 National collaborations

Nationally, the NICHD works in collaboration with the FOHS, BGU of the Negev; Department of Physical Therapy, Sackler School of Medicine, Tel Aviv University; Autism Center, Assaf HaRofeh Medical Center; National Rett and PKU Centers at Chaim Sheba Medical Center, Tel HaShomer; Department of Physiotherapy, Haifa University; Department of Education, Bar Ilan University, Ramat Gan, Faculty of Social Sciences and Health Sciences; College of Judea and Samaria in Ariel; and in 2011, in affiliation with Center for Pediatric Chronic Diseases and Center for Down Syndrome, Department of Pediatrics, Hadassah-Hebrew University Medical Center, Mount Scopus Campus, Jerusalem.

25.5 International collaborations

Internationally, the NICHD works in collaboration with the Department of Disability and Human Development, College of Applied Health Sciences, University of Illinois at Chicago; Strong Center for Developmental Disabilities, Golisano Children's Hospital at Strong, University of Rochester School of Medicine and Dentistry, New York; Center on Intellectual Disabilities, University of Albany, New York; Centre for Chronic Disease Prevention and Control, Health Canada, Ottawa; Chandler Medical Center and Children's Hospital, Kentucky Children's Hospital, Section of Adolescent Medicine, University of Kentucky, Lexington; Chronic Disease Prevention and Control Research Center, Baylor College of Medicine, Houston, Texas; Division of Neuroscience, Department of Psychiatry, Columbia University, New York; Institute for the Study of Disadvantage and Disability, Atlanta; Center for Autism and Related Disorders, Department Psychiatry, Children's Hospital Boston, Boston; Department of Paediatrics, Child Health and Adolescent Medicine, Children's Hospital at Westmead, Westmead, Australia; International Centre for the Study of Occupational and Mental Health, Düsseldorf, Germany; Centre for Advanced Studies in Nursing, Department of General Practice and Primary Care, University of Aberdeen, Aberdeen, United Kingdom; Quality of Life Research Center, Copenhagen, Denmark; Nordic School of Public Health, Gottenburg, Sweden; Scandinavian Institute of Quality of Working Life, Oslo, Norway; Centre for Quality of Life of the Hong Kong Institute of Asia-Pacific Studies and School of Social Work, Chinese University, Hong Kong.

25.6 Targets

Our focus is on research, international collaborations, clinical work, teaching, and policy in health, disability, and human development, as well as establishing the NICHD as a permanent institute at one of the residential care centers for persons with intellectual disability in Israel in order to conduct model research and, together with the four university schools of public health/medicine in Israel, establish a national master and doctoral program in disability and human development at the institute to secure the next generation of professionals working in this often nonprestigious/low-status field of work.

Contact

Joav Merrick, MD, MMedSc, DMSc
Professor of Pediatrics, Child Health and Human Development
Medical Director, Health Services, Division for Intellectual and Developmental Disabilities, Ministry of Social Affairs and Social Services, POB 1260, IL-91012 Jerusalem, Israel
E-mail: jmerrick@zahav.net.il

26 About the book series Health, Medicine and Human Development

Health is a key component of human development, growth, and quality of life. The Health, Medicine and Human Development book series aims to provide a public forum for book publications from a multidisciplinary group of researchers, practitioners, and clinicians for an international professional forum interested in the broad spectrum of health, medicine, and human development. We welcome research on a wide variety of substantive areas that will promote and impact healthy human development including prevention, intervention, and care also among people in vulnerable conditions.

- Derevensky JL, Shek DTL, Merrick J, eds. Youth gambling: The hidden addiction. Berlin: Walter de Gruyter, 2011.
- Bricker JT, Omar HA, Merrick J, eds. Adults with childhood illnesses: Considerations for practice. Berlin: Walter de Gruyter, 2011.
- Greydanus DE, Patel DR, Omar HA, Feucht C, Merrick J, eds. Adolescent medicine: Pharmacotherapeutics in general, mental and sexual health. Berlin: Walter de Gruyter, 2012.
- Greydanus DE, Patel DR, Omar HA, Feucht C, Merrick J, eds. Adolescent medicine: Pharmacotherapeutics in medical disorders. Berlin: Walter de Gruyter, 2012.
- Tareen RS, Greydanus DE, Jafferany M, Patel DR, Merrick J, eds. Pediatric psychodermatology: A clinical manual of child and adolescent psychocutaneous disorders. Berlin: Walter de Gruyter, 2012.

Contact

Professor Joav Merrick, MD, MMedSc, DMSc
Medical Director, Medical Services
Division for Intellectual and Developmental Disabilities
Ministry of Social Affairs and Social Services
P.O. Box 1260, IL-91012 Jerusalem, Israel
E-mail: jmerrick@zahav.net.il
Website: http://www.degruyter.com/view/serial/129333

Index

Printed and bound by CPI Group (UK) Ltd, Croydon, CR0 4YY
13/09/2026
14960852-0005